Colorectal Cancers: From Present Problems to Future Solutions

Colorectal Cancers: From Present Problems to Future Solutions

Editor

Heike Allgayer

MDPI • Basel • Beijing • Wuhan • Barcelona • Belgrade • Manchester • Tokyo • Cluj • Tianjin

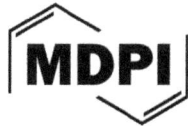

Editor
Prof. Dr. Dr. med. Heike Allgayer
Ruprecht Karls University of
Heidelberg
Germany

Editorial Office
MDPI
St. Alban-Anlage 66
4052 Basel, Switzerland

This is a reprint of articles from the Special Issue published online in the open access journal *Cancers* (ISSN 2072-6694) (available at: https://www.mdpi.com/journal/cancers/special_issues/Colorectal_Cancers_From_Present_Problems_Future_Solutions).

For citation purposes, cite each article independently as indicated on the article page online and as indicated below:

LastName, A.A.; LastName, B.B.; LastName, C.C. Article Title. *Journal Name* **Year**, *Volume Number*, Page Range.

ISBN 978-3-0365-4727-5 (Hbk)
ISBN 978-3-0365-4728-2 (PDF)

© 2022 by the authors. Articles in this book are Open Access and distributed under the Creative Commons Attribution (CC BY) license, which allows users to download, copy and build upon published articles, as long as the author and publisher are properly credited, which ensures maximum dissemination and a wider impact of our publications.

The book as a whole is distributed by MDPI under the terms and conditions of the Creative Commons license CC BY-NC-ND.

Contents

Heike Allgayer
An Editorial View on the Special Issue "Colorectal Cancers: From Present Problems to Future Solutions"
Reprinted from: *Cancers* **2022**, *14*, 975, doi:10.3390/cancers14040975 1

Marlen Keil, Theresia Conrad, Michael Becker, Ulrich Keilholz, Marie-Laure Yaspo, Hans Lehrach, Moritz Schütte, Johannes Haybaeck and Jens Hoffmann
Modeling of Personalized Treatments in Colon Cancer Based on Preclinical Genomic and Drug Sensitivity Data
Reprinted from: *Cancers* **2021**, *13*, 6018, doi:10.3390/cancers13236018 5

Tanja Groll, Franziska Schopf, Daniela Denk, Carolin Mogler, Ulrike Schwittlick, Heike Aupperle-Lellbach, Sabrina Rim Jahan Sarker, Nicole Pfarr, Wilko Weichert, Kaspar Matiasek, Moritz Jesinghaus and Katja Steiger
Bridging the Species Gap: Morphological and Molecular Comparison of Feline and Human Intestinal Carcinomas
Reprinted from: *Cancers* **2021**, *13*, 5941, doi:10.3390/cancers13235941 19

Ethel-Michele de Villiers and Harald zur Hausen
Bovine Meat and Milk Factors (BMMFs): Their Proposed Role in Common Human Cancers and Type 2 Diabetes Mellitus
Reprinted from: *Cancers* **2021**, *13*, 5407, doi:10.3390/cancers13215407 37

Luigi Marongiu, Markus Burkard, Sascha Venturelli and Heike Allgayer
Dietary Modulation of Bacteriophages as an Additional Player in Inflammation and Cancer
Reprinted from: *Cancers* **2021**, *13*, 2036, doi:10.3390/cancers13092036 51

Artur Mezheyeuski, Patrick Micke, Alfonso Martín-Bernabé, Max Backman, Ina Hrynchyk, Klara Hammarström, Simon Ström, Joakim Ekström, Per-Henrik Edqvist, Magnus Sundström, Fredrik Ponten, Karin Leandersson, Bengt Glimelius and Tobias Sjöblom
The Immune Landscape of Colorectal Cancer
Reprinted from: *Cancers* **2021**, *13*, 5545, doi:10.3390/cancers13215545 73

Nitin Patil, Mohammed L. Abba, Chan Zhou, Shujian Chang, Timo Gaiser, Jörg H. Leupold and Heike Allgayer
Changes in Methylation across Structural and MicroRNA Genes Relevant for Progression and Metastasis in Colorectal Cancer
Reprinted from: *Cancers* **2021**, *13*, 5951, doi:10.3390/cancers13235951 87

Mathias Dahlmann, Anne Monks, Erik D. Harris, Dennis Kobelt, Marc Osterland, Fadi Khaireddine, Pia Herrmann, Wolfgang Kemmner, Susen Burock, Wolfgang Walther, Robert H. Shoemaker and Ulrike Stein
Combination of Wnt/β-Catenin Targets S100A4 and DKK1 Improves Prognosis of Human Colorectal Cancer
Reprinted from: *Cancers* **2022**, *14*, 37, doi:10.3390/cancers14010037 107

Zahra Pezeshkian, Stefania Nobili, Noshad Peyravian, Bahador Shojaee, Haniye Nazari, Hiva Soleimani, Hamid Asadzadeh-Aghdaei, Maziar Ashrafian Bonab, Ehsan Nazemalhosseini-Mojarad and Enrico Mini
Insights into the Role of Matrix Metalloproteinases in Precancerous Conditions and in Colorectal Cancer
Reprinted from: *Cancers* **2021**, *13*, 6226, doi:10.3390/cancers13246226 131

Fabian Lang, María F. Contreras-Gerenas, Márton Gelléri, Jan Neumann, Ole Kröger,
Filip Sadlo, Krzysztof Berniak, Alexander Marx, Christoph Cremer,
Hans-Achim Wagenknecht and Heike Allgayer
Tackling Tumour Cell Heterogeneity at the Super-Resolution Level in Human Colorectal Cancer Tissue
Reprinted from: *Cancers* **2021**, *13*, 3692, doi:10.3390/cancers13153692 . . . . **151**

Isabel Heidrich, Thaer S. A. Abdalla, Matthias Reeh and Klaus Pantel
Clinical Applications of Circulating Tumor Cells and Circulating Tumor DNA as a Liquid Biopsy Marker in Colorectal Cancer
Reprinted from: *Cancers* **2021**, *13*, 4500, doi:10.3390/cancers13184500 . . . . **173**

Thibault Mazard, Laure Cayrefourcq, Françoise Perriard, Hélène Senellart, Benjamin Linot,
Christelle de la Fouchardière, Eric Terrebonne, Eric François, Stéphane Obled,
Rosine Guimbaud, Laurent Mineur, Marianne Fonck, Jean-Pierre Daurès, Marc Ychou,
Eric Assenat and Catherine Alix-Panabières
Clinical Relevance of Viable Circulating Tumor Cells in Patients with Metastatic Colorectal Cancer: The COLOSPOT Prospective Study
Reprinted from: *Cancers* **2021**, *13*, 2966, doi:10.3390/cancers13122966 . . . . **187**

Caroline Himbert, Jane C. Figueiredo, David Shibata, Jennifer Ose, Tengda Lin, Lyen C. Huang, Anita R. Peoples, Courtney L. Scaife, Bartley Pickron, Laura Lambert, Jessica N. Cohan, Mary Bronner, Seth Felder, Julian Sanchez, Sophie Dessureault, Domenico Coppola, David M. Hoffman, Yosef F. Nasseri, Robert W. Decker, Karen Zaghiyan, Zuri A. Murrell, Andrew Hendifar, Jun Gong, Eiman Firoozmand, Alexandra Gangi, Beth A. Moore, Kyle G. Cologne, Maryliza S. El-Masry, Nathan Hinkle, Justin Monroe, Matthew Mutch, Cory Bernadt, Deyali Chatterjee, Mika Sinanan, Stacey A. Cohen, Ulrike Wallin, William M. Grady, Paul D. Lampe, Deepti Reddi, Mukta Krane, Alessandro Fichera, Ravi Moonka, Esther Herpel, Peter Schirmacher, Matthias Kloor, Magnus von Knebel-Doeberitz, Johanna Nattenmueller, Hans-Ulrich Kauczor, Eric Swanson, Jolanta Jedrzkiewicz, Stephanie L. Schmit, Biljana Gigic, Alexis B. Ulrich, Adetunji T. Toriola, Erin M. Siegel,
Christopher I. Li, Cornelia M. Ulrich and Sheetal Hardikar
Clinical Characteristics and Outcomes of Colorectal Cancer in the ColoCare Study: Differences by Age of Onset
Reprinted from: *Cancers* **2021**, *13*, 3817, doi:10.3390/cancers13153817 . . . . **199**

Barbara Schuster, Markus Hecht, Manfred Schmidt, Marlen Haderlein, Tina Jost,
Maike Büttner-Herold, Klaus Weber, Axel Denz, Robert Grützmann,
Arndt Hartmann, Hans Geinitz, Rainer Fietkau and Luitpold V. Distel
Influence of Gender on Radiosensitivity during Radiochemotherapy of Advanced Rectal Cancer
Reprinted from: *Cancers* **2022**, *14*, 148, doi:10.3390/cancers14010148 . . . . **213**

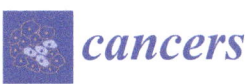

Editorial

An Editorial View on the Special Issue "Colorectal Cancers: From Present Problems to Future Solutions"

Heike Allgayer

Department of Experimental Surgery—Cancer Metastasis, Mannheim Medical Faculty, Ruprecht Karls University of Heidelberg, 68167 Mannheim, Germany; heike.allgayer@medma.uni-heidelberg.de; Tel.: +49-(0)621-383-71630 or +49-(0)621-383-71635; Fax: +49-(0)621-383-71631

Keywords: colorectal cancer; (molecular) carcinogenesis; cancer progression; metastasis; (single) cancer cell heterogeneity; models; infectious agents; (targeted) therapy; personalized medicine

Citation: Allgayer, H. An Editorial View on the Special Issue "Colorectal Cancers: From Present Problems to Future Solutions". *Cancers* **2022**, *14*, 975. https://doi.org/10.3390/cancers14040975

Received: 28 January 2022
Accepted: 11 February 2022
Published: 15 February 2022

Publisher's Note: MDPI stays neutral with regard to jurisdictional claims in published maps and institutional affiliations.

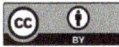

Copyright: © 2022 by the author. Licensee MDPI, Basel, Switzerland. This article is an open access article distributed under the terms and conditions of the Creative Commons Attribution (CC BY) license (https://creativecommons.org/licenses/by/4.0/).

Colorectal cancer (CRC) represents one of the most frequent human cancer entities and is still amongst the "top killers" in human cancer, although fundamental progress has been made in recent years in CRC prevention, early diagnosis, basic and translational research, and (targeted) therapy. The current Special Issue, "Colorectal cancers: from present problems to future solutions", presents 13 highly timely articles, 9 original articles and 4 reviews, which give insights into, and highlight, the latest developments within the scientific, translational and clinical CRC community, presenting views and work of several internationally highly recognized experts in the field. To this end, the special issue covers exciting novel discoveries in basic and mechanistic research that help to understand CRC carcinogenesis, progression and metastasis, tumor cell heterogeneity, and novel microenvironmental components in CRC. It also covers clinical parameters that modify CRC characteristics and therapy response, and tools and models with a high innovative potential to open new chapters in the differential diagnosis of CRC heterogeneity and response to therapy.

Several articles present advances or novel, in part provocative, hypotheses on causes of CRC carcinogenesis, progression, metastasis, and/or CRC interaction with the (micro-) environment. In an exciting review, Nobel Laureate Harald zur Hausen and Ethel-Michele de Villiers give an intriguing overview on a potential, completely novel class of infectious agents, which might open new avenues to our understanding of indirect carcinogenesis, but also further chronic diseases, such as type 2 diabetes, as (co-) caused by bovine meat and milk factors (BMMFs) [1]. BMMFs represent a recently discovered class of infectious species with self-replicating capacity, isolated by the authors from bovine milk and meat, the structure of BMMFs being rather plasmid-like. Initial data from the authors suggest that BMMFs, taken up by nutrition, give rise to chronic inflammation and immune stimulation, thereby contributing to a rather unspecific and indirect means of local (CRC) carcinogenesis but, over and above, to a systemic priming of inflammatory contributions to the development of further malignant tumor and chronic diseases, e.g., type 2 diabetes. This discovery certainly not only widens our understanding of carcinogenesis and chronic disease in general, but bears the potential to revolutionize views on human nutrition, in particular on the milk and meat industry. Adding to potential inflammatory or infectious (co-)factors of CRC carcinogenesis or progression, a review of our own group, together with nutritional experts, discusses novel hypotheses on bacteriophages and their potential contributions to colorectal (chronic) inflammatory conditions and CRC, as modulated by particular components of human nutrition and an associated priming of intestinal microbial microenvironments [2]. Adding to novel microenvironmental insights into CRC, in the currently largest case number study of CRC patients, an exciting original article by Sjöblom and his group [3] systematically analyzes the spatial immune landscape of multiplexed

CRC tissue immunofluorescence panels. The article shows exciting changes in the type of immune cells, representing both adaptive and innate immunity, between different types of CRC. To this end, CRCs of the right colon show an enrichment of most T-cell types and M2 macrophages, whereas rectal cancer is rich in dendritic cells. In this study, M2 macrophages accumulated in CRCs of the elderly, and CD8+ cells, were able to predict a more favorable survival in stages UICC I-III of CRC, in contrast to metastatic (UICC IV) stages, in which CD4+ cells had the strongest impact on survival. Interestingly, immune infiltrates repopulated after rectal irradiation therapy. Taken together, this article opens timely new perspectives on the microenvironmental interaction of CRCs with immune cells and inflammatory components, extends ongoing efforts of additional CRC classifications into particular immune phenotypes, and suggests putative clinical, diagnostic, and therapeutic conclusions. Focusing back at biological changes in CRC tumor cells in a further original article, our own group presents a systematic whole-genome analysis of epigenetic changes across structural and, in particular, microRNA (miR) genes [4] in CRC. We suggest methylation changes in CRC, as compared to the normal colon or rectum, to occur especially in open sea regions and islands, and found that protein coding genes, but in particular genes of miRs that have been shown to be important within CRC progression and metastasis pathways, harbor significant methylation changes in primary CRCs. This adds to our knowledge of miR-regulation in cancer, since, up to now, rather transcriptional and genetic mechanisms of miR-deregulation in cancer, (CRC) progression and metastasis have been elucidated extensively. In a further original article, the group by Ulrike Stein et al. [5] extends our mechanistic knowledge on Wnt/catenin signaling, which is essential in CRC cell invasion and metastasis. They demonstrate an exciting novel means of transcriptional cross-regulation of S100A4 (which is a pro-metastatic Wnt target) and DKK1 (which is a Wnt antagonist) that includes an S100A4-induced feedback loop, which sustains Wnt signaling and associated metastatic properties. Thus, a combined measurement of S100A4 and DKK1 might be powerful as a biomarker for a more precise identification of high-risk patients in precision medicine. Finally, Pezeshkian, Nobili, Mini, and coauthors provide a comprehensive and timely overview on the current status of matrix metalloproteinases (MMPs) in their differential functions for CRC carcinogenesis, the transition from precancerous lesions to tumors, and CRC progression [6].

The issue of tumor cell heterogeneity is certainly still one of the most unresolved problems we are facing when it comes to (colorectal) cancer individual diagnosis, prediction, risk classification, and therapy. Ideally, we would like to aim at scenarios and early diagnostic tools that enable us to predict, for every single patient, the likelihood to develop later progressive disease or metastasis, before this actually happens macroscopically. Therefore, methods to identify metastatically "dangerous" tumor cell clones in any primary tumor, or within single disseminated tumor cells that can be identified in, e.g., the blood of cancer patients, would open tremendous opportunities for a more individualized risk prediction and (preventive) therapy stratification. In an interdisciplinary consortium of molecular translational oncology researchers, optical physicists, and chemists, the groups of H.A. Wagenknecht, C. Cremer, and our own group recently succeeded in establishing a first-in-field approach for quantitative single-cell, single molecule localization microscopy (SMLM) at the nanoscale, within resected human CRC tissues [7]. We specifically show examples of changes in chromatin nanostructure and intracellular distribution of microRNAs between individual (cancer) cells in the resected CRC patient tissue context. Such methodologies have a high potential to enable single-cell differential diagnosis between (cancer) cell clones of different mechanistic capabilities within individual tissues and tumors of patients in the future, aiming at a broadening of current macroscopic clinical imaging methods by microscopic and molecular imaging. Along the same lines, more and more sophisticated methods to (systematically) analyze single circulating (tumor) cells, or CTCs, within individual patients have an equally powerful potential for precision medicine. In an exciting review, Klaus Pantel and his group [8] present an actual status of CTC diagnosis and circulating DNA in the blood of CRC patients, and discuss their still increasing potential as easily accessible liquid biopsy markers able to indicate, e.g., response or resistance to therapy, for the prediction, monitoring, and management of CRC. A specific example of CRC monitoring within a prospective clinical study is impressively demonstrated by C. Alix-Panabieres and her group, in her original article which contributed to this Special Issue [9]. These colleagues show that CTC kinetics, as evaluated by the novel EPISPOT assay, are able to predict prognosis and, most likely, therapy response before and in the course of treatment in metastatic CRC, in a prospective, multicenter study (COLOSPOT). Taken together, all of these articles suggest that tackling tumor cell heterogeneity and single-cell diagnosis have higher chances than ever to enter clinically relevant settings.

Two further articles of this Special Issue show actual clinical study data, illustrating how, up to now rather neglected clinical characteristics (age and gender), can have an impact on clinical courses and outcomes in CRC, and, potentially, response to therapy. During recent years, it has been observed that sporadic CRC has been increasing, also, in younger patients. In an attempt to address potential causes for this, in a large multinational cohort of over 2100 newly diagnosed CRC patients, Himbert et al., together with many colleagues involved in the ColoCare study, analyzed patient, demographic, and lifestyle characteristics, compared between age of onset younger than, or over, 50 years [10]. The results of this study will help in guiding further research on CRC, especially in younger patients with no evidence of hereditary disease components. In another clinical study, Schuster et al. explore the impact of gender on the sensitivity to radio-chemotherapy in advanced rectal cancer [11]. Although these colleagues could not detect a significant difference in response between male and female patients, it is still interesting that female patients experienced an increased deterioration in quality of life following radio-chemotherapy, an observation that needs to be taken into account for future studies and therapy design. Moreover, the data can build a ground for further (re-) translational research on gender differences, in the response or resistance to particular therapies in CRC.

Translational, and re-translational, research in CRC, and its success and impact for clinical consequences will, ultimately, also depend on the availability of the right models that are able to reflect the situation within a CRC patient as authentically as possible. Therefore, two articles in this special issue introduce novel, and timely, means of modelling colorectal cancer. A highly interesting article by Jens Hoffmann and his group [12] introduces powerful patient-derived xenograft (PDX) models that are excellently suited to model personalized treatment in CRC, within defined molecular human patient subgroups, the genomic/molecular characteristics of the tumors being analyzed by systems biology approaches. The article demonstrates how biomarkers, or biomarker panels, can be developed for single drugs, or drug combinations, within these CRC PDX models, or how, for example, alternative therapeutic strategies could be suggested in the individual case, depending on individual oncogenic pathway analysis. Finally, the original article by Katja Steiger and her group [13] introduces amazing similarities in morphology and molecular pathways between human and feline CRC, clearly inviting us to broaden our perspectives to other species of our planet, when attempting to understand, and conquer, human diseases such as CRC. I, personally, think that this is an article coming at the right time, given our actual global alert on the threats of climate change, the increasing extinction of whole species by humankind, and the several-fold overdone exploitation of our planet by the human species. Perhaps, also, this article can encourage us to be more modest and respectful to other species on Earth, since there might be a number of species, some of them maybe already extinguished by us, of whom we could learn a lot for our own life and diseases, such as cancer. With this, the article again builds the bridge to zur Hausen's and de Villiers's review on, up to now, undiscovered species, discussed at the beginning of this Editorial.

Taken together, with this Special Issue, "Colorectal Cancers: From Present Problems to Future Solutions", we hope to present an exciting compilation of articles, by well-known international experts, which can deepen discussions and ideas amongst colleagues in all kinds of disciplines working at CRC and beyond. I hope it can encourage, and intensify, even more translational and interdisciplinary collaborations, aiming at an ultimate understanding of strategies to defeat, and prevent, colorectal cancer, its progression and metastasis, and all the suffering and death resulting from it.

Acknowledgments: The author is grateful to Joerg Leupold for his support in the formal editing of the manuscript.

Conflicts of Interest: The author declares no conflict of interest.

References

1. De Villiers, E.M.; Zur Hausen, H. Bovine Meat and Milk Factors (BMMFs): Their Proposed Role in Common Human Cancers and Type 2 Diabetes Mellitus. *Cancers* **2021**, *13*, 5407. [CrossRef] [PubMed]
2. Marongiu, L.; Burkard, M.; Venturelli, S.; Allgayer, H. Dietary Modulation of Bacteriophages as an Additional Player in Inflammation and Cancer. *Cancers* **2021**, *13*, 2036. [CrossRef] [PubMed]
3. Mezheyeuski, A.; Micke, P.; Martin-Bernabe, A.; Backman, M.; Hrynchyk, I.; Hammarstrom, K.; Strom, S.; Ekstrom, J.; Edqvist, P.H.; Sundstrom, M.; et al. The Immune Landscape of Colorectal Cancer. *Cancers* **2021**, *13*, 5545. [CrossRef] [PubMed]
4. Patil, N.; Abba, M.L.; Zhou, C.; Chang, S.; Gaiser, T.; Leupold, J.H.; Allgayer, H. Changes in Methylation across Structural and MicroRNA Genes Relevant for Progression and Metastasis in Colorectal Cancer. *Cancers* **2021**, *13*, 5951. [CrossRef] [PubMed]
5. Dahlmann, M.; Monks, A.; Harris, E.D.; Kobelt, D.; Osterland, M.; Khaireddine, F.; Herrmann, P.; Kemmner, W.; Burock, S.; Walther, W.; et al. Combination of Wnt/beta-Catenin Targets S100A4 and DKK1 Improves Prognosis of Human Colorectal Cancer. *Cancers* **2021**, *14*, 37. [CrossRef] [PubMed]
6. Pezeshkian, Z.; Nobili, S.; Peyravian, N.; Shojaee, B.; Nazari, H.; Soleimani, H.; Asadzadeh-Aghdaei, H.; Ashrafian Bonab, M.; Nazemalhosseini-Mojarad, E.; Mini, E. Insights into the Role of Matrix Metalloproteinases in Precancerous Conditions and in Colorectal Cancer. *Cancers* **2021**, *13*, 6226. [CrossRef] [PubMed]
7. Lang, F.; Contreras-Gerenas, M.F.; Gelleri, M.; Neumann, J.; Kroger, O.; Sadlo, F.; Berniak, K.; Marx, A.; Cremer, C.; Wagenknecht, H.A.; et al. Tackling Tumour Cell Heterogeneity at the Super-Resolution Level in Human Colorectal Cancer Tissue. *Cancers* **2021**, *13*, 3692. [CrossRef] [PubMed]
8. Heidrich, I.; Abdalla, T.S.A.; Reeh, M.; Pantel, K. Clinical Applications of Circulating Tumor Cells and Circulating Tumor DNA as a Liquid Biopsy Marker in Colorectal Cancer. *Cancers* **2021**, *13*, 4500. [CrossRef] [PubMed]
9. Mazard, T.; Cayrefourcq, L.; Perriard, F.; Senellart, H.; Linot, B.; de la Fouchardiere, C.; Terrebonne, E.; Francois, E.; Obled, S.; Guimbaud, R.; et al. Clinical Relevance of Viable Circulating Tumor Cells in Patients with Metastatic Colorectal Cancer: The COLOSPOT Prospective Study. *Cancers* **2021**, *13*, 2966. [CrossRef] [PubMed]
10. Himbert, C.; Figueiredo, J.C.; Shibata, D.; Ose, J.; Lin, T.; Huang, L.C.; Peoples, A.R.; Scaife, C.L.; Pickron, B.; Lambert, L.; et al. Clinical Characteristics and Outcomes of Colorectal Cancer in the ColoCare Study: Differences by Age of Onset. *Cancers* **2021**, *13*, 3817. [CrossRef] [PubMed]
11. Schuster, B.; Hecht, M.; Schmidt, M.; Haderlein, M.; Jost, T.; Buttner-Herold, M.; Weber, K.; Denz, A.; Grutzmann, R.; Hartmann, A.; et al. Influence of Gender on Radiosensitivity during Radiochemotherapy of Advanced Rectal Cancer. *Cancers* **2021**, *14*, 148. [CrossRef] [PubMed]
12. Keil, M.; Conrad, T.; Becker, M.; Keilholz, U.; Yaspo, M.L.; Lehrach, H.; Schutte, M.; Haybaeck, J.; Hoffmann, J. Modeling of Personalized Treatments in Colon Cancer Based on Preclinical Genomic and Drug Sensitivity Data. *Cancers* **2021**, *13*, 6018. [CrossRef] [PubMed]
13. Groll, T.; Schopf, F.; Denk, D.; Mogler, C.; Schwittlick, U.; Aupperle-Lellbach, H.; Sarker, S.R.J.; Pfarr, N.; Weichert, W.; Matiasek, K.; et al. Bridging the Species Gap: Morphological and Molecular Comparison of Feline and Human Intestinal Carcinomas. *Cancers* **2021**, *13*, 5941. [CrossRef] [PubMed]

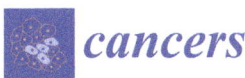

Article

Modeling of Personalized Treatments in Colon Cancer Based on Preclinical Genomic and Drug Sensitivity Data

Marlen Keil [1], Theresia Conrad [1], Michael Becker [1], Ulrich Keilholz [2], Marie-Laure Yaspo [3], Hans Lehrach [3], Moritz Schütte [4], Johannes Haybaeck [5,6] and Jens Hoffmann [1,*]

[1] Experimental Pharmacology and Oncology Berlin-Buch GmbH (EPO), Robert-Roessle-Str. 10, 13125 Berlin, Germany; m.keil@epo-berlin.com (M.K.); theresia.conrad@epo-berlin.com (T.C.); mibecker@epo-berlin.com (M.B.)
[2] Comprehensive Cancer Center, Charite-Universitätsmedizin, Charfitéplatz 1, 10117 Berlin, Germany; ulrich.keilholz@charite.de
[3] Department of Computational Molecular Biology and Department of Vertebrate Genomics/Otto Warburg Laboratory Gene Regulation and Systems Biology of Cancer, Max Planck Institute for Molecular Genetics, Ihnestraße 73, 14195 Berlin, Germany; yaspo@molgen.mpg.de (M.-L.Y.); lehrach@molgen.mpg.de (H.L.)
[4] Alacris Theranostics GmbH, Max-Planck-Straße 3, 12489 Berlin, Germany; m.schuette@alacris.de
[5] Institute of Pathology, Neuropathology, and Molecular Pathology, Medical University of Innsbruck, 6020 Innsbruck, Austria; johannes.haybaeck@i-med.ac.at
[6] Diagnostic & Research Center for Molecular Biomedicine, Institute of Pathology, Medical University of Graz, 8036 Graz, Austria
* Correspondence: jens.hoffmann@epo-berlin.com; Tel.: +49-30-94894440

Simple Summary: This experimental preclinical study developed a strategy to identify signatures for the personalized treatment of colon cancer focusing on target-specific drug combinations. Tumor growth inhibition was analyzed in a preclinical phase II study using 25 patient-derived xenograft models (PDX) treated with drug combinations blocking alternatively activated oncogenic pathways. Results reveal an improved response by combinatorial treatment in some defined molecular subgroups and potential alternative treatment options in KRAS- and BRAF-mutated colon cancer.

Abstract: The current standard therapies for advanced, recurrent or metastatic colon cancer are the 5-fluorouracil and oxaliplatin or irinotecan schedules (FOxFI) +/− targeted drugs cetuximab or bevacizumab. Treatment with the FOxFI cytotoxic chemotherapy regimens causes significant toxicity and might induce secondary cancers. The overall low efficacy of the targeted drugs seen in colon cancer patients still is hindering the substitution of the chemotherapy. The ONCOTRACK project developed a strategy to identify predictive biomarkers based on a systems biology approach, using omics technologies to identify signatures for personalized treatment based on single drug response data. Here, we describe a follow-up project focusing on target-specific drug combinations. Background for this experimental preclinical study was that, by analyzing the tumor growth inhibition in the PDX models by cetuximab treatment, a broad heterogenic response from complete regression to tumor growth stimulation was observed. To provide confirmation of the hypothesis that drug combinations blocking alternatively activated oncogenic pathways may improve therapy outcomes, 25 models out of the well-characterized ONCOTRACK PDX panel were subjected to treatment with a drug combination scheme using four approved, targeted cancer drugs.

Keywords: colon cancer; personalized treatment; drug combinations

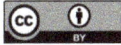

1. Introduction

Although KRAS and BRAF mutations have been established as biomarkers for cetuximab resistance in colorectal cancer (CRC), the predictive value is not satisfying. Approximately 35% of the KRAS wild-type (wt) population does not respond to cetuximab, while there is growing evidence that some mutant tumors might respond to the treatment.

As cetuximab is usually combined with FOxFI, it is difficult to define the contribution to the overall response [1]. However, in some colon cancer PDX models treated with single cetuximab, almost complete regressions were observed [2], raising questions as to whether the combination with FOxFI is mandatory for all patients.

Within the ONCOTRACK project [2], drug sensitivity to the EGFR antibody cetuximab was determined in a cohort of 58 colon cancer PDX models, derived from 58 patients with primary or metastatic cancer. In parallel, these PDX models were treated with the recently approved VEGF and multikinase inhibitor regorafenib and two further investigational drugs targeting the mammalian target of rapamycin (mTOR) and mitogen-activated protein kinase (MAP) pathways, an experimental mTOR inhibitor (BI mTOR FR), and the experimental MEK inhibitor AZD6244. However, no drug combination effects were evaluated in this project.

To identify a rationale for drug combinations, we selected a subpanel of 25 PDX models from the ONCOTRACK cohort with a heterogeneous genetic profile as well as sensitivity towards the four drugs for further analysis.

When comparing the response to the four drugs, the following questions were raised:

1. There is a population of PDX where a strong response to cetuximab is observed—would this group of tumors still require combination therapy, and is there an additional molecular predictor for this subgroup other than the KRAS or BRAF wt phenotype?
2. A second group of PDX seems to significantly benefit from one of the treatments, but still slowly progressing in growth—the most obvious question for this subgroup is will they profit from a combination?
3. Lastly, there is the group of treatment-resistant tumors mainly with mutant KRAS or BRAF and usually worse prognoses—are there any new hypotheses/rationales for a combination of treatments?

To address these questions, a pilot drug combination study was initiated using 25 PDX models representing each of the three response groups. As, during the ONCOTRACK project, two experimental drugs were used, which are not available for clinical routine, we decided to perform the combination study with the approved drugs cetuximab (targeting EGFR), trametinib (targeting MEK), regorafenib (targeting multiple kinases, i.e., VEGFR1/2/3, TIE2, KIT, RET, BRAF, BRAFV600E and FGFR-1, PDGFR-ß), and everolimus (targeting mTOR) (Figure 1). The use of clinically approved drugs should allow the better translation of the experimental results to the clinical setting.

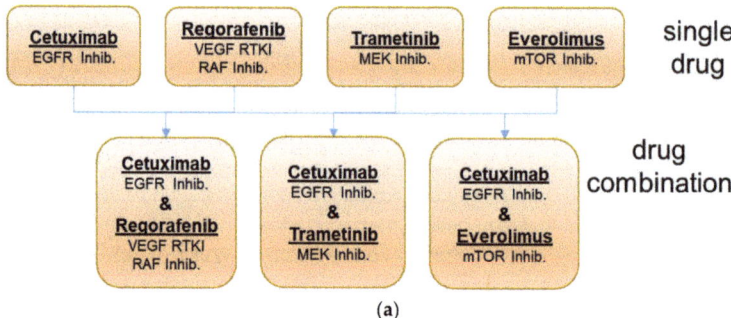

Figure 1. Cont.

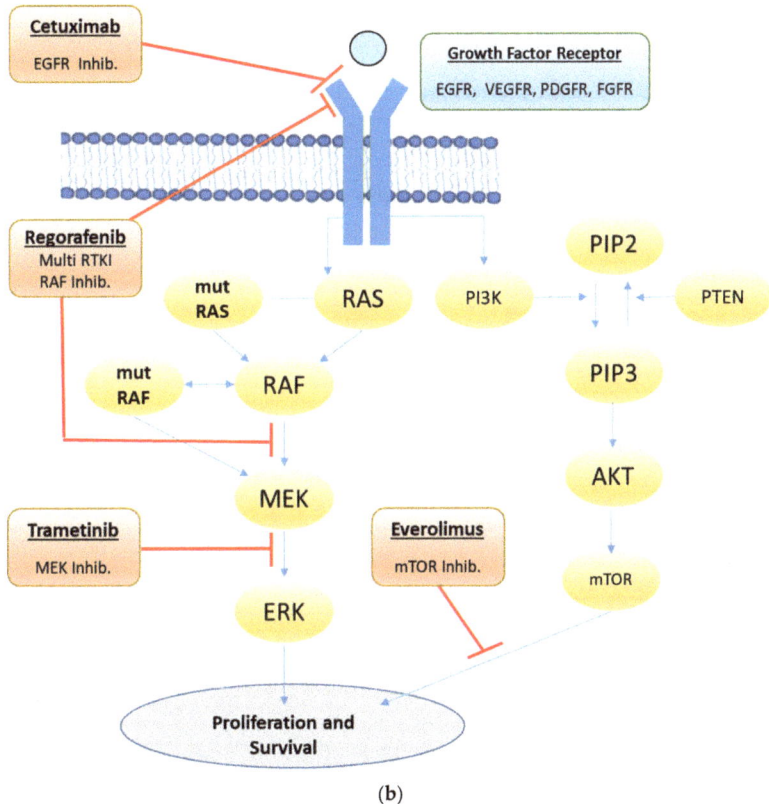

Figure 1. Drug combinations (**a**) and pathways blocked by the different targeted drugs (**b**).

2. Materials and Methods

2.1. Patient Samples

Patient samples were obtained as described by Schütte et al. [2]. Samples were obtained and stored according to the current good clinical practice (GCP) guidelines. Informed consent was obtained from all human subjects included in the study. The study was approved by the local Institutional Review Board of Charité University Medicine (Charité Ethics Cie: Charitéplatz 1, 10117 Berlin, Germany (EA 1/069/11)) and the ethics committee of the Medical University of Graz (Ethic commission of the Medical University of Graz, Auenbruggerplatz 2, 8036 Graz, Austria), confirmed by the ethics committee of the St. John of God Hospital Graz (23-015 ex 10/11).

2.2. Development and Characterization of Patient-Derived Xenografts (PDX)

Development of the PDX models was described in detail by Schütte et al. [2]. In brief, resected tumor tissues were transplanted to immunodeficient mice (NMRI nude or NOG, Taconic, Bomholtgard, DK-Tac: NMRI-Foxn1nu, females, 6–8 weeks at start of transplantation). Animal experiments were carried out in accordance with the United Kingdom Coordinating Committee on Cancer Research regulations for the Welfare of Animals and of the German Animal Protection Law and approved by the local responsible authorities. Mice were monitored 3 times weekly for tumor engraftment for up to 3 months. Engrafted tumors at a size of approximately 1 cm^3 were surgically excised and smaller fragments re-transplanted to naive NMRI nu/nu mice for further passage. Within passage 1 to 3, numerous samples were cryo-conserved (dimethylsulfoxide medium) for further experiments.

Tumors were passaged no more than 6 times. For confirmation of tumor histology, tumor tissue was formalin-fixed and paraffin-embedded (FFPE) and 5 μm sections were prepared. Samples were stained according to a standard protocol for hematoxilin, eosin, and Ki67 to ensure xenograft comparability to the original specimen. Cases with changed histological pattern were sent for pathological review and outgrowth of lymphoproliferative disorders was excluded.

2.3. Molecular Characterization

Molecular characterization was performed within the ONCOTRACK project as described by Schütte et al. [2] and data were used in this study. In brief, DNA and RNA obtained from the PDX tumor sample were analyzed for gene expression, copy number variants, somatic SNVs, gene fusions [2]. Microsatellite status was analyzed using the five monomorphic markers BAT25, BAT26, NR21, NR24, and NR27 and pentaplex polymerase chain reactions (PCR) [2].

2.4. In Vivo Drug Response Testing of the Xenografts

Twenty-five xenografts of the 58 PDX models from the ONCOTRACK cohort were included in the drug combination studies. Response to the selected compounds and combinations was evaluated in early passages using the design of a preclinical phase II study. Tumor fragments of similar size were transplanted subcutaneously to a cohort of mice. At palpable tumor size (80–150 mm^3), mice were randomized to treatment or control groups consisting of 3 animals each. Doses and schedules were chosen according to previous experience in animal experiments and represent maximum tolerated or efficient doses. The following drugs, doses, and schedules for single and combination treatments were used:

1. Cetuximab (Merck KGA), 30 mg/kg biweekly intraperitoneally, in saline;
2. Regorafenib (Bayer AG), 10 mg/kg once daily orally, in pluronic F68 and PEG400;
3. Everolimus (Novartis), 3 mg/kg once daily orally, in Tween 80 and saline;
4. Trametinib (Selleckchem), 3 mg/kg once daily orally, in hydroxypropylmethylcellulose and Tween 80 in water for injection.

Drugs were obtained from the pharmacy or Selleckchem, Houston, TX, USA. The injection volume was 0.1 mL/20 g body weight. In case of therapy resistance (no regression or stable disease), selected mice received all four drugs until further progression for another 4 weeks. Treatment was continued till tumor size exceeded 1.5 cm^3 or animals showed loss of >15% body weight. From the first treatment day onwards, the tumor volumes and body weights were recorded twice weekly. At the end of the treatment period, animals were sacrificed, and blood and tumor samples were collected and stored in liquid nitrogen immediately.

Animal welfare was controlled twice daily. Tumor volume (TV) was calculated from the length and width of subcutaneous tumors (TV = (length × [width]^2)/2). Sensitivity to the tested compounds was determined as tumor growth inhibition by treatment in comparison to the control (T/C) at each measurement point. Efficacy of the tested drugs in PDX models was classified using the adopted clinical response criteria (RECIST). We calculated the relative tumor volume (RTV) as the ratio of the TV on the last day before the study ended or start of quadruple treatment/TV on the first day of treatment.

The response criteria, taking as reference the baseline sum diameters, were defined as follows:

1. Strong Response: (RTV < 1.6);
2. Moderate Response: (RTV < 2.5);
3. Minor Response: (RTV < 5.5);
4. Resistance: (RTV > 5.5).

As RTV is a condensed summary parameter, no standard deviation values for replicate measurements are given in the Supplementary Figures S1–S4; these values have been determined and are available in the raw data.

2.5. Statistical Analyses of Mutational Load and Drug Sensitivity Values

Statistical and graphical analyses were performed with Prism version 9.1.0 (GraphPad Software, San Diego, CA, USA). Statistical differences were analyzed by unpaired t tests with Welch's correction (comparison of the mutational load in MSI and MSS PDX models), Kruskal–Wallis test with Dunn's multiple comparisons post-test, and one-way ANOVA with Holm–Šídák's multiple comparisons post-test (comparison of treatment-dependent RTV values in the respective subgroups). Regarding the comparison of treatment-dependent RTV values in subgroup I, PDX Co11672-327 was excluded from the analysis, since it was the sample with an activating BRAF mutation. p values are displayed as follows: p value > 0.05 ns; p value $\leq$ 0.05 *; p value $\leq$ 0.01 **; p value $\leq$ 0.001 ***.

3. Results

The selected panel of 25 colon cancer PDX models with heterogeneous sensitivity towards cetuximab was tested for response to the single drugs and the drug combinations with cetuximab and trametinib, cetuximab and regorafenib, and cetuximab with everolimus. These combinations should provide a parallel blockade of targets in the downstream MAP kinase pathway or the PI3K/AKT pathway (Figure 1). Mice were treated for up to 4 weeks to determine the initial response to the mono- and dual combination therapies. Responses (RTVs) to the single drug and drug combination treatments are summarized in Figure 2. In the case of therapy resistance (no regression or stable disease), selected mice received all four drugs until further progression for another 4 weeks. General health status and body weights were recorded on a regular basis daily or twice weekly as toxicity of drug combinations has been reported frequently. In our studies, the drugs were well-tolerated in the groups treated with cetuximab, regorafenib, and trametinib. Everolimus has caused a reversible minor body weight loss of between 5 and 10% in some studies. The drug combination treatments were tolerated without additional toxicity (representative data are shown in Supplementary Figures S1–S3).

Based on the analysis of a panel of 65 genes most frequently mutated in the selected 25 PDX models, four molecular subgroups were determined (Figures 2 and 3). The Consensus Molecular Subtype (CMS) classification describes four CRC subtypes with distinct biological characteristics that show prognostic and potential predictive value in the clinical setting. As already described by Schuette et al. [2] for the ONCOTRACK panel of colon cancer PDX models, the CMS classification cannot be transferred directly to the colon cancer PDX models as the immune cell components are missed by xenotransplantation in immune-suppressed mice. Nevertheless, our groups shared some similar characteristics to the annotation within the CRC consensus molecular group labels (CMS1 to CMS4) [3].

The first group (n = 5) is characterized by microsatellite instability (MSI) status, accompanied by a statistically significant higher mutational load in the selected panel of 65 genes (>10 mutations in the panel) compared to PDX models with microsatellite stability (MSS) status (Figure 2). However, in contrast to CMS1, we found a BRAF mutation in only 2 out of these 5 PDX models. In the second cohort (n = 5), all colon cancers had a BRAF V600E mutation; however, again, in contrast to CMS1, all tumors were MSS and had otherwise a very low frequency of mutations ($\leq$3 mutations in the panel). The third group (n = 7) was KRAS and BRAF wt, characterized by adenomatous polyposis coli (APC) and p53 mutations and a low frequency of other mutations (Figure 2). This group seemed to correspond with the CMS2 (canonical) subgroup characteristics. The last group (n = 8) had KRAS mutations and some frequent co-mutations (Figure 2). This group was MSS and included characteristics from both the CMS3 and CMS4 subgroups (Figure 3).

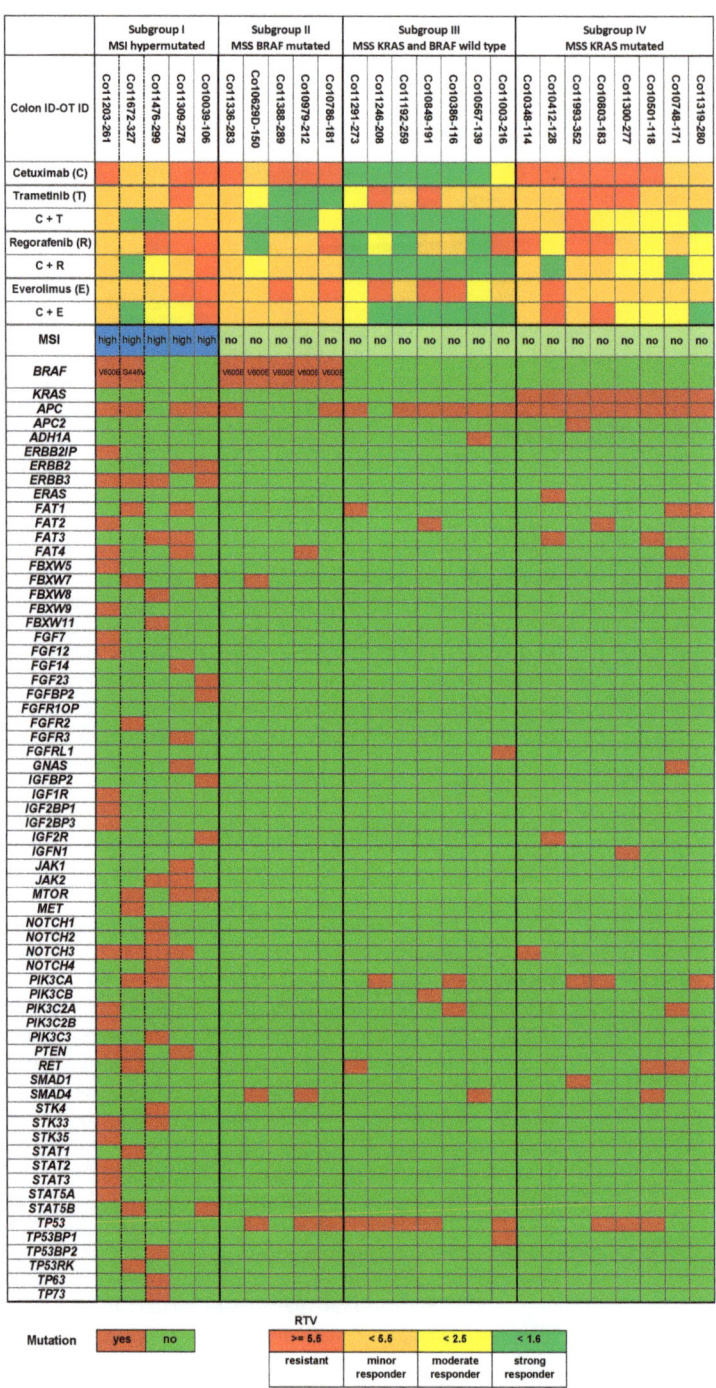

Figure 2. Response of 25 colon cancer PDX to cetuximab, regorafenib, trametinib, and everolimus in correlation with genetic mutation profile. Response data are provided as RTV values (RTV = quote of TV on the last day before study ended or start of quadruple treatment/TV on the first day of treatment).

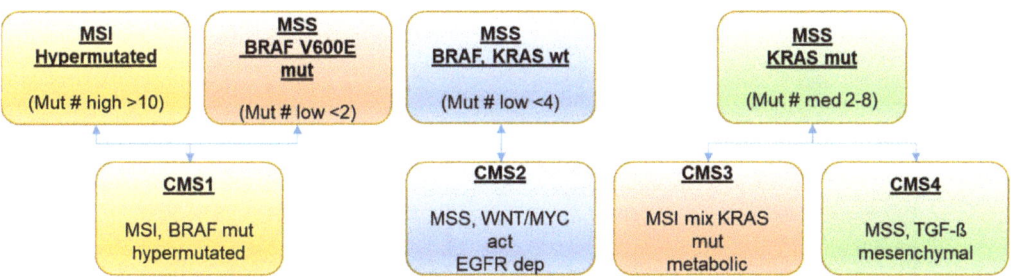

Figure 3. Genomic classification of colon cancer subgroups.

3.1. Patterns of Drug Response in Colon Cancer PDX Models in Relation to the Four Molecular Subgroups

To understand potential synergies by the combination treatments in correlation to the molecular subgroups, drug response evaluation was performed for each described subgroup.

3.1.1. Subgroup I—MSI Hypermutated

Subgroup I with MSI and high mutation frequency is mainly resistant to the four targeted drugs, with only some minor responses. Although there is a trend for synergistic effects by the combination of cetuximab and trametinib, these differences are not statistically relevant (Figure 4a). Taken together, this molecular subgroup is rather resistant to both single and combination treatment with targeted drugs (Supplementary Figure S1).

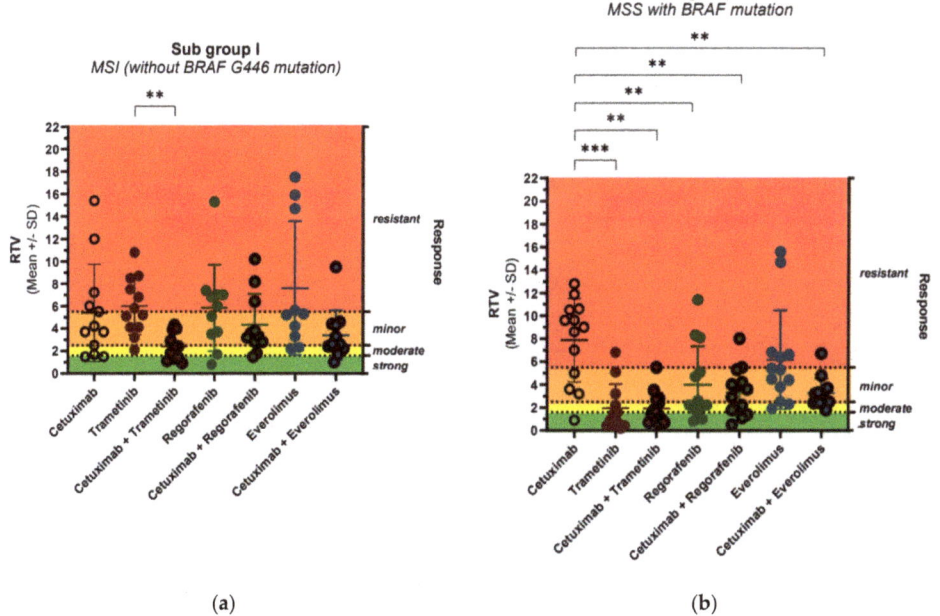

Figure 4. *Cont.*

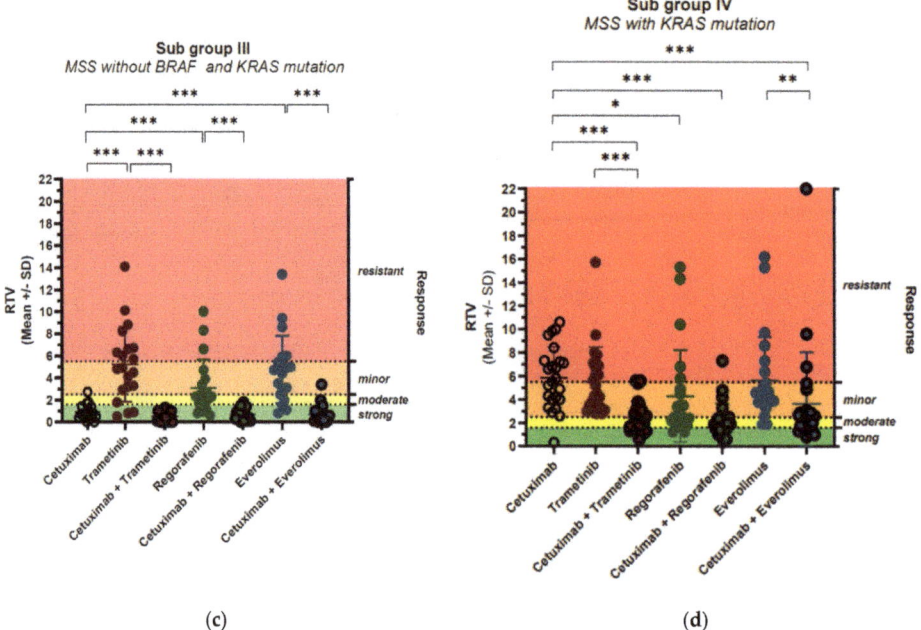

Figure 4. Effects of single treatments in comparison to drug combinations in: Subgroup I with MSI hypermutated colon cancer (**a**), Subgroup II with MSS and BRAF-mutated colon cancer (**b**), Subgroup III with MSS and KRAS and BRAF wild-type colon cancer (**c**), Subgroup IV with MSS and KRAS-mutated colon cancer (**d**) (p values are displayed as follows: p value > 0.05 ns; p value ≤ 0.05 *; p value ≤ 0.01 **; p value ≤ 0.001 ***).

The PDX model Co11672-327 seems to be an exceptional model in this subgroup due to the uncommon kinase impaired BRAF G446V mutation. Hence, it was excluded from the above-mentioned analyses of treatment responses (Figure 4a). However, this model is very sensitive toward all three combinations. It has been reported that other PDX with this BRAF mutation have been sensitive to EGFR and MEK inhibition with even stronger activity of combinations [4].

3.1.2. Subgroup II—MSS BRAF-Mutated

Subgroup II is characterized by the BRAF V600E mutation. However, all five PDX are MSS and have a low frequency of mutations, a rather uncommon combination when compared to the classification in CMS1. Interestingly, all models are resistant to cetuximab, but rather sensitive to the MEK inhibitor trametinib, with a significant difference in terms of responses (Figure 4b). The effect of trametinib in 4 out of 5 PDX models—Co10629-150, Co10786-181, Co10979-212, Co11388-289—is long-lasting disease stabilization with partial regression for up to 3 months (Supplementary Figure S2). Regorafenib and everolimus as single drugs have some minor activity, which is, however, only for regorafenib statistically significant different from cetuximab. The combination of cetuximab with both drugs has synergistic effects and is significantly better. Combination of trametinib with cetuximab does not improve response in the four strongly responding models; however, it has synergistic effects in Co11336-283, the model with only a minor response to trametinib (Supplementary Figure S2).

3.1.3. Subgroup III—MSS KRAS and BRAF Wild-Type

The third group is MSS and does not have prominent oncogenic mutations in the MAP kinase pathway (KRAS and BRAF). All seven colon cancers share common molecular characteristics, with a generally low number of mutations, mainly APC and p53 and three models with PIK3CA/B mutations. All seven colon cancers are highly sensitive to cetuximab, with a strong response. Surprisingly, all models are rather resistant to trametinib and everolimus. The combination with the three other drugs in general did not further improve the response (Figure 4c). However, in selected models, combination with trametinib (Co10849-191, Co11192-259) exerted synergistic effects and complete tumor regressions were observed (Supplementary Figure S3). The combination of cetuximab with everolimus (mTOR inhibition) showed a tendency for synergistic effects in the same two colon cancer PDX models, where, in particular, two complete regressions were remarkable.

The colon cancer model Co11291-273 is characterized by a RET mutation. While both drugs cetuximab or regorafenib alone can induce a strong response, the combination, however, shows synergistic effects with partial to complete regression of the tumors (Supplementary Figure S3).

3.1.4. Subgroup IV—MSS KRAS-Mutated

The fourth subgroup consists of eight colon cancer models with KRAS mutations, and all of them are MSS. Besides the KRAS mutations, these eight colon cancer PDX models do share other common molecular characteristics: some have mutations in PI3K (4), in RET (2), and SMAD4 (1). In general, the number of mutations is higher when compared to Subgroup II.

All models are resistant to treatment with cetuximab and to the inhibition of the MAPK pathway by the MEK inhibitor trametinib. However, a statistically significant synergistic activity of the combination of cetuximab with trametinib was reported in this subgroup (Figure 4). The combination achieved four stable disease states—Co11319-280, Co10748-171, Co10501-118, Co10803-183—and two minor responses—Co11300-277 and Co10412-128—in these otherwise highly resistant tumors (Supplementary Figure S4).

Whereas everolimus is not active in any of these models, response to regorafenib is heterogeneous, with three colon cancers showing a response Co11319-280, Co10501-118, Co11300-277, and Co10412-128, whereas the other four are resistant. Combination with cetuximab seems to provide some significant synergistic effects in selected models. The PDX model Co11993-352, for example, is rather resistant to all single treatments and combinations, except for cetuximab and regorafenib (Supplementary Figure S4).

4. Discussion

Whereas, in the "pre-" personalized medicine area, doublet chemotherapy was seen as the standard of care for advanced or metastatic colon cancer, the identification of activated signaling via the MAPK pathway or the VEGF receptor family in colon cancer has introduced new treatment opportunities with monoclonal antibodies or kinase inhibitors [5]. As per current clinical guidelines, pan-RAS, BRAF, HER2, and mismatch repair (MMR) status are established molecular markers for selection of patient treatment [6]. However, it has been realized that the predictive value of these biomarkers has limitations. From the group of patients without mutations in the MAP kinase pathway members KRAS and BRAF, significant sub-fractions do not benefit from EGFR antibody treatment.

Patients with KRAS or BRAF mutations continue to have a very poor prognosis, often with median survival of less than 12 months, and treatment options are still limited [5]. Approximately 7–10% of CRC patients have a mutation of the BRAF gene, with 90% of them displaying the V600E [7–9]. There are three classes of BRAF mutations; while class I and II, i.e., with the most common mutation—V600E—have a notably worse prognosis, class III has impaired kinase activity and better prognosis. Thus, for patients with BRAF- or KRAS-mutated colon cancer, alternative targeted treatment strategies still need to be developed [10]. Before the era of targeted therapy combinations, intense chemotherapy with anti-VEGF was the standard of care in patients with BRAF class I and II mutations [11]. While KRAS has been, until recently, seen to be undruggable and the new KRAS inhibitors target only the less frequent mutation G12C [12], several BRAF and MEK kinase inhibitors have been developed and tested also in colon cancer patients. The effects of BRAF inhibitors such as vemurafenib in melanoma treatment raised some expectations for the treatment of colon cancer patients. However, inhibition of the MAPK pathway with single BRAF inhibitors such as vemurafenib or dabrafenib has not demonstrated therapeutic benefits in clinical trials [13,14]. It has become clear that BRAF inhibition in colon cancer can lead to activation of EGFR through an ERK-dependent negative feedback loop and induce further upregulation of other receptor tyrosine kinases, including the other human epidermal growth factor receptors, or activation of the phosphoinositide 3-kinase (PI3K)/AKT/mTOR pathway [15,16]. Activation of the PI3K/AKT/mTOR pathway has also been implicated in BRAF inhibition resistance [17].

Based on these findings, we have evaluated combination therapies blocking both pathways with four different drugs in our representative preclinical models to generate new hypotheses for treatments that will overcome resistance and improve response in selected colon cancer patient subgroups (Figure 1). As colon cancers express high levels of activated EGFR, a combined blockade of EGFR and BRAF or even downstream MEK may work synergistically and could be a potential therapeutic opportunity in CRC. As the combination of cetuximab with vemurafenib has not been very effective, we chose either the approved MEK inhibitor trametinib or the (pan) BRAF and VEGF kinase inhibitor regorafenib for the combination experiments. Regorafenib inhibits, next to the main targets, several other kinases, such as TIE2, KIT, RET, RAF-1, BRAFV600E, PDGFR, and FGFR.

As mentioned earlier, activation of the PI3K/AKT/mTOR pathway by negative feedback is one potential pathway in cetuximab resistance. We therefore included the mTOR inhibitor everolimus as the third combination partner in the studies.

The BEACON trial [18] first demonstrated that both a dual therapy targeting BRAF (encorafenib) and EGFR (cetuximab) and especially a triple combination targeting BRAF (encorafenib), MEK (binimetinib), and EGFR (cetuximab) can increase the survival of colon cancer patients compared to the current standard of care (SoC). We observed that tumors in Subgroup II with BAF V600E as a potential single driver mutation strongly responded to trametinib. The combination of trametinib with cetuximab seemed to further increase the overall response in this colon cancer subgroup. Our findings are in line with the results from the BEACON study; however, they provide additional findings that might be of clinical relevance for the treatment of these patients.

For selection of the optimal treatment of colon cancer patients with BRAF mutations, the MSI status might be considered as an additional biomarker. BRAF mutations have been observed in 30–50% of MSI-high CRC, compared with 10% in microsatellite stable tumors [19,20]. According to our data, tumors with BRAF V600E mutations and MSS status (low mutational rate) seem to strongly benefit from the combination of trametinib (MEK inhibition) and cetuximab (EGFR inhibition), whereas MSI tumors seem not to have a benefit, although the number of models in this cohort is too low for statistically significant conclusions.

Colon cancers without KRAS and BRAF mutations strongly respond to treatment with cetuximab and are rather resistant to the other three treatments. However, findings of mutations in other oncogenic pathways have been reported in this subgroup. For example, RET is altered in 2.94% of colorectal carcinoma patients [21] and, further, PI3K signaling can be activated by direct mutation or amplification of PIK3CA or loss of PTEN. Approximately 40% of CRC have been shown to have alterations in PI3K pathway genes, which are almost always mutually exclusive from each other [22].

We observed, in selected models, synergistic effects and complete tumor regressions by the combination of cetuximab with everolimus—for example, in model Co11192-259 with a mutation in PIK3CB. These findings lead to the hypothesis that the combination of cetuximab with PI3K or mTOR inhibition might be of benefit for a subgroup with wt KRAS and BRAF, but activation of the PI3K pathway.

The combination of cetuximab with regorafenib (RAF, VEGF, and RET inhibition) did show synergistic effects in model Co11291-273 with RET mutation. This combination might be a potential therapeutic option for the subgroup of patients with RET as a driver mutation, as we observed complete regressions under this treatment combination (Supplementary Figure S2).

All PDX models with KRAS mutations tested in our study were resistant to treatment with cetuximab, confirming, in this case, the good predictivity of KRAS mutations as a biomarker for cetuximab in colon cancer patients. Similarly, the inhibition of the MAPK pathway by the MEK inhibitor trametinib was not effective. The most surprising outcome in this subgroup was the statistically significant synergistic activity of the combination of cetuximab with trametinib. The combination achieved four stable disease cases and two minor responses in these otherwise highly resistant tumors (Supplementary Figure S4). As there are currently no other treatment alternatives for this colon cancer subgroup, in cases with MSS status, further evaluation of this combination inhibiting EGFR and MEK might be considered.

The MSI-high subgroup with or without BRAF mutation is resistant to the tested targeted drugs. Based on the MSI and the hypermutated profile, this group would be better treated with chemo- or immune therapies. Data from the ONCOTRACK project confirm this hypothesis at least in part, as strong sensitivity to the SoC chemotherapies 5-FU or irinotecan has been observed in 4 out these 5 models [2]. A combination of chemotherapy with a PARP inhibitor has recently shown activity in preclinical models of peritoneal metastases of colorectal cancer with a similar molecular profile [23] and might be an alternative opportunity for this subgroup of patients. Currently, immunotherapy is evaluated as a therapeutic option in these subtypes [24]. As immunotherapies cannot be evaluated in the common PDX models on immunodeficient mice, further studies in humanized mouse models might be required [25].

5. Conclusions

- Molecular profiling allows the identification of colon cancer subgroups for personalized treatment.
- PDX models of CRC enable preclinical screening of targeted drugs and identification of synergistic combinations in correlation with molecular profiles.
- Microsatellite stable colon cancer models with BRAF or KRAS mutations in Subgroups II and IV have shown responses to the combination of EGFR (cetuximab), MEK (trametinib), and/or RAF (regorafenib) inhibition, providing a strong hypothesis for further evaluation.
- PI3K, mTOR (everolimus), and RET (regorafenib) inhibition seem to be synergistic with EGFR (cetuximab) inhibition in selected colon cancers with those activated pathways.
- Although the small preclinical phase II-like sample size precludes firm conclusions, the results of the study have revealed interesting potential relations, which either might be followed up in a larger preclinical panel or translated in personalized clinical trials.

Supplementary Materials: The following are available online at https://www.mdpi.com/article/10.3390/cancers13236018/s1; Figure S1: Effects of single treatments in comparison to drug combinations in the subgroup I with MSI hypermutated colon cancer; Figure S2: Effects of single treatments in comparison to drug combinations in the subgroup II with MSS and BRAF mutated colon cancer; Figure S3: Effects of single treatments in comparison to drug combinations in the subgroup III with MSS and KRAS and BRAF wild type colon cancer; Figure S4: Effects of single treatments in comparison to drug combinations in the subgroup IV, MSS and KRAS mutated colon cancer.

Author Contributions: The clinical cohort was managed and recruited and tissue samples were distributed by U.K., J.H. (Johannes Haybaeck) and colleagues. NGS data generation and analysis, data processing and genome analyses: M.S., M.-L.Y., H.L. and colleagues. Experimental models: xenograft establishment and drug response data were provided by M.K. and J.H. (Jens Hoffmann). Correlation of drug responses with genetic landscape was performed by T.C. and M.B., J.H. (Jens Hoffmann) conceptualized the project and contributed to the interpretation of the data and wrote the manuscript. The manuscript was communicated to all authors and all had the opportunity to comment on and approved the paper. All authors have read and agreed to the published version of the manuscript.

Funding: The research leading to these results has received support from the Innovative Medicines Initiative Joint Undertaking under grant agreement no. 115234 (OncoTrack).

Institutional Review Board Statement: The study was approved by the local Institutional Review Board of Charité University Medicine (Charité Ethics Cie: Charitéplatz 1, 10117 Berlin), Germany (EA 1/069/11) and the ethics committee of the Medical University of Graz (Ethic commission of the Medical University of Graz, Auenbruggerplatz 2, 8036 Graz, Austria), confirmed by the ethics committee of the St. John of God Hospital Graz (23-015 ex 10/11).

Informed Consent Statement: Informed consent was obtained from all subjects involved in the study.

Data Availability Statement: The complete set of NGS data for patient tumors has been published by Schütte et al. [2] and is available in the European Genome-Phenome Archive (EGA) of the EBI data repository under accession number EGAS00001001752.

Acknowledgments: We thank the NGS technical team of the MPI MG Berlin and the Alacris Theranostics GmbH Berlin for generating the NGS data used for this study. We also thank Diana Anders and Katharina Scholl for technical assistance. We thank the teams from the Charite Universitätsmedizin Berlin, the University Graz Hospital, the surgical department of the St. John of God Hospital Graz, and the Department of Pathology of the General Hospital Graz Süd-West (Austria), for helping in collecting clinical samples.

Conflicts of Interest: J.H., T.C., M.B. and M.K. are employed by EPO Berlin-Buch GmbH. The study was funded by the EPO Berlin-Buch GmbH. The funder had no role in the design of the study; in the collection, analyses, or interpretation of data; in the writing of the manuscript, or in the decision to publish the results. The other authors declare no conflict of interest.

References

1. Stintzing, S.; Modest, D.P.; Rossius, L.; Lerch, M.M.; von Weikersthal, L.F.; Decker, T.; Kiani, A.; Vehling-Kaiser, U.; Al-Batran, S.-E.; Heintges, T.; et al. FOLFIRI plus cetuximab versus FOLFIRI plus bevacizumab for metastatic colorectal cancer (FIRE-3): A post-hoc analysis of tumour dynamics in the final RAS wild-type subgroup of this randomised open-label phase 3 trial. *Lancet Oncol.* **2016**, *17*, 1426–1434. [CrossRef]
2. Schütte, M.; Risch, T.; Abdavi-Azar, N.; Boehnke, K.; Schumacher, D.; Keil, M.; Yildiriman, R.; Jandrasits, C.; Borodina, T.; Amstislavskiy, V.; et al. Molecular dissection of colorectal cancer in pre-clinical models identifies biomarkers predicting sensitivity to EGFR inhibitors. *Nat. Commun.* **2017**, *8*, 14262. [CrossRef]
3. Guinney, J.; Dienstmann, R.; Wang, X.; De Reyniès, A.; Schlicker, A.; Soneson, C.; Marisa, L.; Roepman, P.; Nyamundanda, G.; Angelino, P.; et al. The consensus molecular subtypes of colorectal cancer. *Nat. Med.* **2015**, *21*, 1350–1356. [CrossRef]
4. Yao, Z.; Yaeger, R.; Rodrik-Outmezguine, V.S.; Tao, A.; Torres, N.M.; Chang, M.T.; Drosten, M.; Zhao, H.; Cecchi, F.; Hembrough, T.; et al. Tumours with class 3 BRAF mutants are sensitive to the inhibition of activated RAS. *Nat. Cell Biol.* **2017**, *548*, 234–238. [CrossRef]
5. Loree, J.M.; Kopetz, S. Recent developments in the treatment of metastatic colorectal cancer. *Ther. Adv. Med. Oncol.* **2017**, *9*, 551–564. [CrossRef] [PubMed]
6. Van Cutsem, E.; Cervantes, A.; Adam, R.; Sobrero, A.; van Krieken, J.H.; Aderka, D.; Aguilar, E.A.; Bardelli, A.; Benson, A.; Bodoky, G.; et al. ESMO consensus guidelines for the management of patients with metastatic colorectal cancer. *Ann. Oncol.* **2016**, *27*, 1386–1422. [CrossRef]
7. BRAF Gene. COSMIC. 2018. Available online: https://cancer.sanger.ac.uk/cosmic/gene/analysis?ln=BRAF (accessed on 28 November 2021).
8. Tie, J.; Gibbs, P.; Lipton, L.; Christie, M.; Jorissen, R.N.; Burgess, A.W.; Croxford, M.; Jones, I.; Langland, R.; Kosmider, S.; et al. Optimizing targeted therapeutic development: Analysis of a colorectal cancer patient population with the BRAF(V600E) mutation. *Int. J. Cancer* **2011**, *128*, 2075–2084. [CrossRef]
9. Morris, V.; Overman, M.J.; Jiang, Z.Q.; Garrett, C.; Agarwal, S.; Eng, C.; Kee, B.; Fogelman, D.; Dasari, A.; Wolff, R.; et al. Progression-free survival remains poor over se-quential lines of systemic therapy in patients with BRAF-mutated colorectal cancer. *Clin. Colorectal Cancer* **2014**, *13*, 164–171. [CrossRef] [PubMed]
10. Luu, L.-J.; Price, T.J. BRAF Mutation and Its Importance in Colorectal Cancer. In *Advances in the Molecu-lar Understanding of Colorectal Cancer, Eva Segelov*; IntechOpen: London, UK, 2019. [CrossRef]

11. Cremolini, C.; Loupakis, F.; Antoniotti, C.; Lupi, C.; Sensi, E.; Lonardi, S.; Mezi, S.; Tomasello, G.; Ronzoni, M.; Zaniboni, A.; et al. FOLFOXIRI plus bevacizumab versus FOLFIRI plus bevacizumab as first-line treatment of patients with metastatic colorectal cancer: Updated overall survival and molecular subgroup analyses of the open-label, phase 3 TRIBE study. *Lancet Oncol.* **2015**, *16*, 1306–1315. [CrossRef]
12. Rhett, J.M.; Khan, I.; O'Bryan, J.P. Biology, pathology, and therapeutic targeting of RAS. *Adv. Cancer Res.* **2020**, *148*, 69–146. [CrossRef]
13. Kopetz, S.; Desai, J.; Chan, E.; Hecht, J.R.; O'Dwyer, P.J.; Maru, D.; Morris, V.; Janku, F.; Dasari, A.; Chung, W.; et al. Phase II pilot study of vemurafenib in patients with meta-static BRAF-mutated colorectal cancer. *J. Clin. Oncol.* **2015**, *33*, 4032–4038. [CrossRef] [PubMed]
14. Hyman, D.M.; Puzanov, I.; Subbiah, V.; Faris, J.E.; Chau, I.; Blay, J.-Y.; Wolf, J.L.; Raje, N.S.; Diamond, E.; Hollebecque, A.; et al. Vemurafenib in Multiple Nonmelanoma Cancers with BRAF V600 Mutations. *N. Engl. J. Med.* **2015**, *373*, 726–736. [CrossRef] [PubMed]
15. Prahallad, A.; Sun, C.; Huang, S.; Di Nicolantonio, F.; Salazar, R.; Zecchin, D.; Beijersbergen, R.L.; Bardelli, A.; Bernards, R. Unresponsiveness of colon cancer to BRAF(V600E) inhibition through feedback activation of EGFR. *Nat. Cell Biol.* **2012**, *483*, 100–103. [CrossRef] [PubMed]
16. Herr, R.; Halbach, S.; Heizmann, M.; Busch, H.; Boerries, M.; Brummer, T. BRAF inhibition upregulates a variety of receptor tyro-sine kinases and their downstream effector Gab2 in colorectal cancer cell lines. *Oncogene* **2018**, *37*, 1576–1593. [CrossRef] [PubMed]
17. Mao, M.; Tian, F.; Mariadason, J.; Tsao, C.C.; Lemos, R.; Dayyani, F.; Gopal, Y.V.; Jiang, Z.-Q.; Wistuba, I.I.; Tang, X.M.; et al. Resistance to BRAF Inhibition in BRAF-Mutant Colon Cancer Can Be Overcome with PI3K Inhibition or Demethylating Agents. *Clin. Cancer Res.* **2012**, *19*, 657–667. [CrossRef] [PubMed]
18. Shahjehan, F.; Kamatham, S.; Chandrasekharan, C.; Kasi, P. Binimetinib, encorafenib and cetuximab (BEACON Trial) combination therapy for patients with BRAF V600E-mutant metastatic colorectal cancer. *Drugs Today* **2019**, *55*, 683–693. [CrossRef] [PubMed]
19. Tran, B.; Kopetz, S.; Tie, J.; Gibbs, P.; Jiang, Z.-Q.; Lieu, C.H.; Agarwal, A.; Maru, D.M.; Sieber, O.; Desai, J. Impact of BRAF mutation and microsatellite instability on the pattern of metastatic spread and prognosis in metastatic colorectal cancer. *Cancer* **2011**, *117*, 4623–4632. [CrossRef]
20. Sinicrope, F.A.; Mahoney, M.R.; Smyrk, T.C.; Thibodeau, S.N.; Warren, R.S.; Bertagnolli, M.M.; Nelson, G.D.; Goldberg, R.M.; Sargent, D.J.; Alberts, S.R. Prognostic impact of deficient DNA mismatch repair in patients with stage III colon cancer from a randomized trial of FOLFOX-based adjuvant chemo-therapy. *J. Clin. Oncol.* **2013**, *31*, 3664–3672. [CrossRef]
21. The AACR Project GENIE Consortium. AACR Project GENIE: Powering precision medicine through an international con-sortium. *Cancer Discov.* **2017**, *7*, 818–831. [CrossRef]
22. Parsons, D.W.; Wang, T.L.; Samuels, Y.; Bardelli, A.; Cummins, J.M.; DeLong, L.; Silliman, N.; Ptak, J.; Szabo, S.; Willson, J.K.; et al. Colorectal cancer: Mutations in a signalling pathway. *Nature* **2005**, *436*, 792. [CrossRef]
23. Dahlmann, M.; Gambara, G.; Brzezicha, B.; Popp, O.; Pachmayr, E.; Wedeken, L.; Pflaume, A.; Mokritzkij, M.; Gül-Klein, S.; Brandl, A.; et al. Peritoneal metastasis of colorectal cancer (pmCRC): Identification of predictive molecular signatures by a novel preclinical platform of matching pmCRC PDX/PD3D models. *Mol. Cancer* **2021**, *20*, 1–8. [CrossRef] [PubMed]
24. Lenz, H.-J.; Van Cutsem, E.; Limon, M.L.; Wong, K.Y.M.; Hendlisz, A.; Aglietta, M.; García-Alfonso, P.; Neyns, B.; Luppi, G.; Cardin, D.B.; et al. First-Line Nivolumab Plus Low-Dose Ipilimumab for Microsatellite Instability-High/Mismatch Repair-Deficient Metastatic Colorectal Cancer: The Phase II CheckMate 142 Study. *J. Clin. Oncol.* **2021**. [CrossRef]
25. Stecklum, M.; Wulf-Goldenberg, A.; Brzezicha, B.; Fichtner, I.; Hoffmann, J. Humanized immune-oncology mouse models. *Immunology* **2017**, *77*, 1697. [CrossRef]

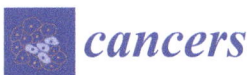

Article

Bridging the Species Gap: Morphological and Molecular Comparison of Feline and Human Intestinal Carcinomas

Tanja Groll [1,2,3], Franziska Schopf [1,2], Daniela Denk [1,2,3], Carolin Mogler [1,2], Ulrike Schwittlick [4], Heike Aupperle-Lellbach [4], Sabrina Rim Jahan Sarker [1,2], Nicole Pfarr [1], Wilko Weichert [1], Kaspar Matiasek [3], Moritz Jesinghaus [1,5] and Katja Steiger [1,2,*]

[1] Institute of Pathology, School of Medicine, Technical University of Munich (TUM), 81675 Munich, Germany; tanja.groll@tum.de (T.G.); f.schopf@campus.lmu.de (F.S.); daniela.denk@patho.vetmed.uni-muenchen.de (D.D.); carolin.mogler@tum.de (C.M.); sabrina.sarker@tum.de (S.R.J.S.); nicole.pfarr@tum.de (N.P.); wilko.weichert@tum.de (W.W.); moritz.jesinghaus@uni-marburg.de (M.J.)

[2] Comparative Experimental Pathology, School of Medicine, Technical University of Munich (TUM), 81675 Munich, Germany

[3] Institute of Veterinary Pathology, Center for Clinical Veterinary Medicine, Ludwig-Maximilians-Universitaet (LMU), 80539 Munich, Germany; kaspar.matiasek@neuropathologie.de

[4] LABOKLIN GmbH & Co. KG, 97688 Bad Kissingen, Germany; schwittlick@laboklin.com (U.S.); aupperle@laboklin.com (H.A.-L.)

[5] Department of Pathology, University Hospital Marburg, 35043 Marburg, Germany

* Correspondence: katja.steiger@tum.de; Tel.: +49-89-4140-6075; Fax: +49-89-4140-4865

Simple Summary: Colorectal cancer (CRC) is the second leading cause of cancer deaths in humans (2020) but modeling late-stage human CRC, including high tumor budding and metastatic activity, experimentally in mouse models is a major challenge. In the present study, histopathological, immunohistochemical and molecular features of spontaneous intestinal carcinomas in cats were evaluated with a special focus on their potential applicability as a valuable model for human CRC. Feline intestinal tumors display aggressive growth patterns and adequately model invasive late-stage human CRC. They exhibit the same histological subtypes and display strikingly high tumor budding activity, both of which are highly significant prognostic factors in human CRC. Moreover, human and feline colorectal tumors harbor the same mutations of the *CTNNB1* gene, encoding β-catenin. Our data indicate that feline intestinal carcinomas constitute a valuable and promising in vivo model for human CRC. Further comparative oncological research, and especially investigation of the molecular landscape of feline intestinal neoplasms, is imperative.

Citation: Groll, T.; Schopf, F.; Denk, D.; Mogler, C.; Schwittlick, U.; Aupperle-Lellbach, H.; Sarker, S.R.J.; Pfarr, N.; Weichert, W.; Matiasek, K.; et al. Bridging the Species Gap: Morphological and Molecular Comparison of Feline and Human Intestinal Carcinomas. *Cancers* **2021**, *13*, 5941. https://doi.org/10.3390/cancers13235941

Academic Editor: Heike Allgayer

Received: 8 November 2021
Accepted: 22 November 2021
Published: 25 November 2021

Publisher's Note: MDPI stays neutral with regard to jurisdictional claims in published maps and institutional affiliations.

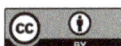

Copyright: © 2021 by the authors. Licensee MDPI, Basel, Switzerland. This article is an open access article distributed under the terms and conditions of the Creative Commons Attribution (CC BY) license (https://creativecommons.org/licenses/by/4.0/).

Abstract: Limited availability of in vivo experimental models for invasive colorectal cancer (CRC) including metastasis and high tumor budding activity is a major problem in colorectal cancer research. In order to compare feline and human intestinal carcinomas, tumors of 49 cats were histologically subtyped, graded and further characterized according to the human WHO classification. Subsequently, feline tumors were compared to a cohort of 1004 human CRC cases. Feline intestinal tumors closely resembled the human phenotype on a histomorphological level. In both species, adenocarcinoma not otherwise specified (ANOS) was the most common WHO subtype. In cats, the second most common subtype of the colon (36.4%), serrated adenocarcinoma (SAC), was overrepresented compared to human CRC (8.7%). Mucinous adenocarcinoma (MAC) was the second most common subtype of the small intestine (12.5%). Intriguingly, feline carcinomas, particularly small intestinal, were generally of high tumor budding (Bd) status (Bd3), which is designated an independent prognostic key factor in human CRC. We also investigated the relevance of feline *CTNNB1* exon 2 alterations by Sanger sequencing. In four cases of feline colonic malignancies (3 ANOS, 1 SAC), somatic missense mutations of feline *CTNNB1* (p.D32G, p.D32N, p.G34R, and p.S37F) were detected, indicating that mutational alterations of the WNT/β-catenin signaling pathway potentially play an essential role in feline intestinal tumorigenesis comparable to humans and dogs. These results indicate that spontaneous intestinal tumors of cats constitute a useful but so far underutilized model for human CRC. Our study provides a solid foundation for advanced comparative oncology studies and emphasizes the need for further (molecular) characterization of feline intestinal carcinomas.

Keywords: spontaneous feline intestinal tumors; comparative oncology; colorectal cancer; tumor budding; CTNNB1

1. Introduction

Worldwide, colon cancer is the third most common cancer type in humans, with an estimated 1.9 million new cases in 2020 and it is the second leading cause of cancer deaths [1]. To date, the most frequently used animal models in colon cancer research are mice with experimentally induced intestinal cancer; however, modeling late stages of human CRC is a major challenge as several mouse models tend to develop a high tumor burden, but no metastasis, leading to preliminary death. Invasively growing, metastasizing tumors of the large intestine, comparable with late-stage human CRC, are difficult to model in clean-housed experimental animal models, particularly genetically engineered mouse models (GEMM) [2–5]. Similarly, other animal models, e.g., rats or pigs, lack the ability to model metastasis and invasive carcinoma [3]. Moreover, the genotype of human tumors appears to be more heterogeneous than the one of experimentally induced murine tumors [6]. Spontaneously arising intestinal tumors of companion animals (pets) thus are of special interest for comparative research, especially since companion animals share their living environment with humans [7].

At present, there are only few studies of feline intestinal cancer, its biological behavior, clinical, histopathological, and molecular features. In cats, lymphoma is the most common intestinal neoplasm followed by intestinal carcinoma with a study-dependent incidence varying from 17 to 31.5% among gastrointestinal neoplasias [8–10]. Feline intestinal carcinomas are more prevalent than canine ones [11] and occur in both the large and small intestine. The available literature provides contradictory statements regarding the most commonly affected site in cats [8,9,11–14]. Feline intestinal carcinomas are more frequent in older animals with increasing risk starting from the age of seven [8,9] and either a breed predisposition of Siamese cats [9,11,13] or no breed predisposition [8,12] has been reported. Tumors metastasize frequently, rapidly, and most often within the peritoneum or to local lymph nodes, but also to distant sites (lung, liver, spleen) [8,11,13,15]. Subtotal colectomy via laparotomy is the current standard treatment but mean overall survival time of cat patients is generally low (68 to 274 days), as recurrence and metastases are common [11,15,16].

The aim of the present study was to characterize sporadic primary feline intestinal carcinomas histologically and molecularly in order to further compare them to human CRC. WHO subtype, tumor grading and tumor budding status are valuable prognostic tools in human CRC [17,18] and feline tumors were characterized according to the current human WHO classification [19].

Mutations, which stabilize the CTNNB1 gene encoding for β-catenin and thus activate the canonical WNT/β-catenin signaling pathway, play a pivotal role in the pathogenesis of human [20,21] and canine [22] intestinal cancer. Based on previous immunohistochemical findings of other authors, showing that dysregulated and nuclear translocated β-catenin was present in spontaneous feline intestinal carcinomas [12], we shed light on the mutational status of feline CTNNB1 by performing Sanger sequencing of feline CTNNB1 exon 2 for the first time.

2. Materials and Methods

2.1. Feline Study Cohort

Thirty-three cases of spontaneous feline colorectal and sixteen cases of feline small intestinal carcinoma were collected from the tissue archive of LABOKLIN GmbH & Co. KG

(Bad Kissingen, Germany) between the years 2013 and 2020. All samples (7 full-thickness biopsies and 42 surgical specimens) were obtained during laparotomy, submitted for pathological routine diagnostics, and reviewed retrospectively. In 20/49 cases, additional lymph node samples were available.

Intestinal tumor samples originated from cats of different breeds including 31 European Shorthair (ESH) cats (63.3%), 4 British Shorthair cats (8.2%), 3 Persian cats (6.1%), 2 Chartreux cats (4.1%), 2 Maine Coon cats (4.1%), 1 Exotic Shorthair cat (2%), 1 Norwegian Forest cat (2%), 1 Oriental Shorthair cat (2%), 1 Siamese cat (2%) and 3 mixed cat breeds (6.2%). The study set included 26 males (53.1%; 20/26 castrated) and 23 females (46.9%; 15/23 spayed), and the age at the time of diagnosis ranged from 4 to 17 years. Mean age ($\pm$ SD) was 11.51 years ($\pm$ 3.31 years). Detailed information on the feline cohort is provided in Tables S1 and S2.

2.1.1. Tissue Processing

Tissue samples were fixed in 10% neutral-buffered formalin and routinely processed for histology. Hematoxylin and eosin (H&E) staining was carried out following standard protocols. A Periodic Acid Schiff (PAS) reaction was performed on six selected cases in order to visualize intracytoplasmic mucin for validating the diagnosis of signet-ring cell carcinoma (SRCC). All slides were scanned in $40\times$ magnification using a high-throughput slide scanner (Aperio AT2, Leica Biosystems, Wetzlar, Germany). The histological classification of tumors was based on H&E and PAS-stained slides and carried out by a trainee veterinary pathologist (T.G.) under the supervision of experienced board-certified human (M.J., C.M.) and veterinary pathologists (D.D., K.S.). Immunohistochemistry (IHC) for β-catenin, Ki-67, Pan-cytokeratin and CD31 was performed. Detailed information on the IHC protocols and primary antibodies is provided in Table S3. Representative images were taken using Aperio ImageScope $\times 64$ (v.12.4.0.7018, Leica Biosystems, Wetzlar, Germany).

2.1.2. Histomorphological Characterization

For comparative reasons, the histological subtype classification of feline tumors was performed based on the current human WHO classification guidelines [19]. The following human WHO subtypes were identifiable amongst the feline intestinal carcinomas: adenocarcinoma not otherwise specified (ANOS), serrated adenocarcinoma (SAC), mucinous adenocarcinoma (MAC), micropapillary adenocarcinoma (MPC), and signet-ring cell carcinoma (SRCC). ANOS is considered a malignant epithelial neoplasia displaying glandular differentiation. SAC is characterized by glandular serration and consists of tumor cells with a low nucleus-to-cytoplasm ratio, which may be mixed with mucinous areas. MAC is defined by significant pools of extracellular mucin that contain tumor cells and form >50% of the tumor. MPC consists of $\geq$5% of small tumor cell clusters surrounded by stromal spaces, morphologically mimicking lymphatic or vascular channels, and therefore displays typical retraction artefacts [23]. SRCC consists of signet-ring cells forming >50% of the tumor, and containing prominent intracytoplasmic mucin, characteristically impressing and partially displacing the nucleus to the periphery. Carcinomas of all types with <50% areas containing mucin are designated as having a mucinous component [19].

The International Tumor Budding Consensus Conference (ITBCC) of 2016 achieved standardized classification for tumor budding in human colon cancer, establishing a clearly delineated tumor budding scoring scheme. Tumor buds were defined as individual or clusters of up to four cancer cells detached from the main tumor mass and counted in one hotspot area (0.785 mm^2) at the invasive front on an H&E slide ($20\times$). Clinically relevant cut-off values were defined in a 3-tier system as low (0–4 buds), intermediate (5–9 buds) and high ($\geq$10 buds), and termed Bd1, Bd2, and Bd3, respectively [18] (Figure S1). Tumor budding assessment was carried out for feline tumors in the same manner (Figure 1).

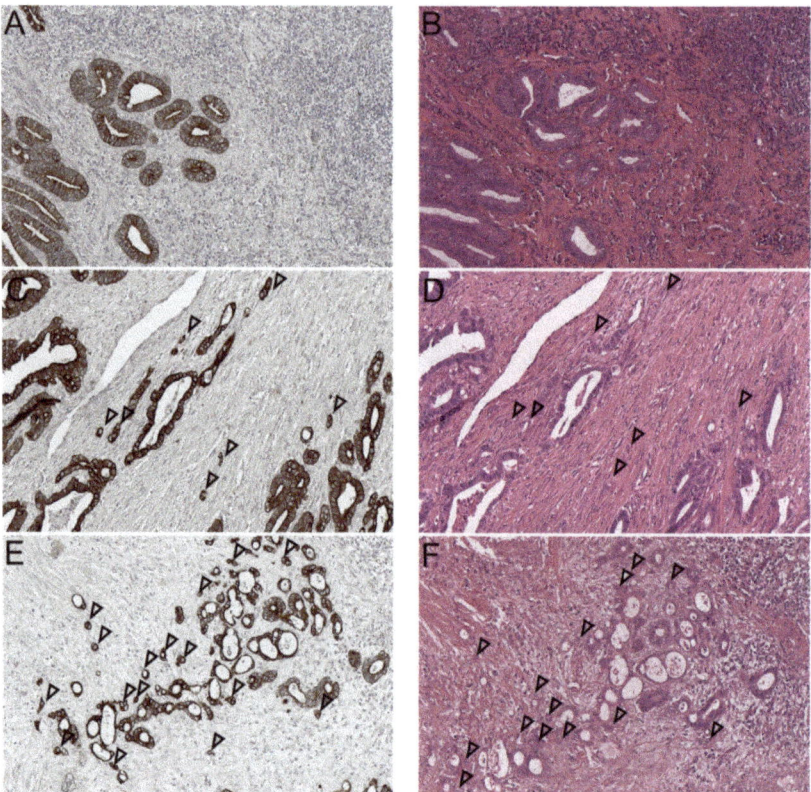

Figure 1. Tumor budding (TB) in the invasive front of feline intestinal carcinomas according to the 3-tier-system for budding assessment of human CRC (left: Pan-cytokeratin, right: H&E, consecutive sections, 20×). Tumor buds are indicated by arrow heads; (**A**) Low TB activity (Bd1, Pan-cytokeratin); (**B**) Low TB activity (Bd1, H&E); (**C**) Moderate TB activity (Bd2, Pan-cytokeratin); (**D**) Moderate TB activity (Bd2, H&E); (**E**) High TB activity (Bd3, Pan-cytokeratin); and (**F**) High TB activity (Bd3, H&E). For corresponding human H&E sections see Figure S1.

Adapted from the human WHO classification of 2019, a 2-tiered grading of feline intestinal tumor was based on the differentiation degree of cellular gland formations in the least differentiated tumor area. In consequence, the neoplasms were categorized as either "low-grade" ($\geq$50% gland formation; well to moderately differentiated) or "high-grade" (<50% gland formation; poorly differentiated) [19].

All neoplasms were scored for 10 additional histological parameters including vascular and lymphatic invasion, perineural growth, invasion depth, lymph node metastasis, inflammatory cell infiltration, scirrhous reaction, presence of osseous metaplasia, a mucinous component and mucosal ulceration. Vascular (extra- and intra-mural) and lymphatic invasion as well as perineural growth were assessed as either absent (0) or present (1). Invasion depth was scored as infiltrating the lamina muscularis propria (1), the tunica muscularis (2), or the serosa or greater omentum (3). A cumulative score of invasiveness, including vascular (1), lymphatic (1), perineural (1), and serosal (1) infiltration was calculated (max. score of 4). Regional lymph nodes were available for histological evaluation of metastasis in 20/49 cases. Cellular immune response was measured semi-quantitatively by scoring the inflammatory infiltrate in the tumorous area as either absent (0), mild (1; mucosal), moderate (2; mucosal, submucosal and partly involving the tunica muscularis), or severe

(3; involving all intestinal layers). A scirrhous reaction, mucinous component, osseous metaplasia, and mucosal ulceration were determined as either absent (0) or present (1).

Mitotic count (MC) was assessed digitally in an area equaling 10 high-power fields (hpf; 40×) on a standard monitor using Aperio ImageScope X64 (Leica Biosystems). Assuming 2.37 mm^2 was agreed to be the standard field area of 10 hpf and 0.0954 mm^2 was the area of one hpf in the aforementioned setting, 25 40× image fields were counted to equal the standard hpf area. The MC was performed randomly within the most densely cellular areas of the neoplasm and cell poor areas were excluded [24]. The total number of mitoses/10 hpf (2.37 mm^2) were scored as follows: 0–9 mitoses (1); 10–19 mitoses (2); and ≥20 mitoses (3).

2.1.3. Semiquantitative Evaluation and Computer-Assisted Image Analysis

Beta-catenin immunoreactivity, in terms of a nuclear translocation of β-catenin, was scored semiquantitatively: 0 (negative; <5% positive cells); 1 (5–25% positive cells); 2 (26–50% positive cells); and 3 (>50% positive cells) (modified score from Uneyama et al.) [12] (Figure 2).

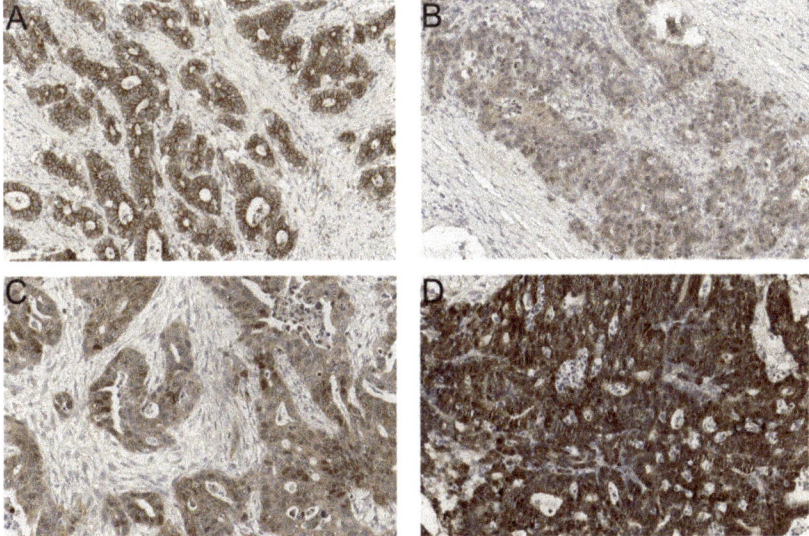

Figure 2. Scoring for nuclear translocated β-catenin in feline intestinal carcinomas (Anti-β-catenin; 20×). (**A**) Tumor with no or scattered (<5%) nuclear β-catenin staining (score 0); (**B**) 5–25% of tumor cells display nuclear positivity for β-catenin (score 1); (**C**) 26–50% of tumor cells display nuclear positivity (score 2); and (**D**) >50% of tumor cells are positive for nuclear β-catenin (score 3). For corresponding human β-catenin stainings see Figure S2.

Regarding proliferative activity, the Ki-67 index was assessed by a computer assisted algorithm. Selected regions of interest (ROI), i.e., tumor areas, were manually annotated by a trainee pathologist (T.G.). The ROI were exported as xml files and transferred into an open-source image analysis software ('QuPath version 0.2.3, https://qupath.github.io, University of Edinburgh, Scotland) for quantification. The default set of parameters of the algorithm was modified according to the stain contrast and intensity of the scanned images. Cell segmentation was performed using the following settings: detection image, optical density sum; requested pixel size 0.5 μm; background radius 8 μm; median filter radius 1 μm; sigma 1.5 μm; minimum cell area 10 μm^2; maximum cell area 400 μm^2, threshold 0.1; and maximum background intensity 2. Cell classification (tumor cells, immune or stromal cells) was completed after training an object classifier using 'Random trees' as a machine learning method [25]. 'Smoothed object features' at a 25 µm radius were added. This was to help with segmenting an image homogeneously so that the classifier performed an accurate classification. As a quality control step, the results of segmentation and correct cell classification were reviewed by a trainee pathologist (T.G.). Finally, the Ki-67 proliferation index was calculated exclusively within the class "tumor cells" as the percentage of cells with positive Ki-67 immunostaining and was scored as follows: <5% (0); 5–30% (1); 31–50% (2); 51–80% (3); and >80% (4).

2.1.4. Sanger Sequencing of Feline *CTNNB1* Exon 2

In order to elucidate the relevance of feline *CTNNB1* exon 2 alterations in intestinal carcinogenesis we established a Sanger sequencing protocol for feline *CTNNB1* gene exon 2 encoding β-catenin. In a first step, we compared and aligned the human (ENST00000349496.11, NM_001904.4, hg19) and feline DNA-sequences of *CTNNB1* (ENSFCAT00000003470.6, Felis_catus_9.0) to identify the corresponding regions of interest in the feline sequence. Human *CTNNB1* exon 3 is known to include a hotspot region of frequent mutations in various cancer entities, e.g., liver, stomach, and colorectal cancer [26]. Therefore, by comparing the two sequences, we identified feline *CTNNB1* exon 2 as homologous to the human nucleotide sequence of exon 3. According to this, a specific primer pair, 5'-AGCTGATCTGATGGAACTGGAC-3' (forward) and 5'-ACACCCTTACCAGCCACTTG-3' (reverse), which amplifies a 237-bp product encompassing feline *CTNNB1* exon 2, was designed. This primer pair was previously established and validated in a pre-study of feline fibrosarcoma ($n = 5$) using tumor samples and matching normal tissue samples. In brief, the DNA was extracted from areas of interest on FFPE sections (tumor tissue and/or normal tissue) by means of a Maxwell® RSC Blood DNA Kit (Promega, Madison, WI, USA) according to the manufacturer's protocol. DNA concentration was afterwards fluorimetrically measured by using a Qubit 4.0 system and the Qubit DNA high sensitivity Assay (both: Thermo Fisher Scientific, Waltham, MA, USA). For amplification of the region of interest (feline *CTNNB1* gene, exon 2) 10–20 ng of DNA was used as input for the polymerase chain reaction (PCR). PCR was performed with AmpliTaq Gold polymerase (Thermo Fisher Scientific, Waltham, MA, USA) in an Eppendorf Mastercycler® Gradient (Eppendorf AG, Hamburg, Germany) with an annealing temperature of 60 °C. Subsequently, the amplification of tumor samples and negative control (non-template control) was validated using agarose gel electrophoresis and visualization on an Amersham Imager 680 detection system (General Electric Company Healthcare Bio-Sciences AB, Uppsala, Sweden). For purification, the PCR products were digested using ExoSAP nuclease (New England Biolabs, Ipswich, MA, USA) for 15 min at 37 °C followed by inhibition of the enzyme at 80 °C for 10 min in an Eppendorf Mastercycler®. Sanger sequencing was performed using the BigDye v1.1 Terminator Mix (Thermo Fisher Scientific, Waltham, MA, USA) according to the manufacturer's protocol in an Eppendorf Mastercycler®. For capillary electrophoresis the sequencing product was purified using the ZR DNA Sequencing Clean-up Kit™ (Zymo Research Europe GmbH, Freiburg, Germany) and loaded on an ABS/Hitachi 3130 genetic analyzer (Thermo Fisher Scientific, Waltham, MA, USA). After sequencing, electropherograms of each tumor sample and corresponding normal tissue were visually analyzed for the occurrence of mutations.

In this study, eleven cases positive for nuclear β-catenin (score 1–3) and containing a sufficient quantity of tumor cells (>30% tumor cell content) were selected for molecular analysis of the feline β-catenin gene exon 2 according to the method described above. Healthy intestinal mucosa from the same animals ($n = 7$) and from other animals ($n = 2$) was used as a negative control in order to confirm the native sequence of feline *CTNNB1*.

2.2. Human Specimen

For comparative purposes, human CRC specimens from the diagnostic archive of the Institute of Pathology of the Technical University of Munich were evaluated. The use of human tissue was approved by the local ethics committee of the Technical University of Munich/Klinikum Rechts der Isar (reference number: 506/17 s).

2.3. Statistical Analysis

Statistical analyses were performed using SPSS software version 27.0.1.0 (SPSS Institute, Chicago, IL, USA). Associations between more than two samples (i.e., WHO subtypes) and the assessed histological features (grade; cumulative score of invasiveness; vascular, lymphatic, and perineural invasion; lymph node metastasis; tumor budding; inflammation; scirrhous reaction; mucinous component; osseous metaplasia; mucosal ulceration; proliferation (MC, Ki-67); and β-catenin translocation) were examined via a Kruskal–Wallis test for nonnormally distributed parameters and a Bonferroni-adjusted post-hoc analysis. Trends between two samples (i.e., grades, tumor localization) were tested via a Mann–Whitney U test. A p value < 0.05 was considered statistically significant for all data sets.

3. Results

3.1. Tumor Site and Frequency

Histomorphological evaluation showed that the majority of examined feline intestinal carcinoma (33/49 cases, 67.3%) was located in the large intestine, whereas 16/49 cases (32.7%) appeared in the small intestine. Due to the striking morphologic similarity with human intestinal neoplasias, we decided to also include small intestinal tumors in the feline study set. In humans, small intestinal neoplasms are rare compared to colonic adenocarcinoma but the subtypes resemble the colonic classification [27].

3.2. Distribution of Histopathological Subtypes of the Feline Intestinal Tumor Cohort

Feline intestinal carcinomas closely resembled human WHO subtypes on a histomorphological level (Figure 3). Of the 16 small intestinal tumors, 12 were classified as ANOS (75%), two as MAC (12.5%), one as SAC (6.3%) and one as MPC (6.3%). Of the 33 tumors of the colon and rectum, 17 were classified as ANOS (51.5%), 12 as SAC (36.4%), 3 as MAC (9.1%), and 1 as SRCC (3%). Overall, ANOS was the most common histological subtype in cats (59.2%) followed by SAC (26.5%). MAC comprised 10.2%, and MPC and SRCC 2% of cases, respectively (Table 1). Other human WHO subtypes, including adenoma-like adenocarcinoma, medullary adenocarcinoma, adenosquamous carcinoma, undifferentiated carcinoma, and carcinoma with sarcomatoid components, were not identified in the investigated feline tumor set.

3.3. Histopathological Features of Feline Intestinal Tumor Subtypes

The majority of small intestinal carcinomas were of high grade (14/16; 87.5%). A mucinous component was found in 10/16 cases (62.5%). Vascular invasion was present in 5/16 cases (31.3%), perineural invasion in 3/16 cases (18.8%) and lymphatic invasion in 9/16 cases (56.3%). Mesenterial lymph nodes were available in 5/16 cases and metastasis was present in 2 of those 5 cases. Serosal infiltration was present in 8/16 cases (50%). Invasiveness was high (score 3) in 5/16 cases (31.3%) and low (score 0) in 3/16 cases (18.8%). Inflammation was mild in 12.5%, moderate in 50% and severe in 37.5% of cases. Mucosal ulceration was present in 13/16 cases (81.3%). A scirrhous reaction was found in 11/16 cases (68.8%). No osseous metaplasia was present. The number of mitotic figures ranged from 1 to 17, mean (± SD) number of mitoses was 6.88 (± 4.573) and the median was 5.5. All small intestinal carcinomas were of the highest budding grade (Bd3).

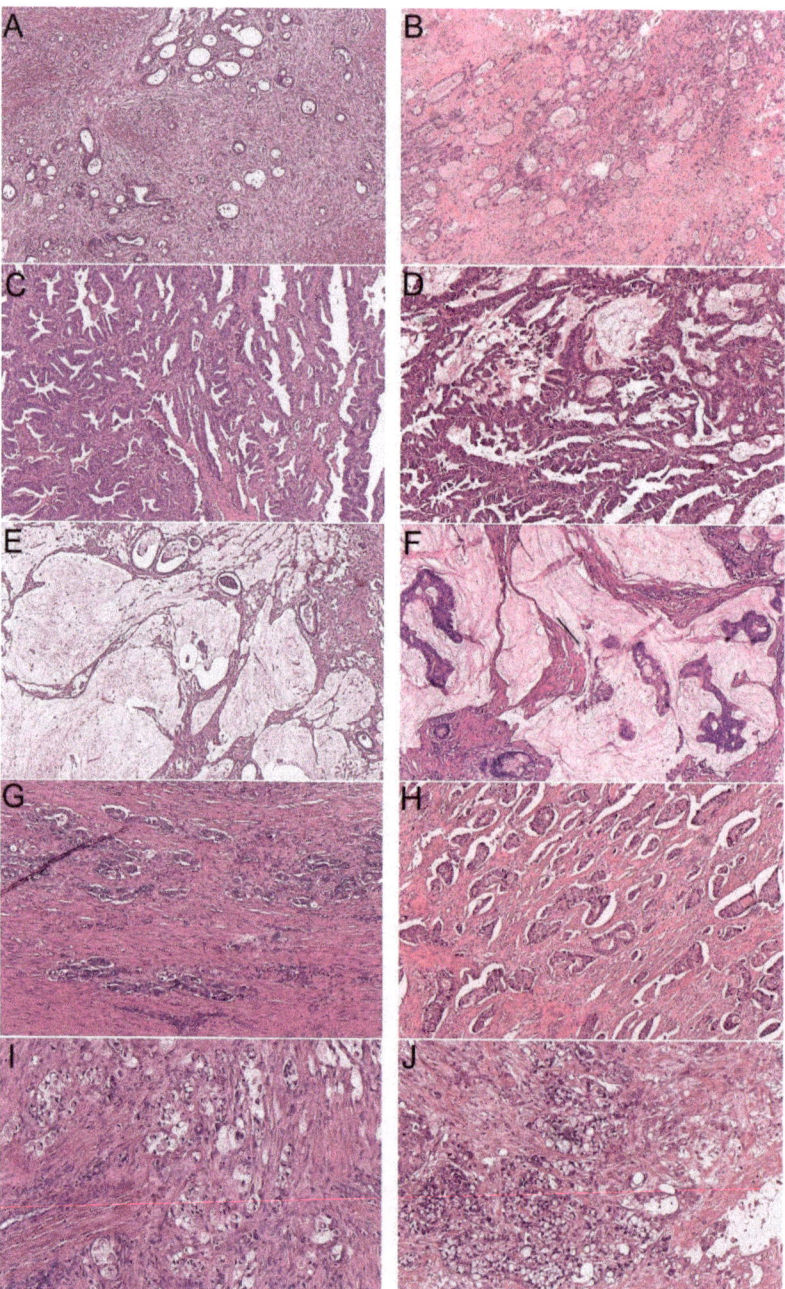

Figure 3. Feline intestinal carcinomas (**left**) closely resemble human WHO subtypes (**right**) (H&E). (**A**) Feline colonic adenocarcinoma not otherwise specified (ANOS, 8×); (**B**) Human colonic ANOS (8×); (**C**) Feline colonic serrated adenocarcinoma (SAC, 8×); (**D**) Human colonic SAC (8×); (**E**) Feline small intestinal mucinous adenocarcinoma (MAC, 8×); (**F**) Human colonic MAC (8×); (**G**) Feline small intestinal micropapillary carcinoma (MPC, 8×); (**H**) Human colonic MPC (8×); (**I**) Feline colonic signet-ring cell carcinoma (SRCC, 20×); and (**J**) Human colonic SRCC (20×).

Table 1. Distribution of histological WHO subtypes of feline intestinal carcinomas.

Cohort	Subtype	n	% of Total
Histological Subtypes (Overall Cohort, n = 49)	ANOS	29	59.18
	SAC	13	26.53
	MAC	5	10.20
	MPC	1	2.04
	SRCC	1	2.04
Histological Subtype (Small Intestinal, n = 16)	ANOS	12	75.00
	SAC	1	6.25
	MAC	2	12.5
	MPC	1	6.25
Histological Subtype (Colonic, n = 33)	ANOS	17	51.52
	SAC	12	36.36
	MAC	3	9.09
	SRCC	1	3.03

ANOS = adenocarcinoma not otherwise specified; SAC = serrated adenocarcinoma; MAC = mucinous adenocarcinoma; MPC = micropapillary carcinoma; SRCC = signet-ring cell carcinoma.

Regarding colonic carcinomas, 54.5% were of low grade and 45.5% of high grade. A mucinous component was identified in 22/33 cases (66.7%). Vascular invasion was present in 13/33 cases (39.4%), perineural invasion in 13/33 cases (39.4%) and lymphatic invasion in 11/33 cases (33.3%). Lymph node metastasis was present in 11 of 15 (73.3%) submitted lymph node samples. Inflammation was mild in 60.6% (20/33), moderate in 15.2% (5/33) and severe in 24.2% (8/33) of the colonic carcinomas. The majority of colonic carcinomas had a scirrhous component (28/33; 84.8%) and osseous metaplasia was present in 7/33 cases (21.2%). The number of mitoses per 10 hpf ranged from 0 to 37, the mean number was 7.42 ($\pm$ 7.87), and the median was 6. The tumor budding status of colonic carcinomas was generally high (84.3% Bd3).

Overall, 20 intestinal tumors were classified as low grade (40.2%) and 29 as high grade (59.8%). Low grade tumors grew significantly less invasive than high grade tumors ($p = 0.025$). A mucinous component was present in 32/49 cases (65.3%) of the investigated neoplasms. Vascular invasion was present in 36.7% ($p = 0.137$), perineural invasion in 32.7% ($p = 0.527$) and lymphatic invasion in 40.8% ($p = 0.141$) of all intestinal carcinomas. Metastases were present in 13 of 20 cases with available lymph nodes. Intestinal tumors penetrated the serosa in 27/49 cases. Mucosal ulceration was present in 37/49 cases (75.5%) (Figure 4). In 44.9% (22/49) of cases inflammation of the tumor area was mild and composed of a mixed inflammatory cell infiltrate. A scirrhous reaction was present in 39/49 (79.6%) and osseous metaplasia in 7/49 (14.3%) cases. In general, the feline tumor budding status was remarkably high (44/49 Bd3, 89.8%). Bd3 tumors had a significantly higher cumulative score of invasiveness ($p = 0.006$) and invaded blood ($p = 0.205$) and lymphatic vessels ($p = 0.152$) more frequently. For the overall cohort, statistical analysis revealed a significant difference between the WHO subtypes regarding the feature invasiveness, represented by a cumulative score of invasiveness ($p = 0.021$). Feline serrated adenocarcinomas grew significantly less invasive than ANOS ($p = 0.014$) (Figure 5). Concordantly, ANOS infiltrated upon the serosa more frequently than SAC ($p = 0.028$). Strikingly, feline intestinal carcinomas generally exhibited an extremely dissociative and aggressively infiltrative growth pattern. For all the other aforementioned criteria no significant trends with regard to the specific histological subtypes could be determined. Detailed information on the relation between histological subtypes and the assessed histological and molecular features of the overall cohort is provided in Table S4.

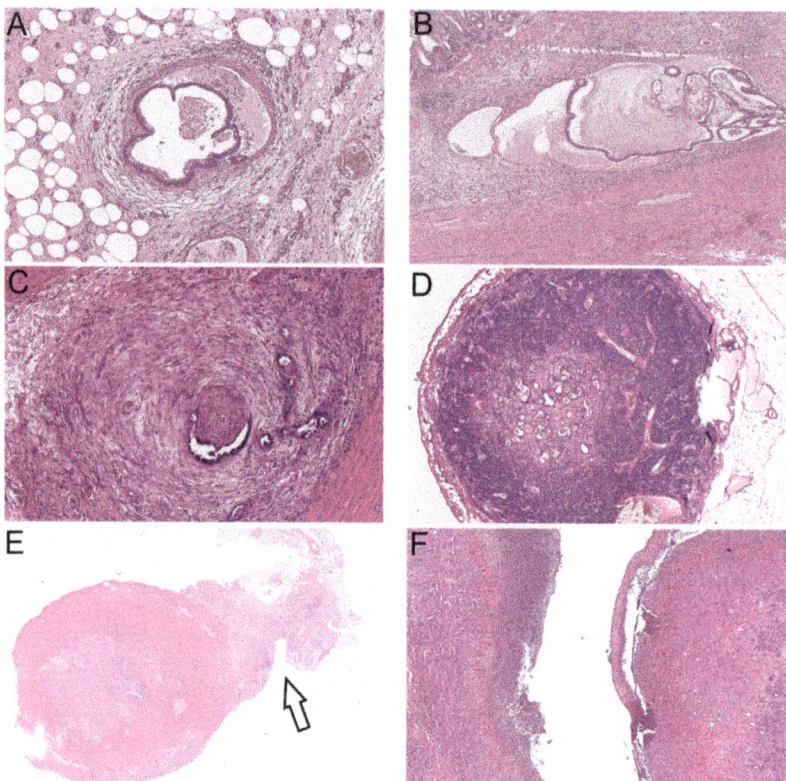

Figure 4. Characteristic malignancy features of feline intestinal tumors (H&E). (**A**) Vascular invasion (10×); (**B**) Lymphangiosis carcinomatosa (4×); (**C**) Perineural invasion (10×); (**D**) Lymph node metastasis (4×); (**E**) Serosal invasion, arrow (1×); and (**F**) Mucosal ulceration (4×).

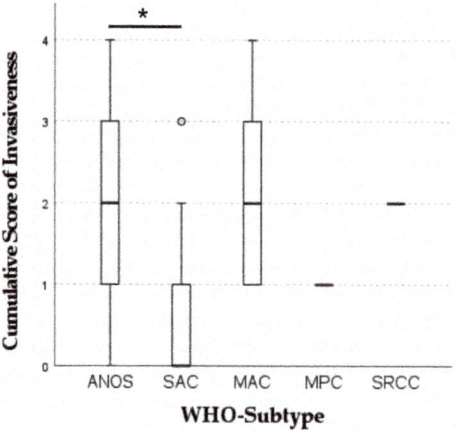

Figure 5. Kruskal–Wallis test of WHO subtypes regarding invasiveness. For the overall cohort, statistical analysis revealed a significant difference between the WHO subtypes regarding the feature invasiveness, represented by a cumulative score of invasiveness (vascular (1), perineural (1), lymphatic (1) and serosal invasion (1), max. score of 4). ($p = 0.021$). The score of invasiveness was significantly higher for ANOS than for SAC (* $p = 0.014$).

3.4. Immunohistochemical Features of the Feline Intestinal Tumor Cohort

Of the 16 small intestinal tumors, 93.8% showed no or scattered nuclear translocation of β-catenin (score 0). Nuclear translocation in 5–25% of tumor cells (score 1) was present in one small intestinal ANOS (6.3%). The 33 colonic carcinomas were positive for nuclear β-catenin to various degrees (69.7% score 0; 24.4% score 1; 3% score 3 or 4, respectively). Out of eight colonic tumors with a score of one, five were of the subtype ANOS, two were SAC and one was MAC. One colonic SAC was a score 2 and one colonic ANOS was a score 3. Taken together, the majority of the examined feline tumors displayed no or scattered nuclear translocation of β-catenin (score 0; 38/49 cases; 77.6%). Nine tumors were a score 1 (18.4%), one colonic tumor a score 2 (2%) and one a score of 3, respectively.

Tumor proliferation (Ki-67) did not differ statistically significant between the histological subtypes ($p = 0.359$) or grades ($p = 0.26$).

3.5. β-Catenin Gene Mutations in Exon 2 of Feline CTNNB1

For 11 tumor samples, which immunohistochemically displayed nuclear translocation of β-catenin (score 1, 2 or 3), Sanger sequencing identified somatic missense mutations in exon 2 of the feline *CTNNB1* gene in 4 colonic tumors (case 14: colonic ANOS score 1; case 20: colonic ANOS score 3; case 22: colonic ANOS score 1; case 31 colonic SAC score 1; 36.4% of all samples). Three of these four mutations were of somatic origin, and in none of the samples germline mutations were detected in exon 2 of the *CTNNB1* gene. In case 20, no matching physiological tissue of the same animal was available, thus, it could not be determined if the mutation was of somatic or of germline origin in this specific case. All identified mutations were exclusively heterozygous, and the mutational spectrum comprised a p.S37F (c.110C>T) (case 14), a p.D32G (c.95A>G) (case 20), a p.D32N (c.94G>A) (case 22), and a p.G34R (c.100G>A) (case 31) mutation (Figure 6). For all of these, an orthologous mutation is known in various human cancers, e.g., CRC, liver and stomach cancer [26]. In the remaining seven samples, a wildtype sequence of *CTNNB1* was identified either exclusively in the tumor tissue ($n = 3$) or in the tumor tissue and normal tissue ($n = 4$). Amplification status of *CTNNB1* could not be determined by Sanger sequencing.

3.6. Comparison of Feline Small Intestinal and Colonic Neoplasias

Small intestinal carcinomas were more often of high grade than colonic carcinomas ($p = 0.005$). Osseous metaplasia was present in the colonic, but not in the small intestinal carcinomas ($p = 0.049$). Nuclear translocation of the β-catenin was proved in one small intestinal ANOS (score 1), but visible to various degrees in 10 colonic tumors ($p = 0.058$). Somatic mutations of *CTNNB1* were exclusively detected in colonic carcinomas ($p = 0.15$). Inflammatory cell infiltration of the neoplastic area appeared to be mild in the majority of colonic cases and moderate to severe in the majority of small intestinal cases ($p = 0.12$). For all other assessed criteria, no statistically significant differences between the small intestinal and colonic carcinomas could be determined.

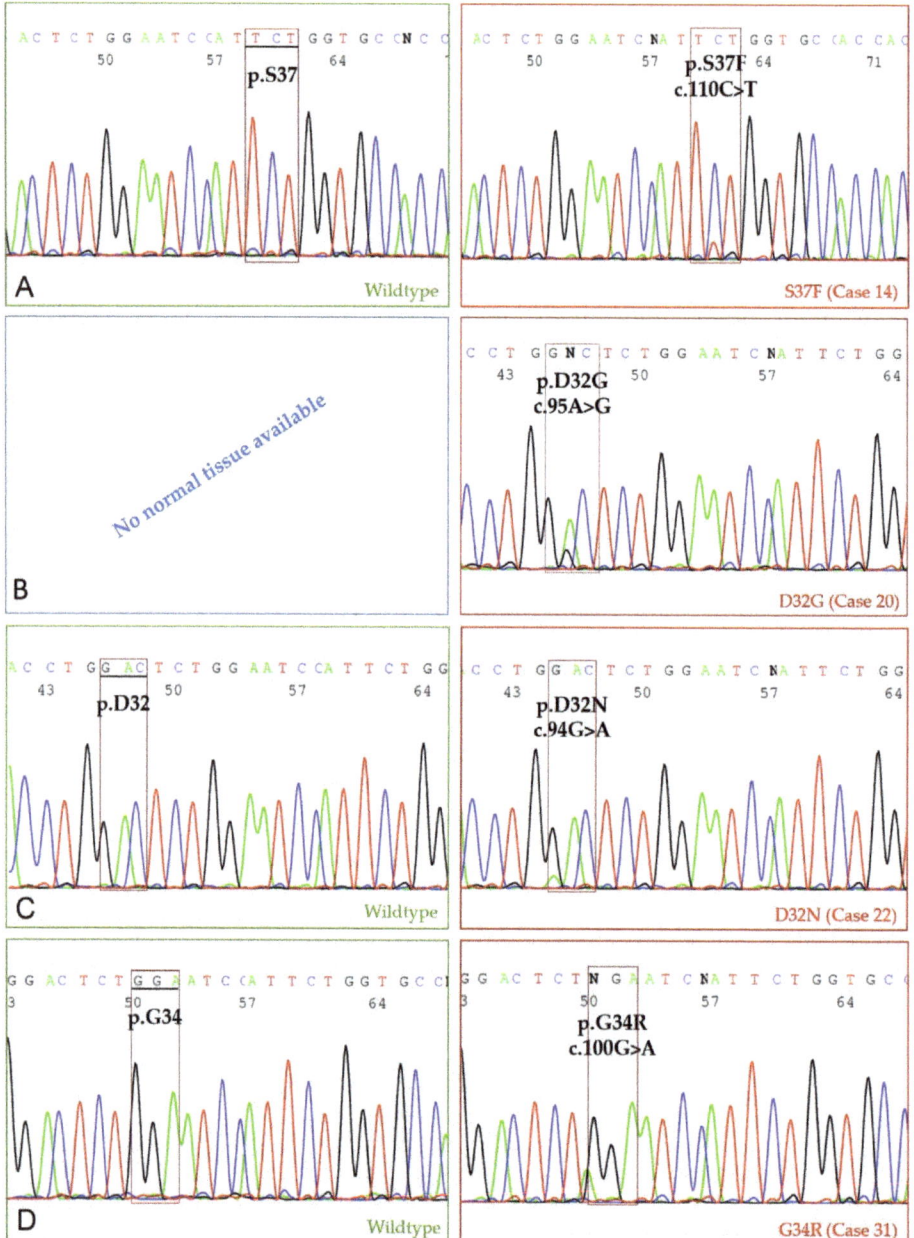

Figure 6. Four distinct somatic missense mutations were detected, each of them in a different case. DNA forward sequences; green: wildtype sequence of normal intestinal tissue (*n* = 3); red: tumor Table S4. (**A**) Cytosine (C) is substituted by Thymine (T), resulting in a missense mutation leading to a replacement of Serine (S) by Phenylalanine (F) on the protein level (colonic ANOS; β-catenin score 1); (**B**) Adenosine (A) is substituted by Guanin (G) resulting in a missense mutation leading to a replacement of Aspartic acid (D) by Glycine (G) (colonic ANOS; score 3). For case 20, no normal tissue was available; (**C**) Guanin (G) is substituted by Adenosine (A) resulting in a replacement of Aspartic acid (D) by Asparagine (N) (colonic ANOS, score 1); (**D**) Guanin (G) is substituted by Adenosine (A) resulting in a replacement of Glycine (G) by Arginine (R) (colonic SAC, score 1).

4. Discussion

The most striking morphological feature of the investigated and described feline cohort was an extremely high tumor budding activity related to a markedly dissociative tumor growth. Since the WHO criteria for human CRC was reclassified in 2019 and tumor budding was added, it is now recognized as a major grading criterion and a highly relevant and independent prognostic factor [17,19] that is generally considered to be a stage-independent predictor of lymph node metastasis in pT1 CRC and of survival in stage II CRC [18]. Tumor budding strongly impacts on all survival parameters and regarding its prognostic significance, it even outperforms WHO grade [17]. This study demonstrates a high budding status in feline intestinal carcinomas (89.8% Bd3) compared to human CRC (20% Bd3) [17]. To the authors' knowledge, no other veterinary studies evaluate feline tumor budding, and further research to establish prognostic data is imperative.

Although many GEMMs are available, researchers frequently face the problem that induced intestinal neoplasms of mice lack the invasive features characteristic for late-stage CRC, e.g., tumor budding. There are orthotopic mouse xenograft models which show tumor budding that are morphologically and immunohistochemically close to what is seen in human CRC; however, these models often have an immunocompromised background and thus are limited in their relevance to the human situation [28,29]. Moreover, the very limited availability of in vivo budding models to date is another drawback [29]. Our study shows the capability of spontaneous feline intestinal carcinomas to serve as an immunocompetent model for elucidating the intestinal tumor budding mechanisms of CRC.

Due to these similarities and the potential use of spontaneously arising feline intestinal tumors for comparative research trials of human CRC, we decided on categorizing feline intestinal tumors according to the human WHO classification of 2019 [19]. Human WHO subtypes were proven to be clinically relevant with a strong impact on overall survival (OS), disease-free survival (DFS), and disease-specific survival (DSS) ($p < 0.001$) and a clear association with WHO grade and budding status. For example, MPC and SRCC are very aggressive subtypes connected to a poor survival prognosis, whereas SAC mostly does not invade perineural or venous and is connected to a better prognosis considering the CRC subtypes [17].

The feline cohort was compared to a large-scale cohort of human colorectal carcinomas recently characterized and published by Jesinghaus et al. in 2021. Most human CRCs are ANOS, defined by an invasive growth pattern breaking the line of the lamina muscularis mucosae and invading the submucosa; a feature which was present in all included feline intestinal tumors. Overall, ANOS was the most common histological subtype (59.2%) in cats, similar to the human cohort (62.7%) [17]. In a recent study of feline intestinal carcinomas, tubular adenocarcinoma was determined to be the most common tumor type (33/50 cases; 66%), morphologically comparable to ANOS [12]. The second most common colonic subtype in the feline cohort was SAC, which was overrepresented compared to human CRCs (8.7%) [17]. Consistent with this, Uneyama et al. found that feline colorectal carcinomas frequently showed glandular serration, and they detected three *KRAS* mutations in seven cases of feline colorectal epithelial tumors [12]. Presuming that *KRAS* gene mutations are frequently involved in human CRC development and particularly in the 'serrated pathway', this pathway may play an important role in feline intestinal carcinogenesis, as it does for human serrated adenocarcinomas [20,30–32]. Although we unfortunately lack survival data for our described feline study set, we were able to show that feline SAC displayed less invasive growth compared to other subtypes, compatible with the rather favorable prognosis of human SAC [17].

A lack of species-specific investigation tools, especially of molecular pathological markers, constitutes a significant challenge in the use of companion animal cancers as human tumor models (e.g., DNA primers). Commercially available and formalin-approved antibodies for cats or dogs are not as readily available as for human and rodent tissue [7] and molecular methods aiming at the detection of specific somatic or germline mutations are infrequently used in companion animal studies. We successfully designed a DNA primer pair appropriate for amplification of the feline *CTNNB1* gene exon 2, which is homologous to the nucleotide sequence of human *CTNNB1* exon 3 and contains a hotspot region of frequent mutations for various human cancers including CRC [26]. Because of this homology, *CTNNB1* mutations located in this DNA-region are most likely to cause similar effects in both species.

Mutations activating the canonical WNT/β-catenin signaling pathway are very frequently involved in the 'classical pathway' of human colorectal carcinogenesis [20]. β-catenin is a highly conserved protein, part of the WNT signaling pathway and plays an important role in cell-adhesion [33]. Alterations of *CTNNB1* that result in disturbed degradation of β-catenin lead to its cytoplasmic accumulation and subsequent translocation into the nucleus, where it acts as an oncogenic player enhancing the expression of several downstream target genes, e.g., *CCND1* (CYCLIN D1) [34,35], *MYC* [20,35,36], and *AXIN2* [35]. On the one hand, stabilizing homozygous *CTNNB1* mutations play a crucial role, especially in human CRC associated with Lynch syndrome [21]. On the other hand, *CTNNB1* mutations are less often (5% non-hypermutated (nHM) CRC; 7% hypermutated (HM) CRC) involved in sporadic human colorectal carcinogenesis than *APC* (Adenomatous polyposis coli) mutations (81% nHM; 53% HM CRC) [20].

From a comparative point of view, in intestinal neoplasms in dogs, *CTNNB1* mutations were proven to be more often causative than *APC* mutations, with *CTNNB1* being mutated in >60% of canine colorectal tumors [22]. Several studies also provide evidence of nuclear β-catenin translocation and accumulation in canine intestinal adenomas and carcinomas [37–39].

Currently, very little is known about the genomic landscape of companion animal cancers [40], and particularly of feline cancers. Because β-catenin score did not correlate with malignancy, Uneyama et al. concluded from their IHC results that dysregulated β-catenin is likely not an important player in feline intestinal tumorigenesis; however, accumulation of β-catenin was evident in 60% of their cases [12]. Our immunohistochemical examination of feline intestinal carcinomas (22.5% of cases positive for nuclear β-catenin) as well as the high expression of active β-catenin in feline mammary tumors compared to healthy tissue [41], prompted us to further investigate the role of this key protein in the entity of feline intestinal cancer.

For the first time, Sanger sequencing of feline *CTNNB1* exon 2 was performed and revealed four somatic missense mutations identical with pathogenic mutations in humans [26]. Human codons most frequently displaying mutations related to CRC are, namely, codons 32, 33, 34, 37, 41, and 45 [26]. Canine mutations were found in codons 32, 34, and 45 [22]. In our study, feline mutations were located at codons 32, 34 and 37, consistent with mutations of human and canine intestinal tumorigenesis. As a result, we strongly challenge the finding that dysregulated WNT/β-catenin signaling is not involved in feline intestinal carcinogenesis.

APC loss-of-function mutations leading to an impacted degradation of β-catenin can also lead to an increase of cytoplasmic and nuclear β-catenin [20]. This could be a possible explanation for the seven cases, which displayed nuclear β-catenin positivity but did not show sequential alterations of *CTNNB1*. Future investigations conducting feline *APC* sequencing (i.e., panel or whole exome sequencing) and including a larger cohort size are required to finally clarify if *APC* mutations also play a role in feline intestinal tumorigenesis. Nevertheless, genomic amplification of the *CTNNB1* gene, which might also be a mechanism for overexpression of the protein in cancer in humans, cannot completely be excluded [42].

The majority (93.8%) of small intestinal tumors displayed no relevant nuclear β-catenin translocation and the only tumor showing a nuclear IHC-signal did not harbor a *CTNNB1* mutation. In contrast to that, colonic tumors displayed various degrees of positivity for nuclear β-catenin ($n = 10$) and mutations of *CTNNB1* ($n = 4$). Although the feline small and large intestinal tumors appear to have histomorphological similarities, small intestinal tumors were almost exclusively of high grade and high tumor budding status. Future investigations are needed to further elucidate the mutational spectrum of feline small intestinal tumors.

A first step has been taken, but much work remains to be done. In order to beneficially integrate the feline model into human CRC research, further investigation of feline cancers' genetics, genome-wide studies as well as genome annotation are imperative. The final ideal of comparative oncology is to include companion animals (pets) with comparative cancer diseases in clinical trials. Educating and informing pet owners and considering ethical standards is a major point here [40].

Our data provides an accurate histological classification system for feline intestinal tumors and a basis for comparative oncology [40] studies by harmonizing histological classification and conducting molecular examination on spontaneously arising intestinal tumors in pet cats. The results indicate that feline intestinal carcinomas constitute a valuable and promising in vivo model for human CRC, worthy of further characterization.

5. Conclusions

In conclusion, the present study evaluates histopathological features and patterns of feline intestinal tumors. It demonstrates two main reasons for the suitability of feline intestinal tumors as a valid spontaneous in vivo model for late-stage human CRC: (1) Feline intestinal carcinomas resemble human subtypes and present with an invasive growth and high tumor budding activity, (2) *CTNNB1* mutations are present in feline intestinal carcinomas, as has been reported in human and canine intestinal tumorigenesis. Sharing two important molecular alterations, namely *KRAS* [12] and *CTNNB1* mutations involved in intestinal carcinogenesis, cats are a valuable model for late-stage sporadic human CRC.

This study provides a solid foundation for the comparison of feline and human CRC, indicates the need to review the available classification schemes for feline intestinal cancers and paves the way for future comparative oncology studies.

Supplementary Materials: The following are available online at https://www.mdpi.com/article/10.3390/cancers13235941/s1, Figure S1: tumor budding (TB) in the invasive front of human CRC, Figure S2: corresponding human β-catenin phenotypes to Figure 2, Table S1: feline cohort SPSS dataset, Table S2: feline cohort information (localization, specimen, breed, sex, age), Table S3: primary antibodies and IHC protocols, Table S4: relationship between histological subtypes and histological and molecular features.

Author Contributions: Conceptualization of the study, T.G., N.P., W.W., K.M., M.J. and K.S.; resources, U.S., H.A.-L., N.P., W.W., M.J. and K.S.; methodology, T.G., F.S., S.R.J.S., N.P., M.J. and K.S.; evaluation of slides, results, T.G., D.D., C.M., U.S., N.P., M.J. and K.S.; critical discussion, T.G., D.D., C.M., U.S., H.A.-L., S.R.J.S., N.P., M.J., K.M. and K.S.; writing—original draft preparation, T.G.; writing—review and editing, T.G., F.S., D.D., U.S., H.A.-L., S.R.J.S., N.P., K.M. and K.S.; All authors have read and agreed to the published version of the manuscript.

Funding: T.G. received a scholarship from the Cusanuswerk, Bischöfliche Studienförderung, Bonn, Germany. S.R.J.S. is supported by the German Research Foundation (Deutsche Forschungsgemeinschaft, DFG, SFB1371-395357507). K.S. is supported by the Germany Research Foundation (DFG, SFB1335-360372040) project Z01.

Institutional Review Board Statement: The use of human tissue was approved by the local ethics committee of the Technical University of Munich/Klinikum Rechts der Isar (reference number: 506/17 s).

Informed Consent Statement: Not applicable.

Data Availability Statement: The raw data of the results presented in this study are available on request from the corresponding author.

Acknowledgments: The authors thank O. Seelbach, A. Jacob, M. Mielke and U. Mühlthaler for their outstanding technical support.

Conflicts of Interest: LABOKLIN GmbH & Co. KG offers histopathological service for routine diagnostics. T.G. presented preliminary parts of this study at the 4th Cutting Edge Pathology Congress 2021. W.W. has attended Advisory Boards and served as speaker for Roche, MSD, BMS, AstraZeneca, Pfizer, Merck, Lilly, Boehringer, Novartis, Takeda, Bayer, Amgen, Astellas, Eisai, Illumina, Siemens, Agilent, ADC, GSK, and Molecular Health. W.W. receives research funding from Roche, MSD, BMS and AstraZeneca. N.P. has attended Advisory Boards and served as speaker for Roche, BMS, AstraZeneca, Lilly, Novartis, Bayer, Illumina, and Thermo Fisher Scientific. K.S. is consultant for Roche Pharma AG, member of the advisory board of TRIMT GmbH and has filed a patent on a radiopharmaceutical. All other authors declare no conflicts of interest.

References

1. Sung, H.; Ferlay, J.; Siegel, R.L.; Laversanne, M.; Soerjomataram, I.; Jemal, A.; Bray, F. Global Cancer Statistics 2020: GLOBOCAN Estimates of Incidence and Mortality Worldwide for 36 Cancers in 185 Countries. *CA Cancer J. Clin.* **2021**, *71*, 209–249. [CrossRef]
2. Washington, M.K.; Powell, A.E.; Sullivan, R.; Sundberg, J.P.; Wright, N.; Coffey, R.J.; Dove, W.F. Pathology of rodent models of intestinal cancer: Progress report and recommendations. *Gastroenterology* **2013**, *144*, 705–717. [CrossRef] [PubMed]
3. Jackstadt, R.; Sansom, O.J. Mouse models of intestinal cancer. *J. Pathol.* **2016**, *238*, 141–151. [CrossRef]
4. Taketo, M.M.; Edelmann, W. Mouse models of colon cancer. *Gastroenterology* **2009**, *136*, 780–798. [CrossRef]
5. McIntyre, R.E.; Buczacki, S.J.; Arends, M.J.; Adams, D.J. Mouse models of colorectal cancer as preclinical models. *Bioessays* **2015**, *37*, 909–920. [CrossRef] [PubMed]
6. McIntyre, R.E.; van der Weyden, L.; Adams, D.J. Cancer gene discovery in the mouse. *Curr. Opin. Genet. Dev.* **2012**, *22*, 14–20. [CrossRef] [PubMed]
7. Vail, D.M.; MacEwen, E.G. Spontaneously occurring tumors of companion animals as models for human cancer. *Cancer Investig.* **2000**, *18*, 781–792. [CrossRef]
8. Schwittlick, U.; Becker, S.; Aupperle-Lellbach, H. Vorkommen und Lokalisation von gastrointestinalen Neoplasien bei 293 Katzen. *Kleintiermedizin* **2020**, *6*, 250–253.
9. Rissetto, K.; Villamil, J.A.; Selting, K.A.; Tyler, J.; Henry, C.J. Recent trends in feline intestinal neoplasia: An epidemiologic study of 1129 cases in the veterinary medical database from 1964 to 2004. *J. Am. Anim. Hosp. Assoc.* **2011**, *47*, 28–36. [CrossRef]
10. Bonfanti, U.; Bertazzolo, W.; Bottero, E.; De Lorenzi, D.; Marconato, L.; Masserdotti, C.; Zatelli, A.; Zini, E. Diagnostic value of cytologic examination of gastrointestinal tract tumors in dogs and cats: 83 cases (2001–2004). *J. Am. Vet. Med. Assoc.* **2006**, *229*, 1130–1133. [CrossRef] [PubMed]
11. Turk, M.A.; Gallina, A.M.; Russell, T.S. Nonhematopoietic gastrointestinal neoplasia in cats: A retrospective study of 44 cases. *Vet. Pathol.* **1981**, *18*, 614–620. [CrossRef]
12. Uneyama, M.; Chambers, J.K.; Nakashima, K.; Uchida, K.; Nakayama, H. Histological Classification and Immunohistochemical Study of Feline Colorectal Epithelial Tumors. *Vet. Pathol.* **2021**, *58*, 305–314. [CrossRef] [PubMed]
13. Patnaik, A.K.; Liu, S.K.; Johnson, G.F. Feline intestinal adenocarcinoma. A clinicopathologic study of 22 cases. *Vet. Pathol.* **1976**, *13*, 1–10. [CrossRef]
14. Manuali, E.; Forte, C.; Vichi, G.; Genovese, D.A.; Mancini, D.; De Leo, A.A.P.; Cavicchioli, L.; Pierucci, P.; Zappulli, V. Tumours in European Shorthair cats: A retrospective study of 680 cases. *J. Feline Med. Surg.* **2020**, *22*, 1095–1102. [CrossRef] [PubMed]
15. Slawienski, M.J.; Mauldin, G.E.; Mauldin, G.N.; Patnaik, A.K. Malignant colonic neoplasia in cats: 46 cases (1990–1996). *J. Am. Vet. Med. Assoc.* **1997**, *211*, 878–881.
16. Hume, D.Z.; Solomon, J.A.; Weisse, C.W. Palliative use of a stent for colonic obstruction caused by adenocarcinoma in two cats. *J. Am. Vet. Med. Assoc.* **2006**, *228*, 392–396. [CrossRef] [PubMed]
17. Jesinghaus, M.; Schmitt, M.; Lang, C.; Reiser, M.; Scheiter, A.; Konukiewitz, B.; Steiger, K.; Silva, M.; Tschurtschenthaler, M.; Lange, S.; et al. Morphology Matters: A Critical Reappraisal of the Clinical Relevance of Morphologic Criteria From the 2019 WHO Classification in a Large Colorectal Cancer Cohort Comprising 1004 Cases. *Am. J. Surg. Pathol.* **2021**, *45*, 969–978. [CrossRef]
18. Lugli, A.; Kirsch, R.; Ajioka, Y.; Bosman, F.; Cathomas, G.; Dawson, H.; El Zimaity, H.; Fléjou, J.F.; Hansen, T.P.; Hartmann, A.; et al. Recommendations for reporting tumor budding in colorectal cancer based on the International Tumor Budding Consensus Conference (ITBCC) 2016. *Mod. Pathol.* **2017**, *30*, 1299–1311. [CrossRef]
19. Nagtegaal, I.; Arends, M.; Odze, R. Tumours of the Colon and Rectum: WHO Classification of Tumours of the Colon and Rectum, TNM Staging of Carcinomas of the Colon and Rectum and the Introduction. In *World Health Organization Classification of Tumours of the Digestive System*; IARC Press: Geneva, Switzerland, 2019; pp. 157–187.
20. Cancer Genome Atlas Network. Comprehensive molecular characterization of human colon and rectal cancer. *Nature* **2012**, *487*, 330–337. [CrossRef]
21. Arnold, A.; Tronser, M.; Sers, C.; Ahadova, A.; Endris, V.; Mamlouk, S.; Horst, D.; Möbs, M.; Bischoff, P.; Kloor, M.; et al. The majority of β-catenin mutations in colorectal cancer is homozygous. *BMC Cancer* **2020**, *20*, 1038. [CrossRef]
22. Wang, J.; Wang, T.; Sun, Y.; Feng, Y.; Kisseberth, W.C.; Henry, C.J.; Mok, I.; Lana, S.E.; Dobbin, K.; Northrup, N.; et al. Proliferative and Invasive Colorectal Tumors in Pet Dogs Provide Unique Insights into Human Colorectal Cancer. *Cancers* **2018**, *10*, 330. [CrossRef]

23. Gonzalez, R.S.; Huh, W.J.; Cates, J.M.; Washington, K.; Beauchamp, R.D.; Coffey, R.J.; Shi, C. Micropapillary colorectal carcinoma: Clinical, pathological and molecular properties, including evidence of epithelial-mesenchymal transition. *Histopathology* **2017**, *70*, 223–231. [CrossRef] [PubMed]
24. Meuten, D.J.; Moore, F.M.; George, J.W. Mitotic Count and the Field of View Area: Time to Standardize. *Vet. Pathol.* **2016**, *53*, 7–9. [CrossRef] [PubMed]
25. Breiman, L. Random Forests. *Mach. Learn.* **2001**, *45*, 5–32. [CrossRef]
26. Tate, J.G.; Bamford, S.; Jubb, H.C.; Sondka, Z.; Beare, D.M.; Bindal, N.; Boutselakis, H.; Cole, C.G.; Creatore, C.; Dawson, E.; et al. COSMIC: The Catalogue of Somatic Mutations in Cancer. *Nucleic Acids Res.* **2019**, *47*, D941–D947. [CrossRef]
27. Salto-Tellez, M.; Rugge, M. Tumours of the Small Intestine and Ampulla. In *World Health Organization Classification of Tumours of the Digestive System*; Salto-Tellez, M., Nagtegaal, I., Rugge, M., Eds.; IARC Press: Geneva, Switzerland, 2019.
28. Prall, F.; Maletzki, C.; Hühns, M.; Krohn, M.; Linnebacher, M. Colorectal carcinoma tumour budding and podia formation in the xenograft microenvironment. *PLoS ONE* **2017**, *12*, e0186271. [CrossRef] [PubMed]
29. Georges, L.M.C.; De Wever, O.; Galván, J.A.; Dawson, H.; Lugli, A.; Demetter, P.; Zlobec, I. Cell Line Derived Xenograft Mouse Models Are a Suitable in vivo Model for Studying Tumor Budding in Colorectal Cancer. *Front. Med.* **2019**, *6*, 139. [CrossRef]
30. Pai, R.K.; Bettington, M.; Srivastava, A.; Rosty, C. An update on the morphology and molecular pathology of serrated colorectal polyps and associated carcinomas. *Mod. Pathol.* **2019**, *32*, 1390–1415. [CrossRef] [PubMed]
31. Jass, J.R. Classification of colorectal cancer based on correlation of clinical, morphological and molecular features. *Histopathology* **2007**, *50*, 113–130. [CrossRef]
32. Rex, D.K.; Ahnen, D.J.; Baron, J.A.; Batts, K.P.; Burke, C.A.; Burt, R.W.; Goldblum, J.R.; Guillem, J.G.; Kahi, C.J.; Kalady, M.F.; et al. Serrated lesions of the colorectum: Review and recommendations from an expert panel. *Am. J. Gastroenterol.* **2012**, *107*, 1315–1329, quiz 1314, 1330. [CrossRef]
33. Valenta, T.; Hausmann, G.; Basler, K. The many faces and functions of β-catenin. *Embo. J.* **2012**, *31*, 2714–2736. [CrossRef]
34. Tetsu, O.; McCormick, F. Beta-catenin regulates expression of cyclin D1 in colon carcinoma cells. *Nature* **1999**, *398*, 422–426. [CrossRef] [PubMed]
35. Herbst, A.; Jurinovic, V.; Krebs, S.; Thieme, S.E.; Blum, H.; Göke, B.; Kolligs, F.T. Comprehensive analysis of β-catenin target genes in colorectal carcinoma cell lines with deregulated Wnt/β-catenin signaling. *BMC Genom.* **2014**, *15*, 74. [CrossRef]
36. He, T.C.; Sparks, A.B.; Rago, C.; Hermeking, H.; Zawel, L.; da Costa, L.T.; Morin, P.J.; Vogelstein, B.; Kinzler, K.W. Identification of c-MYC as a target of the APC pathway. *Science* **1998**, *281*, 1509–1512. [CrossRef] [PubMed]
37. Saito, T.; Chambers, J.K.; Nakashima, K.; Uchida, E.; Ohno, K.; Tsujimoto, H.; Uchida, K.; Nakayama, H. Histopathologic Features of Colorectal Adenoma and Adenocarcinoma Developing Within Inflammatory Polyps in Miniature Dachshunds. *Vet. Pathol.* **2018**, *55*, 654–662. [CrossRef]
38. McEntee, M.F.; Brenneman, K.A. Dysregulation of beta-catenin is common in canine sporadic colorectal tumors. *Vet. Pathol.* **1999**, *36*, 228–236. [CrossRef] [PubMed]
39. Herstad, K.M.V.; Gunnes, G.; Rørtveit, R.; Kolbjørnsen, Ø.; Tran, L.; Skancke, E. Immunohistochemical expression of β-catenin, Ki67, CD3 and CD18 in canine colorectal adenomas and adenocarcinomas. *BMC Vet. Res.* **2021**, *17*, 119. [CrossRef]
40. LeBlanc, A.K.; Breen, M.; Choyke, P.; Dewhirst, M.; Fan, T.M.; Gustafson, D.L.; Helman, L.J.; Kastan, M.B.; Knapp, D.W.; Levin, W.J.; et al. Perspectives from man's best friend: National Academy of Medicine's Workshop on Comparative Oncology. *Sci. Transl. Med.* **2016**, *8*, 324ps325. [CrossRef]
41. Sammarco, A.; Gomiero, C.; Sacchetto, R.; Beffagna, G.; Michieletto, S.; Orvieto, E.; Cavicchioli, L.; Gelain, M.E.; Ferro, S.; Patruno, M.; et al. Wnt/β-Catenin and Hippo Pathway Deregulation in Mammary Tumors of Humans, Dogs, and Cats. *Vet. Pathol.* **2020**, *57*, 774–790. [CrossRef]
42. Suriano, G.; Vrcelj, N.; Senz, J.; Ferreira, P.; Masoudi, H.; Cox, K.; Nabais, S.; Lopes, C.; Machado, J.C.; Seruca, R.; et al. beta-catenin (CTNNB1) gene amplification: A new mechanism of protein overexpression in cancer. *Genes Chromosomes Cancer* **2005**, *42*, 238–246. [CrossRef]

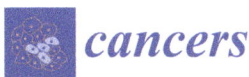

Review

Bovine Meat and Milk Factors (BMMFs): Their Proposed Role in Common Human Cancers and Type 2 Diabetes Mellitus

Ethel-Michele de Villiers * and Harald zur Hausen *

Deutsches Krebsforschungszentrum (DKFZ), Im Neuenheimer Feld 280, 69120 Heidelberg, Germany
* Correspondence: e.devilliers@dkfz.de (E.-M.d.V.); zurhausen@dkfz.de (H.z.H.);
 Tel.: +49-151-4312-3085 (E.-M.d.V.); +49-6221-423850 (H.z.H.)

Simple Summary: This manuscript emphasizes the mechanistic differences of infectious agents contributing to human cancers either by "direct" or "indirect" interactions. The epidemiology of cancers linked to direct carcinogens differs (e.g., response to immunosuppression) from those cancers linked with indirect infectious interactions. We discuss their role in colon, breast, and prostate cancers and type II diabetes mellitus. A brief discussion covers the potential role of BMMF (bovine meat and milk factor) infections in acute myeloid leukemia.

Abstract: Exemplified by infections with bovine meat and milk factors (BMMFs), this manuscript emphasizes the different mechanistic aspects of infectious agents contributing to human cancers by "direct" or "indirect" interactions. The epidemiology of cancers linked to direct carcinogens (e.g., response to immunosuppression) differs from those cancers linked with indirect infectious interactions. Cancers induced by direct infectious carcinogens commonly increase under immunosuppression, whereas the cancer risk by indirect carcinogens is reduced. This influences their responses to preventive and therapeutic interferences. In addition, we discuss their role in colon, breast and prostate cancers and type II diabetes mellitus. A brief discussion covers the potential role of BMMF infections in acute myeloid leukemia.

Keywords: indirect carcinogenesis; bovine meat and milk factors (BMMF); chronic zoonosis

1. Introduction:

Viral, bacterial, or parasitic infections contribute, as causative agents, to a number of human cancers [1]. Most of these reports have noted 14–16% as the global cancer incidence caused by infectious events—many caused by persisting tumor virus infections [2]. Our group calculated slightly higher incidence rates (20–21%) [1]. Basic criteria considered here for definition of a causal role of infections in cancers were:

(1) Persistence of whole genomes or specific genes in certain cancer cells;
(2) Transformed or malignant phenotype of the latter, dependent on the expression and/or function of those genes;
(3) Induction of malignant growth in susceptible animal systems.

These, among others (Figure 1), are common features of *direct carcinogenesis* and evidence for a link between specific infections and cancer [1,3,4]. A few exceptions, however, did not fit these postulates—for instance, the absence of hepatitis C virus in liver cancer cells of patients at high risk after long-time exposure to this persistent virus. In cases where infections lead to chronic inflammation, cancers eventually arise locally, although the infectious agent itself does not persist in the respective cancer cells. Helicobacter pylori infections may lead to chronic inflammation, ulcers and eventually gastric cancers. Parasitic infections of the vascular system in the bladder and liver may eventually lead to bladder and liver cancer, respectively [1]. The role of chronic inflammations emerges as relatively non-specific or indirect by inducing the production of reactive oxygen molecules, leading

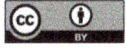

to increased mutagenesis at the respective sites [5,6]. Support for this view originated from observations revealing increased cancer risk in long persisting chronic ulcerations, scar tissue and even in poxvirus vaccination scars [7]. It has been difficult to identify such infectious factors, as well as to understand the mechanism in detail of their contribution to different types of cancers.

Presently established differences between direct and indirect modes of carcinogens are defined in Figure 1 (summarized from [1,3,4,8]). Further evaluation is required to analyze whether the role of hepatitis B infection (hepatitis B in both columns) in carcinogenesis is direct and/or indirect.

Direct carcinogens	**Indirect carcinogens**
Papillomaviruses, polyomaviruses, EBV, HHV-8, Retroviruses, (Hepatitis B).	*Hepatitis-C, (Hepatitis B), HIV 1 and 2, Helicobacter pylori, parasitic infections, Plasmidoses (BMMFs), synergise with various mutagens and specific inherited gene modifications.*
Persistence of genes or whole viral DNA (integrated or episomal) in cancer cells.	
<u>Malignant growth depends on specific expression of these viral genes.</u>	<u>No persistence within the induced cancer cells, frequently, however, in close proximity of the latter.</u>
<u>Increased frequency of the respective cancers under immunosuppression.</u>	<u>Malignant growth results from induction of specific inflammations with production of oxygen radicals inducing random mutations.</u>
Latency periods vary substantially between 3-15 years (EBV, HHV-8) and several decades (Merkel polyomavirus, T-lymphotropic retroviruses).	
Interactions with chemical or physical mutagens best studied in the case of papillomavirus and Hepatitis B virus infections.	<u>Once initiated, malignant growth does not depend on persistence of genes or genomes of the respective agents.</u>
Long-lasting immunosuppressions (e.g. HIV and organ transplant recipients) results in increasing rates of cancers induced by direct carcinogens, but reduce the rates for breast, colon, and prostate cancers.	<u>Long-lasting immuno-suppression interferes with chronic inflammations, blocks oxygen radicals and thereby induction of mutations. This results in a reduced rate of colon, breast, and prostate cancers [summarized in 8]</u>
	Latency periods between initial infection and cancer appearance commonly extend over several decades (except for cancers emerging under immunosuppression)

Figure 1. Mechanisms by which infections contribute to human cancer development. BMMFs (bovine meat and milk factors) represent small single-stranded circular DNA, predominantly isolated from sera and dairy products of Eurasian cattle and subsequently identified in periglandular cells of colon, breast and prostate cancers [6]. These infectious agents share characteristics of both bacterial plasmids and known viruses [9], and are related to two DNA isolates from transmissible spongiform encephalopathies reported by Manuelidis [10].

Recently, several publications reported viral detection after whole-genome DNA sequencing of a large number of different human cancers [11–14]. These studies aimed at identifying hitherto unknown tumor viruses, in part defined by their close relationship to known oncogenic agents. In summary, taking aspects known for direct carcinogenic involvement into consideration, the majority of results failed to identify additional known or unknown foreign DNA sequences in the tumors investigated. This resulted in concluding that at least the majority of infectious agents contributing as direct carcinogens to human cancers is presently known [15]. The authors supported their argument with observations that cancers with persisting foreign DNA are commonly substantially increased in incidence during immunosuppression following organ transplantation or persistent human immunodeficiency infections. This is in remarkable contrast to other common cancers (e.g., colon, breast and prostate cancers), which do not increase under the same conditions [8]. In contrast to cancers linked to direct carcinogens, immunosuppression was even protective against these latter cancers (Figure 1).

2. Bovine Meat and Milk Factors (BMMFs)

Epidemiological studies have pointed to a relationship between colon, breast and prostate cancers and nutritional habits—in particular, to red meat consumption. We evaluated different geographic risks for colon and breast cancers in relation to meat consumption [16]. Surprising results pointed to differences involving consumption of red meat originating from different species of cattle, e.g., Eurasian dairy cattle versus Zebu and Yak breeds [16]. Countries consuming red meat mostly from Eurasian dairy cattle origins revealed high incidences of breast and colon cancers. Mongolia was an outstanding exception [17]. Residents of this country traditionally consume high quantities of red meat (from Yak or Chinese Yellow cattle origin), but incidences of colon and breast cancers are remarkably low. Wide variations in colon cancer incidences have been reported, depending on specific life-style habits [18]. Globocan calculations of 2008 calculate an age-standardized risk in Western populations of <38 per 100,000 inhabitants. In Mongolia the respective data are <3.2 per 100,000 inhabitants. Thus, the difference in incidence seems to exceed a factor of 10. Less conspicuous observations exist in a few other countries. Recently, however, BMMF 1 and 2 sequences were demonstrated in milk from a different aurochs-derived bovine species: water buffalos (*Bubalus arnee f. bubalis*) [19].

Our hypothesis [7,16], linking high-risk regions for colon and breast cancers and preferential consumption of Eurasian dairy cattle meat and milk products, prompted experimental studies searching for possible nutritional infectious factors as responsible carcinogens. Thus, we tried to isolate and identify potential agents linked to colon and breast cancers from the milk, dairy products, and serum of Eurasian dairy cattle [9,20,21]. Based on our previous studies with human TT viruses, we concentrated on the isolation of small circular single-stranded DNA. A large number of these molecules, grouped in at least two clades, all share characteristics attributed to both bacterial plasmids, as well as viruses (Figure 2) [9]. The development of monoclonal antibodies against the protein derived from the largest open reading frame, identified in silico as a replication gene (Rep), proved to be very helpful in analyzing the tissue localization and the cell types expressing this protein (Figure 3) [22].

- Known BMMFs share characteristics with viruses, as well as with bacterial plasmids;
- They adapted to genetic activity and replication in certain bovine and human cells;
- They are classified in two different clades (BMMF1 and BMMF2);
- The majority of the initial isolates originated from sera or dairy products of Eurasian dairy cattle;
- An increasing number of original isolates were recently cloned and sequenced from human tissues;
- Apparently, this DNA does not persist in cancer or premalignant precursor cells;
- Their DNA is, however, found in periglandular stroma cells and in CD68-positive macrophages;
- Presence of BMMF antigens and CD68-positive macrophage foci trigger chronic inflammations;
- Products of oxygen radical DNA-interactions (8-hydroxyguanosin) can be demonstrated;
- Mutations are detectable in adjacent proliferating glandular cells, as well as in BMMF DNA extracted from stromal cells [9].

Figure 2. Present knowledge concerning BMMFs (molecular and immunologic evidence).

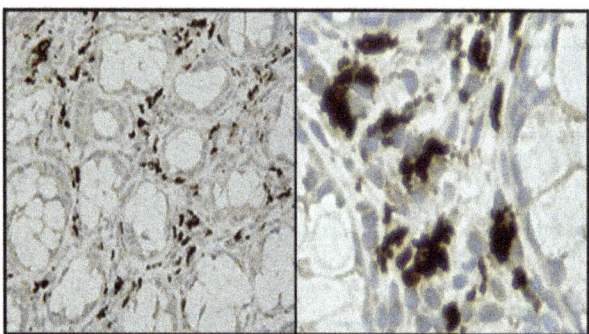

Figure 3. Typical staining pattern of cells expressing the BMMF replication protein, surrounding Lieberkühn crypts of a colon cancer biopsy at 20× and 40× magnification. Photos provided by Timo Bund.

The obtained results (Figure 4) pointed to an indirect mode of BMMF action in carcinogenesis, as previously discussed in detail [6]. In addition, Rep antigen staining occurred in non-glandular tissue of breast and prostate cancer biopsies [23].

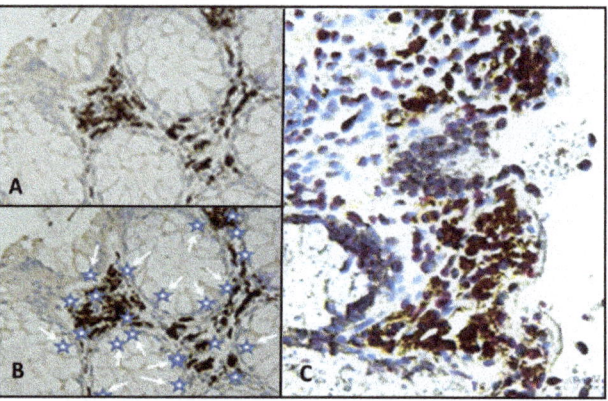

Figure 4. (**A**) Lamina propria cells surrounding Lieberkühn's crypts of the colon, staining positive with monoclonal anti-Rep antibodies. (**B**) Schematic representation of active sites of inflammation-caused oxygen radical activity indicated by white arrows pointing to blue stars. (**C**) Experimental confirmation staining of Rep-positive lamina propria cells with antibodies directed against 8-hydroxy-guanosin as a marker for oxygen radical activity (yellow staining). Reproduced [6] with permission.

In a recent report, Zapatka et al. [14] published a supporting table (without referral in the text) containing contig data of BMMF sequences obtained after sequencing colon, breast, prostate and other cancer biopsies. The authors identified the sequences according to an outdated NCBI databank submission (2014) [14], describing them mainly as "sphinx-related 1.74 or 2.36 contigs". An updated analysis of these sequences showed almost all of them as corresponding to sections of complete BMMF1 or BMMF2 genomes present in all databanks and as previously published [9]. Although not referencing these latter data, Zapatka et al. [14] confirm our colon and breast cancer studies and even extend our data by including a few additional cancers.

3. Potential Consequences of Indirect Carcinogenesis for Strategies in Prevention and Therapy of BMMF-Linked Cancers

In virus-induced direct carcinogenesis, uptake and expression of foreign genes from infectious agents (e.g., cervical cancer, Kaposi's sarcomas, Burkitt's lymphomas and others) lead to growth stimulation and increased mutagenic activity [6]. In addition, the continued interference of one or more viral proteins with growth-regulating host cell genes is a requirement for malignant transition and maintenance of the transformed phenotype [1]. These transformed cells are recognized by the immune system of the respective host, leading to inflammatory infiltrates of tumor-associated macrophages (TAM), in addition to T- and B-lymphocytes, which surround islands of a number of solid human cancers. They seem to act as a natural defense mechanism against uncontrollable cell proliferation [24,25]. The majority of these cancers arise at high frequencies under severe immunosuppression [15].

Cancers resulting from an infectious cause and linked to indirect modes of carcinogenesis follow a different pattern. The sequence of events, as evidenced by BMMF infections and cancer of the colon, was, as previously proposed [6], to be the following (Figure 5):

1. Uptake of infectious agents by nutrition through dairy products and/or meat of Eurasian cattle.
2. Infection by these agents and expression of their antigens in lamina propria cells (stromal mesenchymal cells and CD68-positive macrophages).
3. Macrophage-mediated inflammatory response (reactive oxygen production).
4. Random mutagenesis in DNA-replicating Lieberkühn crypt cells adjacent to infected cells, as well as in replicating single-stranded BMMF-DNA.
5. After long latency periods (commonly more than three decades) "driver"-mutations in genes of specific cells are established and enhanced growth of such clones occurs. These clones undergo further mutations in two or more additional steps, leading to the development of premalignant polyps. Final transformation of these polyps into malignant tumors occurs due to continuing mutagenic activity. This follows a pattern outlined previously and summarized by Greaves and Maley [26] in a quote: "Cancers evolve by a reiterative process of clonal expansion, genetic diversification and clonal selection within the adaptive landscapes of tissue ecosystems".
6. It is evident from the sequence of events described above, that BMMF DNA itself will not be present in the precursor epithelial cells, nor in their malignant progeny. No evidence exists for the frequently quoted "Hit and Run" mechanism [27,28], since infected cells persist in the lamina propria, and oxygen radical production continues. The "Hits" in colon polyps continue from adjacent BMMF-infected cells (Figure 6) [29].

Does this mechanism provide predictable consequences for prevention and even therapy of such cancers?

Present recommendations for the prevention of colon cancer include avoiding consumption of red meat, avoidance of obesity, use of non-steroidal anti-inflammatory drugs, e.g., aspirin, cox-2 inhibitors and others [6]. Secondary prevention relies on colonoscopies, as well as the detection and removal of precursor lesions (colon polyps). Undeniably, this is a successful procedure, reducing the risk for subsequent colon cancer development. It requires, however, in several cases surgical intervention, in particular when removal of the polyp was only partially successful.

Our data point to possibilities for prevention even very early in life. Specific human milk sugars (*2′- and 3′-fucosyllactose* and *disialyl-lacto-N-tetraose*) occur in human, but not in cow milk [6]. These sugars bind to lectin receptors, thereby blocking the binding for several different infectious agents. Initial reports unraveled this effect for agents causing severe gastrointestinal and respiratory infections. Interestingly, where baby formulas had been supplemented with human milk sugars, a risk reduction was observed for acute childhood leukemias, Hodgkin's disease and multiple sclerosis [6] in non-breast-fed or early-weaned babies. Their risk for developing these diseases then approximates to that of breast-fed babies [30]. A small number of mostly short-term studies reported analyses of the protective effects of these sugars when added to the diet of adults; the results remain inconclusive at present.

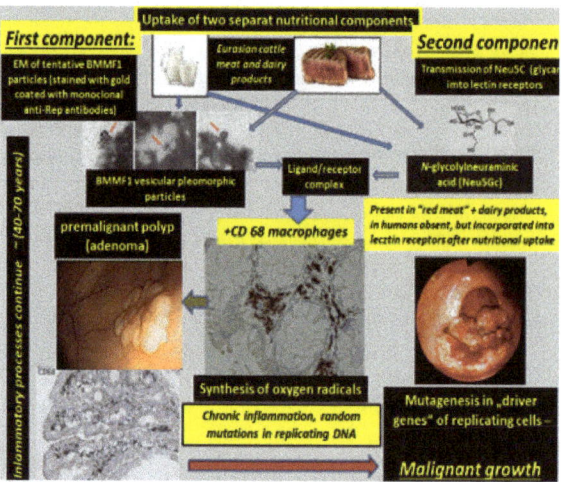

Figure 5. Sequence of events leading to malignant growth in colon. Uptake of two components is required for binding of infectious particles of bovine meat and milk factors (BMMF) to Neu5Gc as a terminal component of lectin receptors. Both are commonly present in Eurasian bovine sera and dairy products. EM—electron microscopy.

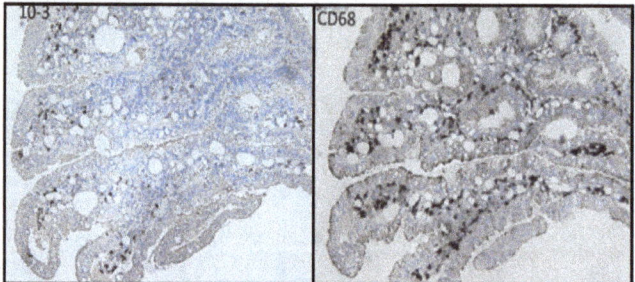

Figure 6. Colon polyps stained with anti-Rep and anti-CD68 monoclonal antibodies. The continuation of inflammation alongside mutagenic activity is evidenced by CD68 presence and Rep expression.

Indirect evidence for activity of the mentioned human sugars in adults originated, however, from follow-up studies of women with multiple pregnancies and breast-feeding periods (Figure 7). A significant reduction in breast cancer, but also in a few additional cancer types occurred in follow-up studies of this group [6]. Human milk sugars appeared in the blood and urine of these women, emerging during the second half of each pregnancy [31,32]. Other groups published similar observations and attempted to link this protective effect to specific hormonal interactions [33]. Yet, in our interpretation, this may provide a hint that prolonged exposure to human sugars in adults probably does not pose a high risk for the recipients and even seems to be protective. Although suggestive, the beneficial effects of the consumption of human milk sugar components at higher ages remain to be evaluated.

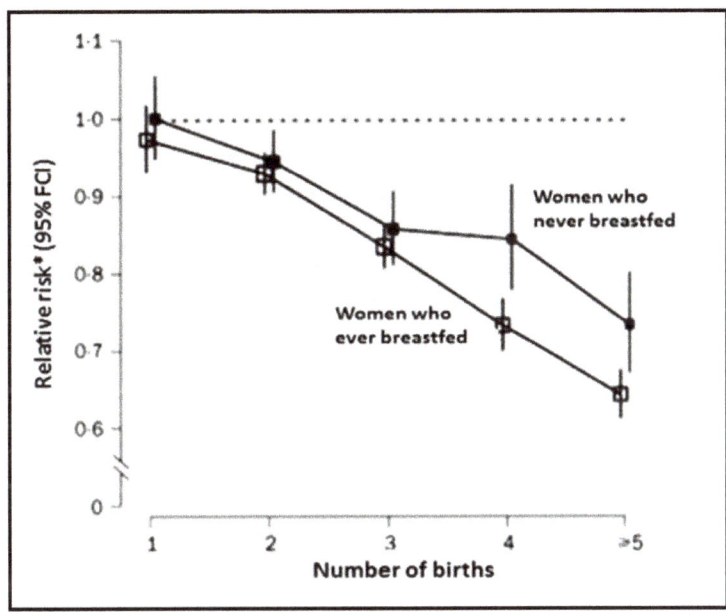

Figure 7. Reduced breast cancer risk after multiple deliveries and breast-feeding periods. Slightly less impressive reductions exist for colon and endometrial cancers (adapted with permission from [6]).

4. N-glycolylneuraminic Acid (Neu5Gc)

As suspected in a previous publication [16] Neu5Gc emerges as a strong candidate, as a terminal glycan of lectin receptors determining the susceptibility for various infections—in particular, those which are prevented by human milk sugars. We proposed blocking effects of the latter (probably due to their high affinity as terminal components of these receptors) for these infections as a mechanism of the observed protective effect of HMOs.

The nutritional transmission of Neu5Gc and the resulting immune response against this glycan [34,35] resulted in the speculation that reactive chronic immune reactions eventually induced mutational modifications in proliferating cells. This was proposed to explain malignant conversions following red meat consumption. The discovery of BMMF genomes and the expression of their Rep proteins in chronic inflammatory lesions of the colon and other tissues binding to the respective receptors added another dimension to these observations.

Among others, two questions emerge with relevance for the prevention of BMMF-linked cancers and other diseases:

Why are the cancers discussed here not at all, or extremely rarely, found in Eurasian dairy cattle, although BMMF infections are very common in their peripheral blood, their udders and in their milk?

The most likely answer seems to be an almost invariable immune tolerance resulting from the continuous conversion of Neu5Ac (N-acetylneuraminic acid) into Neu5Gc. Thus, this stresses the importance of inflammatory lesions in humans—their absence or reduction clearly leads to risk reductions for colon, breast, and prostate cancers. The subsequent chapter stresses this point.

It therefore also renders it difficult to include animal experiments for documenting BMMF carcinogenicity. Cattle, mice and most other mammals, as well as birds (except chicken) produce Neu5Gc endogenously. They are most likely immune tolerant. Thus, BMMF infection per se will not induce chronic inflammatory lesions.

The second question concerns an evolutionary aspect: is the loss of the Neu5Ac–Neu5Gc converting enzyme CMAH (Figure 8) an advantage for human evolution? To provide a clear-cut answer is probably difficult; it is unlikely that malignant tumors, commonly occurring late in life, will influence the selection of Neu5Gc-negative persons. Frequently fatal infections, however, in the first year or years of life, like noro- and rotavirus, gastrointestinal or respiratory tract infections, will almost certainly favor selection of CMAH-negative persons. Other types of prehistoric infections in the early period of human evolution may have added to this development.

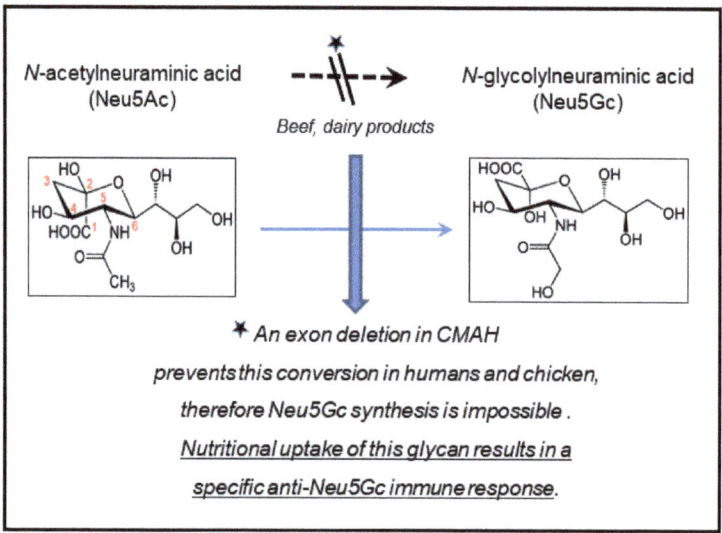

Figure 8. Cytidine monophosphate-N-acetylneuraminic acid hydrolase (CMAH).

Yet, it becomes increasingly clear (if we disregard possibilities of rare vertical transplacenta transmissions) that we are commonly born without BMMF infections. Humans are even devoid of endogenous Neu5Gc, an essential component for binding BMMFs to cellular receptors. Thus, we receive both of these components through nutrition, mainly from dairy products and, in particular, Neu5Gc from dairy products and "red" meat. Both of these components offer possibilities for specific preventive and therapeutic interferences—they need to be further explored.

5. Non-Steroidal Antiphlogistica: Preventive and Immunosuppressive Events

Inflammatory events adjacent to malignant or premalignant tumors have repeatedly been implicated in playing a role in tumor initiation or promotion [5,36–38]. This has been underlined by the tumor-preventive functions of non-steroidal anti-inflammatory drugs (NSAIDs) (Figure 9), as analyzed in a meta-analysis by Harris et al. [39].

The anti-inflammatory function of these drugs results in blocking of the induction of mutagenic events induced by oxygen radicals, as described for the mode of action of indirect carcinogenesis [16,17]. Supporting evidence for this interpretation originates from the reduced risk for colon, breast and prostate cancers after prolonged immunosuppression in organ transplant patients or chronic infections with human immunodeficiency viruses [8]. Long-time intake of NSAIDs, in particular of higher doses of aspirin and related drugs, may cause bleeding risk and requires medical supervision.

Meta-analysis of 91 epidemiological studies [39]:

Decline in the risk with increasing intake of NSAIDs (primarily aspirin or ibuprofen) for 7-10 malignancies including four major types:

colon, breast, lung and prostate cancer

Daily intake of NSAIDs, primarily aspirin,	
risk reductions of	63% for colon
	39% for breast
	36% for lung
	39% for prostate
Significant risk reductions were also observed for esophageal (73%), stomach (62% and ovarian cancer (47%)	

Figure 9. Significance of inflammatory events for specific human cancers, e.g., aspirin, ibuprofen and other Cox-2 inhibitors. Copied from [6] with permission.

6. Type II Diabetes Mellitus and BMMF

As summarized previously, human milk oligosaccharides (HMO)–among other protective effects–also reduce the risk for early onset of diabetes mellitus [16]. A remarkably interesting observation resulted from treating type II diabetes mellitus patients with the glucagon-inhibitor *metformin*: intake of this drug reduced the formation of colon polyps. Based on the knowledge that the latter depends on inflammatory reactions caused by BMMF infections and CD68 macrophages, this stimulates the hypothesis that metformin may act as an inhibitor of BMMF synthesis [40–45]. This question at present remains unresolved. It is, however, an interesting observation that the incidence of several cancers is increased in type II Diabetes mellitus patients (Figure 10) [46–48].

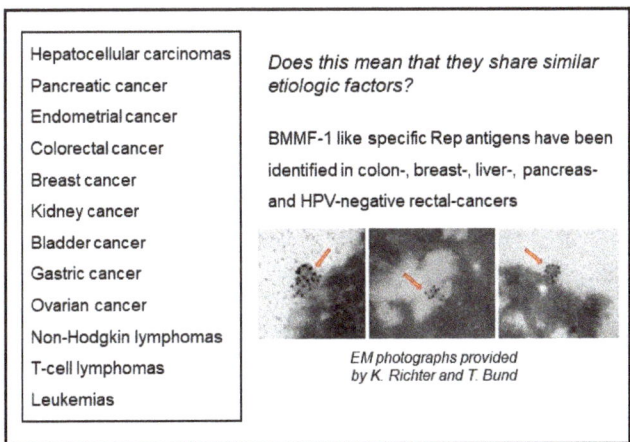

Figure 10. Cancers increased in type II Diabetes mellitus patients (summarized from [46]). The right lower part (red arrows) of the figure shows vesicular pleomorphic structures labelled with Rep antibody-coated gold particles, suspected to represent BMMF-structures.

We previously linked several of these cancers (among them colorectal and breast cancers) to indirect modes of carcinogenesis. We derived this conclusion from the detection and isolation of BMMF genomes from these tissues, or the positive staining for BMMF-1 Rep antigen (the latter also in Hepatitis B- and C-negative liver cancers, in prostate and HPV-negative rectal cancers—not shown in Figure 10).

Are they arising from mutational events triggered by oxygen or nitrogen radicals? Does this suggest common etiologic factors for these cancers? These cancers are clearly very different from those with increased incidence arising under immunosuppression [48].

Many of the outlined preventive or therapeutic interventions require intensive further investigation. Induction of long-lasting immunosuppression, mentioned as a preventive interference, is presently of no practical value for medical applications. Type-specific neutralization of BMMF, removal of BMMF from Eurasian-cattle products, as well as Rep-antibody-directed cytotoxicity of Rep-expressing cells as preventive measures of BMMF also require further experimentation (Figure 11).

Prevention (and treatment) of BMMF infections	Primary prevention of colon cancers
Possible primary prevention of colon, breast and prostate cancers?	
• Prolonged breast-feeding periods (babies)	• Prolonged breast-feeding period (mothers)
• Repeated pregnancies and breast-feeding periods (mothers)	• Multiple pregnancies and breast-feeding periods (mothers)
• Addition of human milk oligosaccharides to formulas after weaning (babies)	• Strictly vegetarian diet, avoiding Eurasian cattle dairy products and meat
• Long-lasting immunosuppression	• Long-lasting immunosuppression (after organ transplantation, persisting HIV-infection
• Type-specific BMMF neutralization	
• BMMF removal from dairy products and meat of Bos taurus-derived domestic cattle	
• Rep-antibody-directed cytotoxicity for Rep-expressing cells (also potential therapy)	• Nonsteroidal anti-inflammatory drugs (e.g. aspirin, ibuprofen, Cox-2 inhibitors)

Figure 11. Several potential and established preventive interventions for colon cancer in comparison to possible preventions of BMMF infections.

Additional existing possibilities deserve an evaluation—as previously discussed. The functional expression of the enzyme CMAH (cytidine-monophosphate-N-acetylneuraminic acid hydrolase) [34], converting acetylneuraminic acid (Neu5Ac) into N-glycolylneuraminic acid (Neu5Gc) [35], was deleted in mice [49]. This deletion corresponds to the natural situation in humans where a mutation in CMAH does not permit Neu5Gc synthesis.

Neu5Gc seems to represent an essential component of receptors for BMMF binding [6,16]. Theoretically, similar CMAH mutations induced by gene manipulation into breeds of Eurasian dairy cattle should result in Neu5Gc-negative cattle. The products from these animals should not pose a risk for BMMF infection of humans in the absence of appropriate receptors.

Rep antibody-directed cytotoxicity may have some therapeutic value, which needs further exploration. A possibly even more interesting alternative would be their use in destroying Rep-positive persistently BMMF-infected carrier cells by this procedure, even at an early stage of life. Prevention of the carrier state could represent a kind of "early stage secondary prevention" in already infected persons.

7. Basal Cell Carcinomas in Pox Vaccination Scars

As previously mentioned, basal cell carcinomas (BCCs) can develop in pox vaccination scars (Figure 12) [7]. They may deserve special interest if a possible relationship to BMMF infections exists. Skin cancers occur in excess of one in three newly diagnosed cancers. BCCs represent the vast majority of skin cancers [7]. Prolonged solar exposure is a major risk factor for the development of actinic keratoses—precursor lesions for this cancer [50]. Occasional reports claim a role for several types of cutaneous papillomaviruses in addition to solar exposure in the pathogenesis of these malignancies. This has then frequently been referred to as a "hit and run" mechanism. This postulate tried to explain inconsistencies—in particular, the absence of persisting viral DNA in these cancer cells [1,27,28]. A few observations on BCCs reported over past decades may provide clues deserving a fresh look; BCCs repeatedly emerged in pox vaccination scars, occasionally as multiple foci, years after inoculation with the vaccine [7].

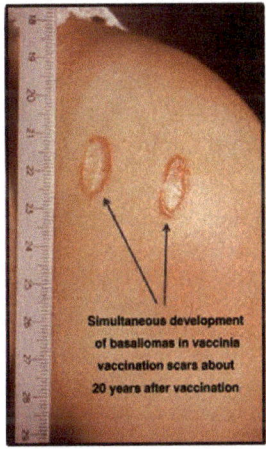

Figure 12. Basal cell carcinoma emerged in a pox vaccination scar. Copied [7] (with permission).

Studies performed by our group during the past decade provide the basis for a different speculation: we demonstrated an almost regular presence of CD68-positive TAMs in foci of BMMF1 Rep-positive peri-tumorous cells [16]. During previous decades, poxvirus vaccines were prepared from inoculation of vaccinia virus preparations into the scratched skin of calves. The initial formation of pox-like pustules subsequently converted to crusts. The copious vaccinia virus crudely purified from these harvested crusts represented the basis for human vaccination.

Presently, we know that the majority of Eurasian cattle are carriers of BMMF infections in various tissues, including peripheral blood [9,17]. BMMF transmission/transfusion into the scratches on the calfskin is highly probable. The intensive local infection occurring after vaccination and the subsequent induction of slow chronic inflammation many years after the inoculation of the vaccine could result in BCCs in the vaccination scars. Other environmental mutagens may synergize with this process [7].

8. Acute Myeloid Leukemia

In addition to the global epidemiological incidence pattern of BMMF infection-linked cancers discussed up to now, one other neoplastic disease deserves further investigation: acute myeloid leukemia (AML). The global incidence of this malignancy is somewhat similar to the global pattern of colon cancer incidence (Figure 13). The figure compares the global pattern of those two cancers with the very different epidemiology of gastric and liver cancers.

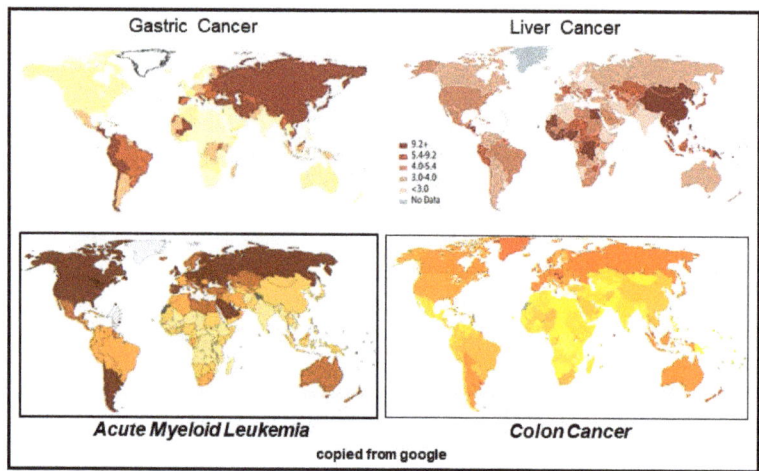

Figure 13. Global epidemiological incidence of AML and colon cancer in comparison to gastric and liver cancers.

RNA-seq data provided evidence for BMMF1 transcription. These sequences differ substantially from the BMMF1 HSB1 in colon cancers [51]. These data seem to be of specific interest for several reasons:

1. To our knowledge, this is the first direct link between a human leukemia and a specific BMMF infection;
2. Since the respective BMMF types have been identified in dairy products, it is likely that the human infection was acquired by consumption of infected nutritional components;
3. AML, as well as acute lymphatic leukemia (ALL), has very often been reported to occur even in the prenatal phase. A further confirmation of their infectious origin implies prenatal trans-placenta transmission during pregnancy, as proposed previously [52,53].

Future transcription analyses of acute lymphatic leukemias searching for BMMF-like infections will be of substantial interest.

9. Conclusions

Except for infection-linked human cancers (EBV, HPV, HBV, HCV, others) our knowledge of agents causally involved in the majority of human cancers is still very limited. This applies for chronic neurological diseases, arteriosclerosis, autoimmune and metabolic diseases as well. A fresh look into indirect mechanisms, as defined now for a few common cancers, may provide surprising results, with far reaching implications for the prevention and therapy of these diseases.

Funding: This research was supported in part by the Deutsches Krebsforschungszentrum (German Cancer Center), as well as an unrestricted grant from Oryx Alpha.

Acknowledgments: The authors thank Timo Bund for providing unpublished images.

Conflicts of Interest: The authors declare no conflict of interest.

References

1. Zur Hausen, H. *Infections Causing Human Cancer*; Wiley-VCH: Weinheim, Germany, 2006; pp. 1–517.
2. De Martel, C.; Georges, D.; Bray, F.; Ferlay, J.; Clifford, G.M. Global burden of cancer attributable to infections in 2018: A worldwide incidence analysis. *Lancet Glob. Health* **2020**, *8*, e180–e190. [CrossRef]
3. Zur Hausen, H. Oncogenic DNA viruses. *Oncogene* **2001**, *20*, 7820–7823. [CrossRef] [PubMed]

4. Zur Hausen, H.; de Villiers, E.M. Cancer "causation" by infections—Individual contributions and synergistic networks. *Semin. Oncol.* **2014**, *41*, 860–875. [CrossRef]
5. Lin, S.; Li, Y.; Zamyatnin, A.A.; Werner, J.; Bazhin, A.V. Reactive oxygen species and colorectal cancer. Review *J. Cell Physiol.* **2018**, *233*, 5119–5132. [CrossRef]
6. Zur Hausen, H.; Bund, T.; de Villiers, E.M. Specific nutritional infections early in life as risk factors for human colon and breast cancers several decades later. *Int. J. Cancer.* **2019**, *144*, 1574–1583. [CrossRef]
7. Zur Hausen, H. The search for infectious causes of human cancers: Where and why. *Virology* **2009**, *392*, 1–10. [CrossRef]
8. Coghill, A.E.; Engels, E.A.; Schymura, M.J.; Mahale, P.; Shiels, M.S. Risk of breast, prostate, and colorectal cancer diagnoses among HIV-infected individuals in the United States. *J. Natl. Cancer Inst.* **2018**, *110*, 959–966. [CrossRef]
9. De Villiers, E.M.; Gunst, K.; Chakraborty, D.; Ernst, C.; Bund, T.; zur Hausen, H. A specific class of infectious agents isolated from bovine serum and dairy products and peritumoral colon cancer tissue. *Emerg. Microbes Infect.* **2019**, *8*, 1205–1218. [CrossRef]
10. Manuelidis, L. Nuclease resistant circular DNAs copurify with infectivity in scrapie and CJD. *J. Neurovirol.* **2011**, *17*, 131–145. [CrossRef] [PubMed]
11. Tae, H.; Karunasena, E.; Bavarva, J.H.; McIver, L.J.; Garner, H.R. Large scale comparison of non-human sequences in human sequencing data. *Genomics* **2014**, *104*, 453–458. [CrossRef]
12. Chen, X.; Kost, J.; Sulovari, A.; Wong, N.; Liang, W.S.; Jian Cao, J.; Li, D. A virome-wide clonal integration analysis platform for discovering cancer viral etiology. *Genome Res.* **2019**, *29*, 819–830. [CrossRef] [PubMed]
13. Kumata, R.; Ito, J.; Tahashi, K.; Suzuki, T.; Sato, K. A tissue level atlas of the healthy human virome. Version 2. *BMC Biol.* **2020**, *18*, 55. [CrossRef] [PubMed]
14. Zapatka, M.; Borozan, I.; Brewer, D.S.; Iskar, M.; Grundhoff, A.; Alawi, M.; Desai, N.; Sültmann, H.; Moch, H.; Cooper, C.S.; et al. The landscape of viral associations in human cancers. *Nat. Genet.* **2020**, *52*, 320–330. [CrossRef] [PubMed]
15. Grulich, A.E.; van Leeuwen, M.T.; Falster, M.O.; Vajdic, C.M. Incidence of cancers in people with HIV/AIDS compared with immunosuppressed transplant recipients: A meta-analysis. *Lancet* **2007**, *370*, 59–67. [CrossRef]
16. Zur Hausen, H.; Bund, T.; de Villiers, E.M. Infectious agents in bovine red meat and milk and their potential role in cancer and other chronic diseases. *Curr. Top. Microbiol. Immunol.* **2017**, *407*, 83–116.
17. Zur Hausen, H. Red meat consumption and cancer: Reasons to suspect involvement of bovine infectious factors in colorectal cancer. *Int. J. Cancer* **2012**, *130*, 2475–2483. [CrossRef]
18. Huxley, R.R.; Ansary-Moghaddam, A.; Clifton, P.; Czernichow, S.; Parr, C.L.; Woodward, M. The impact of dietary and lifestyle risk factors on risk of colorectal cancer: A quantitative overview of the epidemiological evidence. *Int. J. Cancer* **2009**, *125*, 171–180. [CrossRef] [PubMed]
19. König, M.T.; Fux, R.; Link, E.; Sutter, G.; Märtlbauer, E.; Didier, A. Circular Rep-encoding single-stranded DNA sequences in milk from water buffalos (*Bubalus arnee f. bubalis*). *Viruses* **2021**, *13*, 1088. [CrossRef]
20. Whitley, C.; Gunst, K.; Müller, H.; Funk, M.; zur Hausen, H.; de Villiers, E.M. Novel replication-competent circular DNA molecules from healthy cattle serum and milk and multiple sclerosis-affected human brain tissue. *Genome Announc.* **2014**, *2*, e00849-14. [CrossRef] [PubMed]
21. Funk, M.; Gunst, K.; Lucansky, V.; Müller, H.; zur Hausen, H.; de Villiers, E.M. Isolation of protein-associated circular DNA from healthy cattle serum. *Genome Announc.* **2014**, *2*, e00846-14. [CrossRef]
22. Bund, T.; Nikitina, E.; Chakraborty, D.; Ernst, C.; Gunst, K.; Boneva, B.; Tessmer, C.; Volk, N.; Brobeil, A.; Weber, A.; et al. Analysis of chronic inflammatory lesions of the colon for BMMF Rep antigen expression and CD68 macrophage interactions. *Proc. Nat. Acad. Sci. USA* **2021**, *118*, e2025830118. [CrossRef]
23. Bund, T.; de Villiers, E.M.; zur Hausen, H. Detection of BMMF antigen in breast- and prostate cancer biopsies. unpublished.
24. Grivennikov, S.I.; Greten, F.R.; Karin, M. Immunity, inflammation, and cancer. *Rev. Cell.* **2010**, *140*, 883–899. [CrossRef]
25. Candido, J.; Hagemann, T. Cancer-related inflammation. *J. Clin. Immunol.* **2013**, *1*, 579–584. [CrossRef] [PubMed]
26. Greaves, M.; Maley, C.C. Clonal evolution in cancer. *Nature* **2012**, *481*, 306–313. [CrossRef] [PubMed]
27. Lau, C.C.; Gadi, I.K.; Anisowicz, A.; Sager, R. Plasmid-induced "hit-and-run" tumorigenesis in Chinese hamster embryo fibroblast (CHEF) cells. *Proc. Natl. Acad. Sci. USA* **1985**, *82*, 2839–2843. [CrossRef] [PubMed]
28. Scarisbrick, I.A.; Rodriguez, M. Hit-Hit and hit-Run: Viruses in the playing field of multiple sclerosis. *Cur. Neurol. Neurosc. Rep.* **2003**, *3*, 265–271. [CrossRef] [PubMed]
29. Aarons, C.B.; Shanmugan, S.; Bleier, J.I. Management of malignant colon polyps: Current status and controversies. *World J. Gastroenterol.* **2014**, *20*, 16178–16183. [CrossRef] [PubMed]
30. Akkerman, R.; Faas, M.M.; de Vos, P. Non-digestible carbohydrates in infant formula as substitution for human milk oligosaccharide functions: Effects on microbiota and gut maturation. *Crit. Rev. Food Sci. Nutr.* **2019**, *59*, 1486–1497. [CrossRef]
31. Beral, V. Collaborative Group on Hormonal Factors in Breast Cancer. Breast cancer and breastfeeding: Collaborative reanalysis of individual data from 47 epidemiological studies in 30 countries, including 50,302 women with breast cancer and 96,973 women without the disease. *Lancet* **2002**, *360*, 187–195.
32. Faupel-Badger, J.M.; Arcaro, K.F.; Balkam, J.J.; Eliassen, A.H.; Hassiotou, F.; Lebrilla, C.B.; Michels, K.B.; Palmer, J.R.; Schedin, P.; Stuebe, A.M.; et al. Postpartum remodeling, lactation, and breast cancer risk: Summary of a National Cancer Institute-sponsored workshop. *J. Natl. Cancer Inst.* **2013**, *105*, 166–174. [CrossRef]

33. Troisi, R.; Bjørge, T.; Gissler, M.; Grotmol, T.; Kitahara, C.M.; Myrtveit Saether, S.M.; Ording, A.G.; Sköld, C.; Sørensen, H.T.; Trabert, B.; et al. The role of pregnancy, perinatal factors and hormones in maternal cancer risk: A review of the evidence. *J. Intern. Med.* **2018**, *283*, 430–445. [CrossRef]
34. Okerblom, J.; Varki, A. Biochemical, cellular, physiological, and pathological consequences of human loss of N-glycolylneuraminic acid. *Chembiochem.* **2017**, *18*, 1155–1171. [CrossRef]
35. Diaz, S.L.; Padler-Karavani, V.; Ghaderi, D.; Hurtado-Ziola, N.; Yu, H.; Chen, X.; Brinkman-Van der Linden, E.C.M.; Varki, A.; Varki, N.M. Sensitive and specific detection of the non-human sialic acid N-glycolylneuraminic acid in human tissues and biotherapeutic products. *PLoS ONE* **2009**, *4*, e4241. [CrossRef] [PubMed]
36. Wang, K.; Karin, M. Tumor-Elicited Inflammation and Colorectal Cancer. *Adv. Cancer Res.* **2015**, *128*, 173–196.
37. Crusz, S.M.; Balkwill, F.R. Inflammation and cancer: Advances and new agents. *Nat. Rev. Clin. Oncol.* **2015**, *12*, 584–596. [CrossRef]
38. Marelli, G.; Sica, A.; Vannucci, L.; Allavena, P. Inflammation as Target in Cancer Therapy. *Curr. Opin. Pharmacol.* **2017**, *35*, 57–65. [CrossRef]
39. Harris, R.E.; Beebe-Donk, J.; Doss, H.; Burr Doss, D. Aspirin, ibuprofen, and other non-steroidal anti-inflammatory drugs in cancer prevention: A critical review of non-selective COX-2 blockade. *Oncol. Rep.* **2005**, *13*, 559–583. [CrossRef] [PubMed]
40. Eddi, R.; Karki, A.; Shah, A.; DeBari, V.A.; DePasquale, J.R. Association of type 2 diabetes and colon adenomas. *J. Gastrointest. Cancer.* **2012**, *43*, 87–92. [CrossRef]
41. Wang, Z.; Lai, S.T.; Xie, L.; Zhao, J.D.; Ma, N.Y.; Zhu, J.; Ren, Z.G.; Jiang, G.L. Metformin is associated with reduced risk of pancreatic cancer in patients with type 2 diabetes mellitus: A systematic review and meta-analysis. *Diabetes Res. Clin. Pract.* **2014**, *106*, 19–26. [CrossRef]
42. Cho, Y.H.; Ko, B.M.; Kim, S.H.; Myung, Y.S.; Choi, J.H.; Han, J.P.; Hong, S.J.; Jeon, S.R.; Kim, H.G.; Kim, J.O.; et al. Does metformin affect the incidence of colonic polyps and adenomas in patients with type 2 diabetes mellitus? *Intest. Res.* **2014**, *12*, 139–145. [CrossRef]
43. Rokkas, T.; Portincasa, P. Colon neoplasia in patients with type 2 diabetes on metformin: A meta-analysis. *Eur. J. Intern. Med.* **2016**, *33*, 60–66. [CrossRef]
44. Miłek, T.; Forysiński, K.; Myrcha, P.; Ciostek, P. Diabetes association of polyps and colon cancer. *Pol. Przegl. Chir.* **2019**, *91*, 9–12. [CrossRef] [PubMed]
45. Zhang, J.; Wen, L.; Zhou, Q.; He, K.; Teng, L. Preventative and therapeutic effects of metformin in gastric cancer: A new contribution of an old friend. *Cancer Manag. Res.* **2020**, *12*, 8545–8554. [CrossRef]
46. Gallagher, E.J.; LeRoith, D. Does a single nucleotide polymorphism in the FGFR explain the connection between diabetes and cancer? *Cell Metab.* **2013**, *17*, 808–809. [CrossRef]
47. Yan, P.; Wang, Y.; Fu, T.; Liu, Y.; Zhang, Z.-Y. The association between type 1 and 2 diabetes mellitus and the risk of leukemia: A systematic review and meta-analysis of 18 cohort studies. *Endocr. J.* **2021**, *68*, 281–289. [CrossRef]
48. Vajdic, C.M.; Grulich, A.E.; Kaldor, J.M.; Fritschi, L.; Benke, G.; Hughes, A.M.; Kricker, A.; Turner, J.J.; Milliken, S.; Armstrong, B.K. Specific infections, infection-related behavior, and risk of non-Hodgkin lymphoma in adults. *Cancer Epidemiol. Biomark. Prev.* **2006**, *15*, 1102–1108. [CrossRef]
49. Hedlund, M.; Tangvoranuntakul, P.; Takematsu, H.; Long, J.M.; Housley, G.D.; Kozutsumi, Y.; Suzuki, A.; Wynshaw-Boris, A.; Ryan, A.F.; Gallo, R.L.; et al. N-glycolylneuraminic acid deficiency in mice: Implications for human biology and evolution. *Mol. Cell Biol.* **2007**, *27*, 4340–4346. [CrossRef]
50. Khalesi, M.; Whiteman, D.C.; Doi, S.A.; Clark, J.; Kimlin, M.G.; Neale, R.E. Cutaneous markers of photo-damage and risk of Basal cell carcinoma of the skin: A meta-analysis. *Cancer Epidemiol. Biomarkers Prev.* **2013**, *22*, 1483–1489. [CrossRef] [PubMed]
51. Haefele, L.; Feuerbach, L.; Bund, T. RNA-Seq analyses. Unpublished.
52. Zur Hausen, H.; de Villiers, E.M. Virus target cell conditioning model to explain some epidemiologic characteristics of childhood leukemias and lymphomas. *Int. J. Cancer.* **2005**, *115*, 1–5. [CrossRef] [PubMed]
53. Zur Hausen, H. Childhood leukemias and other hematopoietic malignancies: Interdependence between an infectious event and chromosomal modifications. *Int. J. Cancer* **2009**, *125*, 1764–1770. [CrossRef] [PubMed]

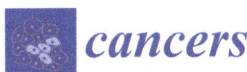

Review

Dietary Modulation of Bacteriophages as an Additional Player in Inflammation and Cancer

Luigi Marongiu [1], Markus Burkard [2], Sascha Venturelli [2,3,*] and Heike Allgayer [1,*]

[1] Department of Experimental Surgery—Cancer Metastasis, Medical Faculty Mannheim, Ruprecht-Karls University of Heidelberg, Ludolf-Krehl-Str. 13-17, 68167 Mannheim, Germany; Luigi.marongiu@medma.uni-heidelberg.de

[2] Department of Biochemistry of Nutrition, University of Hohenheim, Garbenstr. 30, 70599 Stuttgart, Germany; markus.burkard@uni-hohenheim.de

[3] Department of Vegetative and Clinical Physiology, University Hospital of Tuebingen, Otfried-Müllerstr. 27, 72076 Tuebingen, Germany

* Correspondence: sascha.venturelli@uni-hohenheim.de (S.V.); heike.allgayer@medma.uni-heidelberg.de (H.A.); Tel.: +49-(0)711-459-24113 (ext. 24195) (S.V.); +49-(0)621-383-71630 (ext. 71635) (H.A.); Fax: +49-(0)-711-459-23822 (S.V.); +49-(0)-621-383-71631 (H.A.)

Citation: Marongiu, L.; Burkard, M.; Venturelli, S.; Allgayer, H. Dietary Modulation of Bacteriophages as an Additional Player in Inflammation and Cancer. *Cancers* **2021**, *13*, 2036. https://doi.org/10.3390/cancers13092036

Academic Editor: Damián García-Olmo

Received: 9 April 2021
Accepted: 21 April 2021
Published: 23 April 2021

Publisher's Note: MDPI stays neutral with regard to jurisdictional claims in published maps and institutional affiliations.

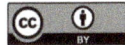

Copyright: © 2021 by the authors. Licensee MDPI, Basel, Switzerland. This article is an open access article distributed under the terms and conditions of the Creative Commons Attribution (CC BY) license (https:// creativecommons.org/licenses/by/ 4.0/).

Simple Summary: The role and function of bacteriophages (phages) in the intestine, its health and microbial homeostasis has been underestimated so far. This interdisciplinary review highlights the effect of dietary compounds on phages and puts this into perspective with putative contributions of phages to gastrointestinal diseases, specifically inflammation, infection, and cancer. The review discusses novel fields of opportunities in this context. These include, but are not limited to, perspectives how a better understanding of modulating the activity of specific phages by particular nutritional components may contribute to reorganizing the microbial network, thus supporting in the combat, or even prevention, of inflammation or even cancer in the gut.

Abstract: Natural compounds such as essential oils and tea have been used successfully in naturopathy and folk medicine for hundreds of years. Current research is unveiling the molecular role of their antibacterial, anti-inflammatory, and anticancer properties. Nevertheless, the effect of these compounds on bacteriophages is still poorly understood. The application of bacteriophages against bacteria has gained a particular interest in recent years due to, e.g., the constant rise of antimicrobial resistance to antibiotics, or an increasing awareness of different types of microbiota and their potential contribution to gastrointestinal diseases, including inflammatory and malignant conditions. Thus, a better knowledge of how dietary products can affect bacteriophages and, in turn, the whole gut microbiome can help maintain healthy homeostasis, reducing the risk of developing diseases such as diverse types of gastroenteritis, inflammatory bowel disease, or even cancer. The present review summarizes the effect of dietary compounds on the physiology of bacteriophages. In a majority of works, the substance class of polyphenols showed a particular activity against bacteriophages, and the primary mechanism of action involved structural damage of the capsid, inhibiting bacteriophage activity and infectivity. Some further dietary compounds such as caffeine, salt or oregano have been shown to induce or suppress prophages, whereas others, such as the natural sweeter stevia, promoted species-specific phage responses. A better understanding of how dietary compounds could selectively, and specifically, modulate the activity of individual phages opens the possibility to reorganize the microbial network as an additional strategy to support in the combat, or in prevention, of gastrointestinal diseases, including inflammation and cancer.

Keywords: Phage; bacteriophages; diet; infection; colorectal; cancer; nutrition

1. Introduction

The impact of the gut bacteriome on the human physiology is currently being investigated and seems to have a significant influence on the development and treatment of various diseases. Collectively, the over one thousand bacterial species residing in the human gut encode 3.3 million genes, expanding the human genome 150 times over [1]. Several studies have demonstrated that microorganisms present in the human gut (the gut microbiome) modulate human physiology at different levels. Intestinal bacteria not only metabolize polysaccharides that would be otherwise indigestible [2], but also regulate peristalsis [3], help to keep a proper intestinal morphology as it has been shown in a gnotobiotic pig model [4], maintain the integrity of the intestinal barrier [5–7], attenuate inflammation [8,9], reduce the virulence of pathogenic species [10], and even influence the action of anticancer drugs [11]. Although it has been proposed to consider the intestinal microorganisms as symbionts rather than simple commensal species [12], our understanding of the dynamics underlying the interactions between host and gut microbiome is still limited [13,14].

Bacteriophages (or phages for short) represent a significant modulator of the gut microbiome [15]. By definition, phages infect bacteria, but more and more data highlight the interrelation between eukaryotic cells and bacterial viruses. Phages can interact directly with the human body since they can translocate inside eukaryotic cells [16] and activate the immune system, exacerbating ongoing colitis symptoms and boosting the antibacterial response [17]. It has recently been proposed to consider phages as human pathogens [18].

In the last few years, phages have become a crucial topic in the medical and microbiological fields because these viruses can be used as a treatment of bacterial infections in the context of the rising problem of antibiotic resistance [19–21]. As our understanding of phage biology increases, the applications of phage therapy also expand. Phages have been applied to treat bacterial infections ever since their discovery, and phage therapy is becoming more and more popular in fields ranging from dentistry to medical microbiology [22–25]. For example, phages are currently being evaluated to fight infections in poultry that are still an economic and health issue [24]. Recent studies suggest that phages can also be applied in antiviral and anticancer therapies. For instance, it has been proposed that phage T4 might be used as a co-treatment for COVID-19 because this phage reduces the immune response, which is an important contributor to the fatality associated with this disease [26]. Furthermore, it has been shown that phages bind to cancerous cells and reduce the size of the tumor mass in different mouse models [17,27,28], opening the possibility of phage-mediated oncolytic virotherapy.

Diet can influence the gut microbiome, and it is actively used as an intervention to reduce the risk of developing diseases [29]. Particular components have been shown to be of benefit in the treatment of even severe disease conditions up to cancer. For example, in own previous studies, it was demonstrated that the plant-derivatives curcumin and artesunate inhibit tumor cell invasion and metastasis, at least in part via regulating the expression of proteolytic enzymes, the molecular cascades involving transcriptional factors and microRNAs, respectively [30–33]. However, there is a lack of studies describing how dietary compounds impact microorganisms in general and phages in particular. Seminal studies in the 1950 s demonstrated the antiviral activity of tannins, which are contained in popular beverages such as tea and coffee, and of acerin, the active component of maple fruit [34,35]. Especially, tea showed broad antimicrobial activity, including inactivation of phages [36]. It is also known that essential oils have antibacterial and antiviral properties as well as anti-inflammatory and regenerative activities [37]. Nevertheless, gaining experimental knowledge on the influence of dietary compounds on phages as modulators of microbiota has not yet been in focus of attention in the research community.

Most of the studies related to the effect of dietary compounds on phages have been focusing on human viruses associated with gastroenteritis. Phages have been used as surrogates for viruses that cannot be easily cultivated, such as norovirus, rather than for studying bacterial virus biology as such. Also, most of the bacteriophage studies so far have been limited to phages infecting *Escherichia coli* (coliphages). Nonetheless, *E. coli* plays an essential role in human health since certain strains of this species, known as Shiga toxin-producing *E. coli* (STEC), are widespread food-borne pathogens. The most prevalent STECs are O157, O26, O45, O103, O111, O121, and O145. These seven serotypes induce diseases ranging from acute diarrhea to hemorrhagic colitis and fatal hemolytic syndrome [38–40].

The main STEC derived virulence factor is shiga-like toxin (Stx), which is encoded by the prophages 933 J (*Stx1*) and 933 W (*Stx2*) [41,42]. Upon activation, these prophages express *Stx*, and they can horizontally spread this gene by transduction [43,44]. Genotoxins, such as cytolethal distending toxins and colibactin, are considered cancer risk factors and can be found in pathogenic *E. coli* strains [45]. Interestingly, many natural compounds have been shown to be bactericidal against pathogens [46], and to suppress the biological activity of toxins, including the cholera and ricin toxins [46–49]. Peas showed to bind with high efficiency Stx, acting as toxic-scavengers, whereas beans can reduce the intake of Stx [50].

We speculate that a better understanding of how phages are activated or inhibited in the human gut might be pivotal in modulating the intestinal microbiome, e.g., to counteract bacterial infections, inflammatory conditions, and even carcinogenesis and cancer progression. Such indirect antibacterial activity is a particularly relevant feature in light of the urgent need to identify alternatives and additional strategies to antibiotics to defeat (therapy-resistant) bacterial infections. The present review will summarize the current knowledge on the effect of dietary compounds on phages, their activity, and infectivity.

2. Interactions between Phages and Bacteria in the Gut Microbiome

Phages were first described by the French-Canadian Félix d'Hérelle, of Institute Pasteur in 1917, who also defined the term 'bacteriophage' ("eater of bacteria"). As a first, pioneering phage-based therapy, he applied bacteriophages to treat *Shigella* infections in soldiers, establishing what became known as phage therapy [51–53]. Phages can be subdivided into two groups: virulent (lytic) and temperate (lysogenic) (Figure 1) [54]. Lytic viruses start the replication process soon after the infection of the bacterial host. Once the progeny virions have assembled in a sufficient number (the burst size), the cell bursts open, releasing the new phages in the surrounding environment. Lysogenic phages have an additional phase: they can integrate as prophages in the bacterial chromosome and undergo a latency period where only a viral transcription suppressor is produced actively. In particular contexts, such as bacterial starvation or DNA damage, the suppression control is relieved, and the prophage enters the lytic phase. Conversely, in the presence of a high number of infected bacteria, phages exit the lytic phase and initiate lysogeny [55]. Both virulent and temperate phages modulate the bacterial population through lysis.

Phages can also modulate the bacterial population, indirectly. It is well known that bacteria must undergo a fierce competition within each ecological niche, and, therefore, some species have developed virulence factors to improve their chances of survival [56]. Moreover, the microbial competition is complex and difficult to predict. For instance, *Lactobacillus delbrueckii* and *L. rhamnosus* inhibit *E. coli* O157, but *L. plantarum* suppresses the commensal strains of *E. coli* but not O157, and *L. paracasei* does not constrain *E. coli* at all [57]. In addition, the suppression of one species might cause the unexpected expansion of a species not apparently associated with the suppressed one. For instance, *E. coli* fosters the growth of *B. fragilis* but represses *B. vulgatus*. Knocking down *E. coli* by phage T4 is, therefore, followed by a contraction of the prevalence of *B. fragilis* and an increased growth of *B. vulgatus*, but also of *Proteus mirabilis* and *Akkermansia muciniphila* [58]. It is also known that commensal species can neutralize toxins, reducing the fitness of the pathogens. For instance, surface proteins of *L. plantarum* can neutralize Stx, reducing the cytotoxicity (and, thus, the fitness) of *E. coli* O157 [59]. Therefore, the alteration of even one species due to phagial predation can have drastic consequences for the microbiome.

Mounting evidence suggests that phages have access to eukaryotic (and human) cells [60]. Even though tissues are expected to be sterile, it has been known for decades that an ingestion of phage preparations during phage therapy is followed by a recovery of phages in human urine and blood within a few minutes from the administration [61,62]. This recovery implies that the viruses had somehow crossed the gastrointestinal barrier. Recent virome studies have identified genes belonging to phages in both blood and brain [63,64]. The circulation of phages in the peripheral blood has been named 'phagemia', but there is a lack of hard evidence for its actual existence in physiological conditions [65]. Furthermore, phages can be actively transported from one side to another of intestinal cells (transcytosis) via the Golgi network [16].

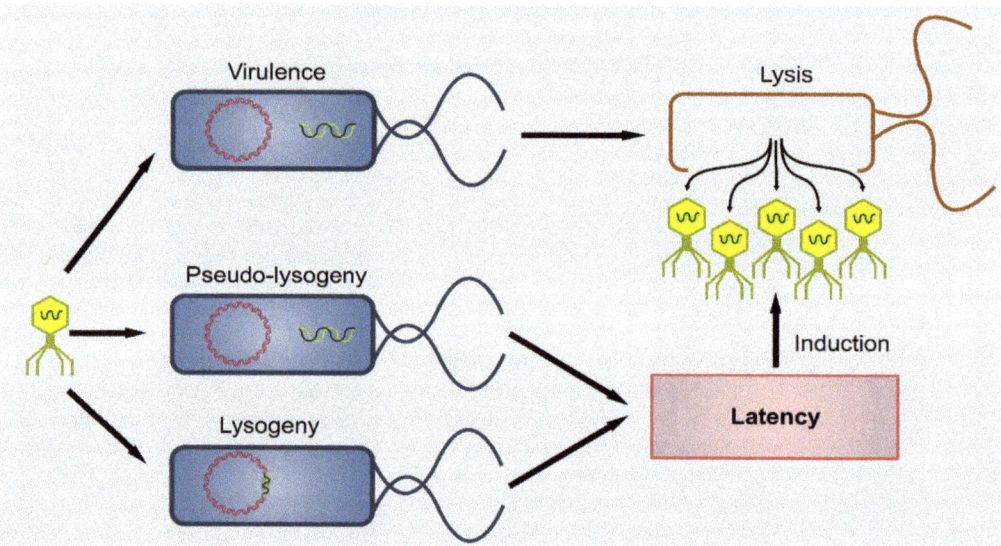

Figure 1. Outcomes of phagial infection of bacteria. A virulent phage (yellow particle on the left) can infect a bacterium (in blue). The replication of the phage leads to lysis of the host cell, releasing the viral progeny (yellow particles on the right). Alternatively, some viral species known as temperate can establish an additional step known as latency. The phagial genome can remain independent from that of the bacterium (pseudo-lysogeny) or become integrated into the host's genome (lysogeny). In both cases, the viral expression is kept to a minimum and there is no virion production until several cellular conditions are met. Upon induction, temperate phages enter the lytic pathway and determine the lysis of the host.

3. Effect of Dietary Compounds on Phages

Several dietary compounds can alter the physiology of phages, as summarized in Figure 2. Although many studies showed a connection between nutrition and intestinal microbiome, there are only a few studies that deal with the effects of nutrition on the activity of phages. Seminal work in the 1960 s indicated that amino acids and vitamins had a different impact on the induction of prophage λ in *E. coli* [66]. For instance, the amino acid cysteine was an inducer, but its oxidized derivative cystine was not. About four decades later, it was shown that essential oils extracted from chamomile, lemongrass, cinnamon, and geranium could greatly reduce the infectivity of *E. coli* T7 and *S. aureus* SA, whereas others (such as angelica, cardamom, lime, and rosemary) affected only the former phage [67]. A recent study reported how different compounds could selectively activate some viruses but not others in bacterial growth and prophage-induction assays [68]. This study demonstrated how stevia, a natural sweetener obtained from the Brazilian shrub *Stevia rebaudiana* [69], could strongly induce prophages present in *Bacteroides thetaiotamicron* and *Staphylococcus aureus* but not in *Enterococcus faecalis*, whereas uva ursi (derived from the shrub plant *Arctostaphylos uva-ursi*), aspartame (a peptide), and propolis (a flavonoid) resulted in the opposite. These data indicate that dietary compounds can modulate the gut virome and, consequently, alter the gut bacteriome.

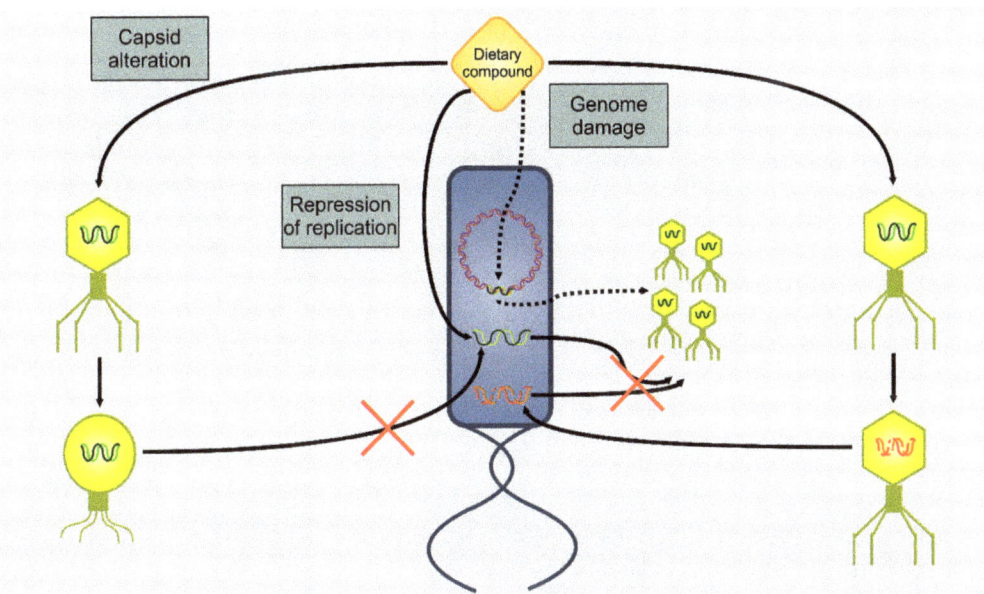

Figure 2. Summary of actions on phages on dietary compounds. There are three main mechanisms of action of dietary compounds upon phages. A dietary compound can modify the capsid, blocking the infectivity of the targeted phage (capsid alteration). Alternatively, dietary compounds can lead to the degradation of nucleic acids (genome damage). In this case, a phage can infect the host, but there will be neither lysis nor viral progeny. However, DNA damage to the host cell's genome triggers the induction of prophages (dotted arrows). A final mechanism of action (repression of replication) involves an interference with the replication of the viral genome. Even in this case, there is infection, but no viral progeny is produced.

Experiments measuring the effect of dietary compounds on phage activity have been based on few classes of compounds, mainly polyphenols. These are molecules that contain one or more phenolic aromatic rings (benzenes with hydroxide moieties). Polyphenols can be subdivided into phenolic acid derivatives and flavonoids [70]. The former can, in turn, be subdivided into derivatives of either hydroxybenzoic acid (for instance, gallic acid) or cinnamic acid (for example, caffeic acid) [71]. Tea, the second most frequently consumed beverage after water, is a primary source for gallic acid [72]. Coffee, whose consumption is increasing worldwide [73], contains chlorogenic acid (a combination of caffeic acid and quinic acid) [71]. Tannic acid, which contains several hydroxybenzoic acid moieties, is particularly abundant in berries; soy is rich in isoflavonoids, such as genistein and daidzein [74]. The exact mechanism of action of these phenol-compounds is not entirely understood. Still, it is known that they can be beneficial for human physiology and have been used in folk medicine since millennia [75]. They are currently being investigated for their anticancer activity [76–78].

The chemical structure of the compounds discussed herein is shown in Figures 3–5. A summary of the activities identified is given in Table 1. The most common outcome of exposure to a given nutrient is a loss of infectivity; this is measured by comparing the plaque-forming units (PFU) of a control and an exposed suspension (measured in mL) of phages. If the control and the exposed suspensions showed, for instance, 10^{10} and 10^9 PFU/mL, then the reduction is said to be one $\log_{10}$. Herein, we will report the results using this notation.

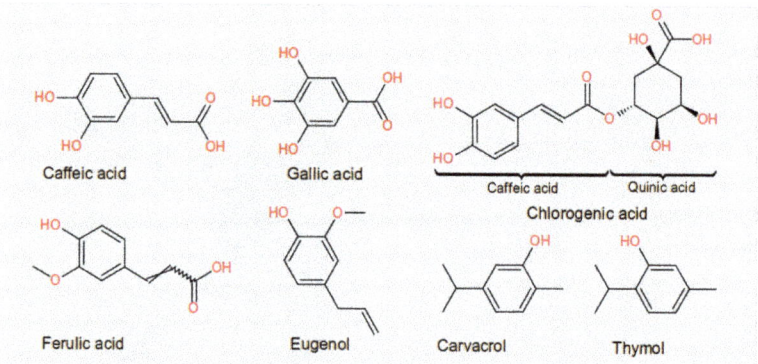

Figure 3. Chemical structures of the phenolic acids reported in the present review.

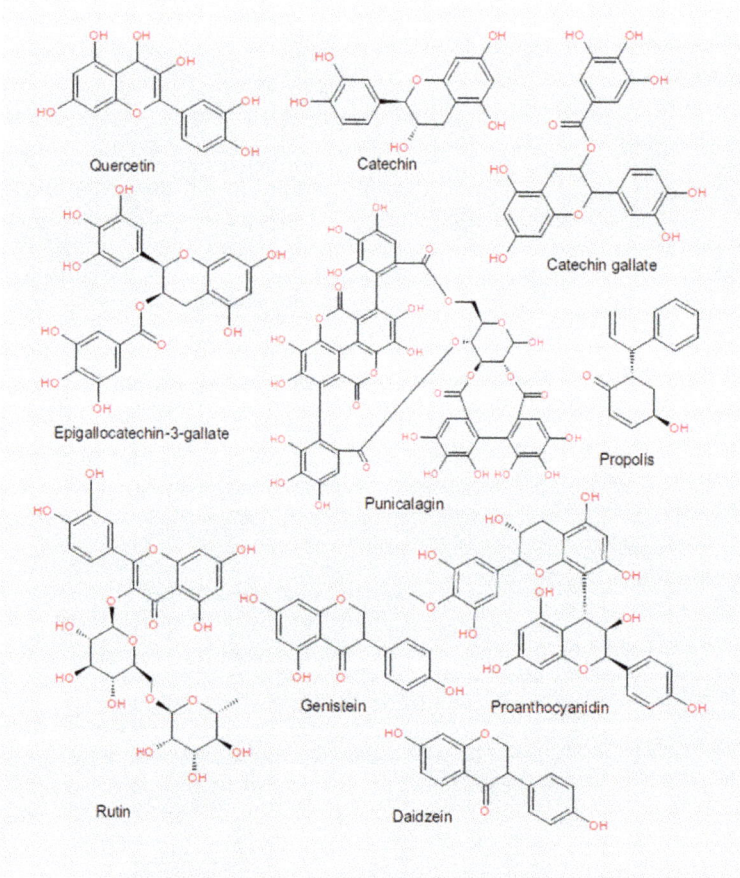

Figure 4. Chemical structures of the flavonoids reported in the present review.

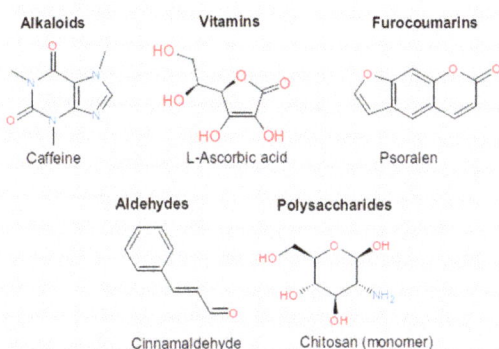

Figure 5. Chemical structures of the other active dietary compounds reported in the present review.

Table 1. Effect of the dietary compounds reported in the present review, stratified by chemical class and viral target. The principle of action is also reported, as far as known so far.

Nutrient	Class	Virus	Effect	Mechanism	References
Caffeic acid (or carbonyls)	Phenolic acids (or hydrocarbons)	λ	Prophage induction	Stress response to DNA damage	[79]
Gallic acid, chlorogenic acid	Phenolic acids	Av-5, MS2	Infectivity reduction	Inhibition of replication	[80]
		Av-5, MS2	Infectivity reduction	Inhibition of replication	[80]
Gallic acid	Phenolic acids	PL-1	Infectivity reduction	Interference to infection	[81]
		MS2	No effect	Unreported	[82]
Carvacrol, thymol	Phenolic acids	933 W	Prophage suppression	Unreported	[83]
Tea extracts	Phenolic acids or flavonoids	Felix 01 and P22	Infectivity reduction	Unreported	[84]
Pomegranate juice (punicalagin)	Phenolic acids or flavonoids	MS2	Infectivity reduction	Interference to infection (Capsid denaturation?)	[85]
Catechins	Flavonoids	T4	Infectivity reduction	Unreported	[86]
EGCG	Flavonoids	933 J	Prophage suppression	Repression of *recA*	[87]
GCG	Flavonoids	933 W	Prophage induction	Stress response to ROS	[88]
Genistein, daidzein	Flavonoids	φX174	Genome protection	Scavenging	[89]
Proanthocyanidin	Flavonoids	MS2, φX174	Infectivity reduction	Capsid denaturation	[90,91]
PJE	Flavonoids	MS2	Infectivity reduction	Capsid denaturation	[92]
GSE	Flavonoids	MS2	Infectivity reduction	Interference to infection (Capsid denaturation?)	[93]
		933 W	Prophage suppression	Unreported	[94]
		T2, T4	Infectivity reduction	Capsid denaturation	[95]
Cranberry juice	Flavonoids				
Propolis	Flavonoids	Unreported	Prophage induction or suppression	Unreported	[68]
Red propolis (formononetin)	Flavonoids	MS2, Av-08	Infectivity reduction	Interference to infection (Capsid denaturation?)	[96]
Cinnamaldehyde (cinnamon)	Essential oil (aldehydes)	933 W	Prophage suppression	Repression of *recA*	[94,97]
Oregano	Essential oil	Unreported	Prophage suppression	Unreported	[68]
Chamomile, lemongrass, cinnamon	Essential oils	T7, SA	Infectivity reduction	Unreported	[67]
Chitosan	Polysaccharide	MS2, φX174	Infectivity reduction	Capsid denaturation	[98]
		1–97 A	Infectivity reduction	Capsid denaturation	[99]
		c2	Infectivity reduction	Capsid denaturation	[100]
		933 W	Infectivity reduction	Unreported	[101]
Ascorbic acid	Vitamin	δA, φX174, T7, P22, D29, PM2, MS2	Infectivity reduction	Genome damage	[88,102–106]
Psoralen	Furocoumarins	MS2	Infectivity reduction	Unreported	[107]
Caffeine	Alkaloids	φX174	Prophage induction	Stress response to DNA damage	[108]
Sodium chloride	Salt	933 W	Prophage induction	Unreported	[109]

3.1. Phenolic Acids

Roasted coffee, but not freshly brewed coffee, has been shown to induce the prophage λ in *E. coli* [79]. However, the λ progeny suffered from aberrant replication, and most of the resulting virions were not infective [110]. Therefore, one hypothesis to explain this is that the compounds produced during the roasting process of coffee beans, such as aliphatic carbonyls or volatile substances [73], can cause DNA damage that, in turn, initiates a stress response and the consequent induction of λ prophages. The DNA damage also would explain why the viral progeny, whose genome is a linear double-stranded DNA (dsDNA) molecule, displays a reduced level of infectivity.

Potatoes are commonly used as food worldwide, particularly in the Western diet [111,112]. Potato peel extracts (PPE) contain a mixture of polyphenols (e.g., gallic acid, chlorogenic acid, caffeic acid, and ferulic acid) and flavonoids (such as quercetin and rutin). Exposure of the *E. coli* O157 phages MS2 and Av-05 to 5 mg/mL of PPE for three hours in vitro resulted in a 2.8 and 3.9 log10 reduction, respectively [113]. Hence, Av-05 was more susceptible than MS2 to PPE exposure. The inhibitory mechanism was probably due to interference with the replication stage. Also, tomatoes contain different polyphenols, mainly in leaves and stems. Although the exact composition of these polyphenols varies, gallic acid and chlorogenic acid belong to the most prevalent. Exposure to 5 mg/mL of tomato leaf extract (TLE) for 12 h reduced the infectivity of both MS2 and Av-05; the magnitude of the reduction depended on the tomato subspecies: the *Pitenza* cultivar reduced the infectivity of MS2 and Av-05 by 3.8 and 5 log10, respectively, compared to 0.57 and 1.6 log10 obtained with the *Floradade* cultivar [80]. Even in this case, the inhibitory mechanism was supposed to be linked to viral replication.

Caffeic acid could also inhibit the cytotoxicity of Stx in a Vero-d2EGFP cell-based assay, in a process independent from the alteration of the induction of 933J and 933W [114]. Gallic and caffeic acids at low concentration (around 10^{-6} mg/mL) and tannins (0.5 mg/mL) reduced the infectivity of PL-1 (infecting *L. casei*) by 80–90% [81]. Others reported that both tannic (0.01–0.1 mg/mL) and gallic (0.1–0.4 mg/mL) acids had negligible action upon the infectivity of MS2, with a reduction that reached a maximum of 0.06 $\log_{10}$ [82].

Zataria multiflora is an aromatic plant native from Iran and Afghanistan that is rich in the monoterpenoids carvacrol (or cymophenol) and thymol [115]. A 0.03% v/v of *Z. multiflora* extracts were bacteriostatic for *E. coli* O157, but sub-inhibitory concentrations reduced the induction of 933 W, measured by quantifying the expression of *Stx2* [83]. Several other compounds, including several derivatives of gallic acid, showed antiviral activity in vitro measured with the MTT method and estimated by the inhibition of viral cytopathic effects [116].

3.2. Flavonoids

Flavonoids also belong to the class of polyphenols. In natural sources, they are usually mixed with other phenolic acids; thus, it is difficult to separate the former's activity from that of the latter. Nevertheless, the active compound of cranberry juice is believed to be proanthocyanidin, a flavonoid [90]. In contrast, the active compounds of pomegranate juice extracts (PJE) were identified in punicalagin, a phenolic acid with antioxidant properties that could also inhibit the influenza virus [117,118]. Flavonoids are classified as antioxidants because they can react with, and remove from the cellular environment, the highly reactive superoxide anions (O_2^-) in a process known as scavenging [119]. Flavonoids include two products, catechin and genistein, with peculiar characteristics. Catechin is the basic block of tannins, found in fruit, tea, and wine; genistein is present in many medicinal plants.

Tea extracts were able to inactivate the *Salmonella* phages Felix 01 and P22, without affecting the growth of the bacterial host [84]. Exposure to 35 mg/mL of catechin for 24 h reduced the infectivity of the coliphage T4 by over two $\log_{10}$ in vitro, whereas the host did not show any reduction in population [86]. In addition, derivatives of catechins extracted from green tea could inhibit prophage induction. Epigallocatechin-3-gallate (EGCG) decreased the expression of *Stx1* but increased that of *Stx2* in *E. coli* O157 [87]. Since the expression of these two toxins is associated with the induction of 933 W in a germ-free mouse model [120], it needs to be assumed that, in this situation, EGCG is able to act as a virus inhibitor. The mechanism of action of EGCG involves the repression of the bacterial gene *recA* [87], an effector of the stress response that is central in the induction of 933 J, whereas the induction of 933 W relies on additional pathways not related to the expression of *recA*. This difference explains why only *Stx1* was reduced upon exposure to EGCG. This nutrient is believed to cause membrane damage that affects the growth of *E. coli* O157 and triggers stress response [87]. Other studies suggested that *Stx1* was still produced upon stimulation with EGCG and gallocatechin gallate (GCG), but the toxin's extracellular release from *E. coli* O157 cultured at 37 °C for 24 h was hampered, probably due to both the galloyl and the hydroxyl moieties of these compounds [121].

Tannic acid is known to have antioxidant properties, since it can bind and remove singlet oxygen ($^1O_2$) from the cellular environment [122]. A 0.3% w/v solution of persimmon, a tannin, could induce a 3.13 $\log_{10}$ reduction in the infectivity of MS2. Electron microscopy confirmed that such exposure caused capsid denaturation [123].

Genistein and daidzein extracted from soybeans could protect the genome of phage φX174 from degradation induced by nitric oxide (NO) or peroxynitrite (ONOO$^-$). Genistein was more effective than daidzein since a 25 µM solution of these dietary compounds protected about 75% and 45% of the viral φX174 DNA molecule confirmed by agarose gel electrophoresis, respectively [89]. This protection might be due to the scavenging properties of the flavonoids [124]. Genistein was also used to protect modified phages containing thymidine kinase derived from Herpes simplex virus during the delivery of this cytotoxin enzyme to tumor cells, thus increasing the targeted elimination of cancer cells [125].

Cranberries are fruits imported from North America and traditionally used by native Americans to treat bacterial infections. Investigations showed that cranberry juice could drastically reduce the growth of *E. coli* O157 in vitro [126]. Exposure for one hour to cranberry juice reduced the infectivity of the coliphages MS2 and φX174 by 1.67 and 1.22 $\log_{10}$, respectively, compared to the 0.05 and 0.29 $\log_{10}$ obtained by orange juice, 0.97 and 1.01 $\log_{10}$ obtained by grape juice, and 1.00 and 2.63 $\log_{10}$ obtained by purified proanthocyanidin [90,91]. Experiments with the coliphages T2 and T4 confirmed a complete and immediate loss of infectivity for these viruses when exposed to cranberry juice purchased from food shops [90,95]. Proanthocyanidin is also contained in blueberries; accordingly, exposure of MS2 to blueberry juice for 21 days induced a 6.32 $\log_{10}$ reduction in its infectivity when compared to incubation in phosphate buffered saline (PBS) [127].

In some studies, pomegranate and grape seed juices, which are rich in both flavonoids and phenolic acids, showed an antiviral activity. PJE at a 4 mg/mL concentration displayed a 0.12–0.32 $\log_{10}$ reduction upon MS2 infectivity in vitro [85,92]. This was in the same order of magnitude of other experiments carried out with pomegranate juice applied for 21 days, which showed a 0.14 $\log_{10}$ reduction in MS2 infectivity. Moreover, pomegranate juice diluted in PBS increased the inactivation to 1.84 $\log_{10}$ [127]. MS2 incubated in 1 mg/mL of grape seed extract (GSE) for two hours showed a 1.66 $\log_{10}$ reduction evaluated by plaque assay [93]. GSE also inhibited the growth of non-O157 *E. coli* serotypes, and GSE at a concentration of 4 mg/mL reduced the production of *Stx2* [83,94,128]. By comparison, pomegranate, grape, and orange juices showed lower, albeit still significant, reduction in phage infectivity in vitro [85,127]. In addition, grape seeds, which contain epicatechin, gallocatechin, GCG, and EGCG, could inactivate the cytotoxicity of Stx [114].

Su and colleagues suggested that cranberry juice in general, and proanthocyanidin in particular, inhibits the attachment phase of infecting phages in vitro, possibly via alterating the capsid [91]. This suggestion has been confirmed by electron microscopy analysis, which revealed that T4 treated with cranberry juice did not attach to their host [95]. Moreover, the feline calicivirus 9 showed structural modification of the capsid upon exposure to cranberry juice [91]. Likewise, apple juice, which is rich in procyanidins, increased the resistance of Vero cells against Stx [129].

Propolis ("bee glue", a mixture of the saliva of honey bees with beeswax and plant exudates) contains flavonoids [130]. As mentioned above, it has been shown to specifically induce prophages in *E. faecalis* but not *B. thetaiotamicron* and *S. aureus* [68]. Brazil is the major producer of propolis and this natural substance can be classified according to its color. Green propolis induced a 3.0 $\log_{10}$ reduction in the infectivity of MS2 and 3.5 log10 in Av-08; red propolis was even more effective in reducing PFU, with a 4.2 and 4.0 log10 reduction for MS2 and Av-08 [96]. The main active molecule of red propolis is formononetin and the suggested mechanism of inhibition was alteration of the structure of the capsid [131].

3.3. Saccharides

Chitosan is a family of polysaccharides present in the exoskeleton of crustaceans and insects as well as in the cell wall of fungi. The members of this family are classified according to their molecular weight [132]. A 0.7% w/v solution of chitosan applied for three hours could decrease the infectivity of MS2 by up to 2.80 $\log_{10}$ (when using a molecule with a molecular mass of 53 kDa) and 5.16 $\log_{10}$ (when using 222 kDa). By increasing the concentration to 1%, only the 222 kDa form could completely inhibit MS2 [98,133,134]. Higher concentrations of both forms (1.5% w/v) were needed to achieve the inactivation of φX174, albeit the magnitude was much smaller than that of MS2 (0.94 $\log_{10}$). Chitosan was also active against *Bacillus thuringiensis* phage 1–97 A [99] and *Lactococcus lactis* phage c2 in vitro [100]. Furthermore, in vivo experiments with mice showed that chitosan was able to reduce Stx expression and the diffusion of induced 933 W progeny into the tissues, and to improve the lifespan of mice infected with enterohemorrhagic *E. coli* [101]. The mechanism of action was hypothesized to be a structural modification of the capsid [134–136]. Moreover, mutagenic effects of a sucrose-rich diet were reported by Dragsted et al. when investigating the colon of Big Blue rats, a specific strain of Fischer rats that carries 40 copies of the lambda phage on chromosome 4. In this study, a sucrose-rich diet resulted in an increase of mutational frequency in the DNA of these colons [137]. Lysozyme, which is widely distributed among prokaryotes and eukaryotes, is expressed by the R gene of phage lambda. Accordingly, the latter is called bacteriophage lambda lysozyme (LaL), and it has been shown to have bacteriolytic capabilities [138]. In contrast to other lysozymes, however, LaL differs regarding the cleavage of the glycosidic bond between N-acetylmuramic acid and N-acetylglucosamine of bacterial peptidoglycan. Duewel and colleagues showed that high concentrations of β(1→4) N-acetyl-D-glucosamine oligomers inhibit LaL but are not cleaved by the enzyme [138]. A similar observation of degrading peptidoglycans into fragments has also been reported for lysates of phage Vi II [139].

3.4. Essential Oils and Vitamins

Several essential oils show antibacterial and antioxidant activity, together with antiviral function [140]. For instance, oregano, thyme, cinnamon, and allspice (a berry from *Pimenta dioica* used commonly in the food industry) extracts, amongst others, can reduce the growth of *E. coli* O157 [141,142]. A 4% v/v solution of cinnamon oil, whose main component is cinnamaldehyde, inhibited the growth of *E. coli* O157 in vitro, but sub-inhibitory doses reduced the expression of *Stx2* and the release of viral progeny [72,94]. As in the case of EGCG, the interference over phage induction was accompanied by down-regulation of the effector of the stress pathway *recA*, but also of the quorum sensing (QS) (*qseB, qseC,* and *luxS*) and oxydative stress (*oxyR, soxR,* and *rpoS*) pathways, as well as the polynucleotide phosphorylase PAP I [94], which is also an inducer of 933 W [143]. These results suggest that cinnamon oil could interfere with 933 W induction as several overlapping levels. Furthermore, cinnamon oil disrupted *E. coli* O156 and *Pseudomonas aeruginosa* biofilms by interfering with the formation of the fimbriae, which are required to make inter-bacterial connections [72,94]. Oregano had a general suppressive action upon prophages, but the effect was stronger in *S. aureus* than in *E. faecalis* or *B. thetaiotamicron* [68]. Eugenol, which is rich in allspice and clove, reduced the induction of both Stx1 and Stx2, and inhibit the growth of *E. coli* O157 in vitro [144].

After a lag phase of few minutes, ascorbic acid (also known as vitamin C), reduced the infectivity of several phages: δA and φX174 (with a genome of ssDNA); T7, P22, D29, and PM2 (dsDNA); and MS2 (ssRNA) in vitro [88,102–106]. Supplementation of ascorbic acid with oxidants such as oxygen and hydrogen peroxide enhanced this effect, whereas antioxidants (for instance thiol compounds), nitrogen gas bubbling, or chelating agents suppressed it [102]. It was postulated that the autoxidation of ascorbic acid produced hydrogen peroxide that damaged the genome of the phages, even though Murata and colleagues found that hydrogen peroxide produced by autoxidation of ascorbic acid did not exert effects on activity of phage δA, in contrast to free radical intermediates [145]. Thus, the scavenging activity provided by thiols and chelating agents was hypothesized to reduce the damage on the viral genome, and the initial delay in the activity of ascorbic acid was interpreted as the time required to internalize this hydrogen peroxide inside the capsid [102]. Subsequent in vitro studies confirmed this hypothesis and showed that ascorbic acid caused the accumulation of nicks in both DNA and RNA genomes, with double-stranded genomes being less affected than single-stranded ones [88,103]. In these studies, the overlap of the nicks determined the formation of double strands breaks, which in fact sometimes appeared after the nicks as a result of the stochastic overlapping of the single-stranded lesions. Furthermore, these damages could be restored by the host's cellular DNA repair system [88].

The oxidized form of vitamin C, dehydroascorbic acid, showed only very limited effects on phage activity and the amount of strand cleavages in ssDNA from phage δA was proportional to ascorbic acid concentration and incubation time. It was significantly increased by Cu2+ or hydrogen peroxide [102,146]. These DNA-damaging properties of the strong reducing combination of ascorbic acid with metal ions (especially Cu^{2+}) [103] can have an impact on the phage population in the intestinal microbiome, but could also have implications in other fields such as the application of high-dose ascorbate in tumor patients. Towards this end, tumor entities like non-small-cell lung cancer and glioblastoma seem to be vulnerable towards the disruption of their intracellular iron metabolism and oxidative damage caused by the formation of hydrogen peroxide and hydroxyl radicals [147].

3.5. Other Compounds

There are very few studies investigating the impact on phages of molecules other than those listed so far. Pioneering work in the late 1950 s demonstrated how hydroquinone and pyrogallol (both derivatives of phenol but not polyphenols) reduced the infectivity of T coliphages [148]. Psoralens belong to the family of furocoumarins, photoactive polyphenols that can induce DNA damage. They are particularly abundant in the peel of limes [149]. Accordingly, a six-hour exposure with lime juice in vitro reduced the infectivity of MS2 by 1.3 $\log_{10}$ even in the absence of photoactivation [107].

Coffee contains not only caffeic acid but also caffeine, an alkaloid; coffee is a beverage on its own and the base for a plethora of soft-drinks [150]. High consumption of coffee and its derivatives has been suggested to confer an increased risk of colorectal cancer, due to its antimicrobial activity that disrupts the intestinal homeostasis [151]. Caffeine is able to induce *E. coli* phage φX174 in mitomycin treated *E. coli* cells [108]. Since caffeine is known to distort DNA and cause mutations [152], its activity is supposedly similar to caffeic acid in terms of inducing a stress signal that starts the lytic process.

Finally, even common salt used for meat preservation has been reported to exert effects on phage biology. Towards this end, a 2% w/v concentration of sodium chloride increased the expression of *Stx2*, as measured by immunoblotting, and the activation of the 933 W, as measured by plaque assay, in *E. coli* O157 [109].

3.6. In Vivo Studies

In contrast to a steadily increasing body of in vitro data that evaluates the interplay of diet or certain nutrients with bacteriophages as discussed in the chapters above, there are still only a few in vivo studies available. However, the possibility to modulate the microbiome by phage application is currently starting to attract more and more attention, especially in the field of inflammatory and malignant diseases. For instance, Zheng and colleagues covalently linked irinotecan-loaded dextran nanoparticles to azide-modified phages that were able to inhibit the growth of *Fusobacterium nucleatum* [153]. After i.v. or oral administration, these phage-guided irinotecan-loaded nanoparticles increased the chemotherapeutic efficacy in mice with colorectal tumors. In another study, a single injection of a lytic bacteriophage cocktail was effective as a rescue treatment for murine severe septic peritonitis, resulting in a significant improvement of the disease state without harming the microbiome [154]. Wild-type phage T4 and the according substrain HAP1, which is characterized by enhanced affinity to melanoma cells, were able to reduce lung metastasis of murine B16 melanoma cells by 47% and 80%, respectively [28]. Moreover, the modulation of the intestinal microbiome and metabolome was investigated using cognate lytic phages in gnotobiotic mice that were colonized with defined human gut commensal bacteria. This approach directly impacted susceptible bacteria, but phage predation also regulated additional bacteria via interbacterial interactions, yielding strong cascading net effects on the gut metabolome [58]. In a gnotobiotic pig model, it was shown that bacteria species are able to affect intestinal morphology as well as the expression of proinflammatory cytokines such as IL-1β and IL-6. Therefore, it can be hypothesized that a modulation of, e.g., neonatal bacterial colonization would have strong implications for a healthy development of the intestine [4]. On the other hand, intestinal inflammation and ulcerative colitis can be aggravated by high levels of certain bacteriophages that induce interferon-γ release [17]. Different phage cocktails (ShigActive™ [155] and ListShield [156]) have been shown to reduce shigella colonization of the murine gut and to decrease *Listeria monocytogenes* in the gastrointestinal tract, respectively. ShigActive™ was found to have comparable therapeutic effects to ampicillin but without the harmful effects on the gut microbiota exerted by the antibiotic [155]. ListShield was applied via oral gavage before mice were orally infected with *Listeria monocytogenes*. Consequently, *Listeria monocytogenes* concentrations were found to be reduced in the liver, spleen, and intestines when compared to controls. Even though, this phage therapy was as effective as the treatment with an antibiotic, it did not result in weight loss of the animals in contrast to infected controls and antibiotic-treated mice [156]. In another study, mice with antibiotic-induced perturbed microbiomes were treated with autochthonous virome transfer and viable phages were effective in reshaping the murine gut microbiota in a way that closely resembled the pre-antibiotic situation [157]. In vivo targeting of specific bacterial pathogens with recombinant or wildtype phages was also investigated for *Clostridium difficile* infections [158], Vancomycin-resistant *Enterococcus faecalis* infections [159], Crohn's disease [160] and even for the attenuation of alcoholic liver disease [161]. The human Bacteriophage for Gastrointestinal Health (PHAGE) study and PHAGE-2 study demonstrated that an application of therapeutic doses of bacteriophages was both safe and tolerable [162–164]. The double-blinded, placebo-controlled crossover PHAGE trial with adults consuming bacteriophages for 28 days (32/43 participants finished the study) also demonstrated that bacteriophages are able to selectively decrease the amount of target organisms, without disrupting the gut microbiome globally [162]. In the randomized, parallel-arm, double-blinded, placebo-controlled PHAGE-2 study (68 participants, four weeks), it could be shown that adding supplemental bacteriophages (PreforPro) to the probiotic *Bifidobacterium animalis* subsp. *lactis* enhanced positive effects on gastrointestinal health [164]. Taken together, there is increasing evidence, in initial in vivo studies, for the high potential of treating different diseases with bacteriophages and for the ability to reshape the gut microbiome via tailored phage cocktails. Still, however, more in vivo studies are needed that investigate the complex interplay between diet and bacteriophages, especially in the context of the prevention and treatment of inflammatory diseases and cancer.

4. Conclusions

In conclusion, the present review shows that many dietary compounds and food ingredients display significant bioactivity with documented effects on phages. The dietary compounds discussed in this review can be consumed directly by diet (as in tea or coffee) or indirectly as food supplements. Still, most of the data reviewed and discussed herein pertain to *E. coli* as the, so far, best studied phage target in humans. Although being a common gut commensal, certain serotypes of this species pose a threat to public health regarding severe infectious and (in part systemic) inflammatory conditions as discussed in the Introduction. A few reports up to now even hypothesized particular *E. coli* strains such as those producing the genotoxin colibactin as potential tumor promoters [165], although their data were restricted to experimental models so far. In own genome data, we have preliminary evidence of sequences of particular *E. coli* strains in human colorectal carcinomas and even metastases (unpublished data based on genomes published in [166]).

The main activity of the dietary compounds discussed in the present review includes inhibitory effects on phages due to the alteration of the capsid, with subsequent reduction of infectivity. In other cases, the viral genome is being damaged, again inhibiting the infectivity of phages. However, some dietary compounds are able to induce (as with common salt or gallocatechin gallate) or repress (as with carvacrol) prophages. More importantly, a few dietary compounds display species-specific activities. For instance, stevia apparently acts as an inducer for *S. aureus* prophages, but not of those present in *E. faecalis*, whereas propolis displays the opposite actions.

Overall, most of the dietary compounds reviewed here, with documented actions towards phages, showed a beneficial effect for the host by interfering with the activity of the pathogens at several levels. Thus, a number of concluding scenaria can be summarized for the putative benefit of nutrients (including the modulation of phages) to human patients and their microbiota (Figure 6A): Several nutritional compounds can directly affect the growth of microbial pathogens, but not that of commensals. Also, dietary compounds are able to inactivate particular toxins produced by pathogens, thus reducing fitness of the latter. More importantly, dietary compounds can inactivate virulent phages, modifying the overall equilibrium of the intestinal microbiome. As a result, phages targeting a commensal species that is a competitor to a pathogen can be removed from the niche. The commensal species will then expand and compete with the pathogen, again reducing the latter's fitness. Finally, dietary compounds might induce prophages present in the pathogen, determining the hosts' lysis and a wave of active virulent phages, which in turn reduce the pathogen's population. Combining all of these inhibitory outcomes will reduce the pathogenicity of invading species and for example, help resolve infections or (chronic) inflammatory conditions.

To better understand how dietary compounds could selectively modulate bacterial infections, we carried out a simulation model (Figure 6b). This model shows that a pathogenic bacterium can wipe out a commensal species, but the selective induction of a prophage can then control the growth of the pathogen, reducing the virulence of the infecting species. The model suggests that it could be possible, in principle, to reorganize the microbial network to fight infections and further disease. Experimental data is required to assess the specificity of particular dietary compounds' action to, effectively and safely, direct such attempts of specific reorganization.

Similar considerations as for phage-directed attempts to counteract infections and inflammatory conditions could be speculated for the field of carcinogenesis and cancer. Interfering with particular commensals within the intestinal microbiome by phages of different activities and properties, with the result of changing the intestinal microenvironment towards a more pro- or anti-carcinogenic condition, could be an exciting novel field of colorectal and other intestinal cancer research, and of treatment development. In parallel, more specific research on particular dietary compounds, chemical components, and associated modulation of phages that exert controllable, specific effects on the microbiome could open exciting new possibilities to interfere with intra-intestinal conditions in ways to foster anti-carcinogenic, more cancer-preventive environments.

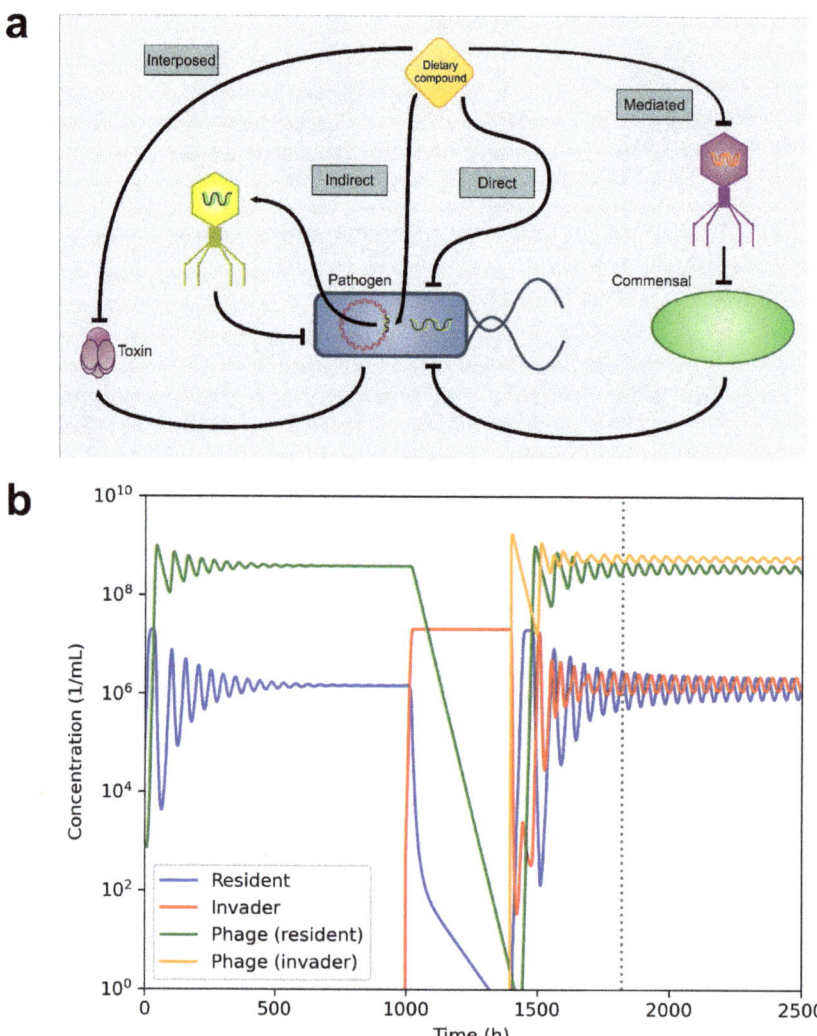

Figure 6. Overall impact of dietary compounds on infections. Dietary compounds can modify the bacterial population indirectly, based on the interaction between phages and bacteria, and by bacterial competition. (**a**) A dietary compound (nutrient) can interfere with the activity of a pathogenic bacterium at different levels by: inactivating a bacterial toxin (interposed inhibition); inducing a prophage already present in the invading bacterium, which then lyses the pathogen (indirect inhibition); acting bactericidal on invading species (direct inhibition); inactivating a lytic phage of an antagonist commensal species that, freed from the phagial burden, can compete with the pathogen (mediated inhibition). (**b**) Simulation of the interaction between bacteria and phages. The model considers the presence of a commensal bacterium (resident) and its phage. These reach an equilibrium where the number of cells or phages remains constant. A pathogenic bacterium (invader) will have virulence factors that favor its replication. As a result, it overgrows the commensal species. The activation of phages, namely through dietary-mediated induction of prophages, reduces the replication rate of the invader and re-establish, as a result, the commensal population. For the simulation, the parameters used were as follows. Carrying capacity: 2.2×10^7. Maximum growth rate, 0.47 (commensal), and 0.72 (invader). Phage adsorption rate: 10^{-9}, Phage lyse rate: 1.0. Phage burst size: 50. Particle loss rate: 0.05. Initial population of commensal bacteria: 50 000 cells. Amount of invader bacteria inoculated: 500 cells. Amount of phages: 1000 particles each. The model was implemented in *Julia* language using the *DifferentialEquations* package.

Author Contributions: L.M., S.V., and H.A. conceptualized this interdisciplinary review. H.A. conceptualized the idea of linking phages, and their contributions to the microbiome and microenvironment, to cancer, carcinogenesis, progression, and metastasis. L.M. did the statistical analyses and carried out the literature research. L.M. and M.B. designed the figures. All of the authors (L.M., M.B., S.V., and H.A.) wrote and carefully revised the manuscript. All authors have read and agreed to the published version of the manuscript.

Funding: H.A. was supported by the Alfried Krupp von Bohlen und Halbach Foundation, Essen; the Deutsche Krebshilfe, Bonn (70112168); the Deutsche Forschungsgemeinschaft (DFG, grant number AL 465/9-1); the HEiKA Initiative (Karlsruhe Institute of Technology/University of Heidelberg collaborative effort); the DKFZ-MOST Cooperation, Heidelberg (grant number CA149); the HIPO/POP-Initiative for Personalized Oncology, Heidelberg (H032 and H027). S.V. and M.B. were supported by a grant from the Else-Uebelmesser-Stiftung (grant no. D.30.21947) and PASCOE Pharmazeutische Praeparate GmbH. We further acknowledge support by Open Access Publishing Fund of University of Tuebingen.

Institutional Review Board Statement: Not applicable.

Informed Consent Statement: Not applicable.

Acknowledgments: We would like to thank Maurizio Grilli, Library of the Medical Faculty Mannheim, Ruprecht Karls University of Heidelberg, Germany, for his support in the literature search of this review. A special thanks goes to Ingo Plag, Institute for English Language and Linguistics of the University of Düsseldorf, for his advice on the adjective 'phagial', which is still not officially recognized.

Conflicts of Interest: The authors declare no conflict of interest.

References

1. Qin, J.; Li, R.; Raes, J.; Arumugam, M.; Burgdorf, K.S.; Manichanh, C.; Nielsen, T.; Pons, N.; Levenez, F.; Yamada, T.; et al. A human gut microbial gene catalogue established by metagenomic sequencing. *Nature* **2010**, *464*, 59–65. [CrossRef] [PubMed]
2. Ramakrishnan, R.; Donahue, H.; Garcia, D.; Tan, J.; Shimizu, N.; Rice, A.P.; Ling, P.D. Epstein-barr virus BART9 miRNA modulates LMP1 levels and affects growth rate of nasal NK T cell lymphomas. *PLoS ONE* **2011**, *6*, e27271. [CrossRef] [PubMed]
3. Bultman, S.J. Interplay between diet, gut microbiota, epigenetic events, and colorectal cancer. *Mol. Nutr. Food Res.* **2017**, *61*, 1500902. [CrossRef] [PubMed]
4. Shirkey, T.W.; Siggers, R.H.; Goldade, B.G.; Marshall, J.K.; Drew, M.D.; Laarveld, B.; Kessel, A.G.V. Effects of commensal bacteria on intestinal morphology and expression of proinflammatory cytokines in the gnotobiotic pig. *Exp. Biol. Med.* **2006**, *231*, 1333–1345. [CrossRef]
5. Pull, S.L.; Doherty, J.M.; Mills, J.C.; Gordon, J.I.; Stappenbeck, T.S. Activated macrophages are an adaptive element of the colonic epithelial progenitor niche necessary for regenerative responses to injury. *Proc. Natl. Acad. Sci. USA* **2005**, *102*, 99–104. [CrossRef]
6. Ukena, S.N.; Singh, A.; Dringenberg, U.; Engelhardt, R.; Seidler, U.; Hansen, W.; Bleich, A.; Bruder, D.; Franzke, A.; Rogler, G.; et al. Probiotic escherichia coli Nissle 1917 inhibits leaky gut by enhancing mucosal integrity. *PLoS ONE* **2007**, *2*, e1308. [CrossRef]
7. Mennigen, R.; Nolte, K.; Rijcken, E.; Utech, M.; Loeffler, B.; Senninger, N.; Bruewer, M. Probiotic mixture VSL # 3 protects the epithelial barrier by maintaining tight junction protein expression and preventing apoptosis in a murine model of colitis. *Am. J. Physiol.* **2009**, *296*, 1140–1149.
8. Kelly, D.; Campbell, J.I.; King, T.P.; Grant, G.; Jansson, E.A.; Coutts, A.G.P.; Pettersson, S.; Conway, S. Commensal anaerobic gut bacteria attenuate inflammation by regulating nuclear-cytoplasmic shutting of PPAR and RelA. *Nat. Immunol.* **2004**, *5*, 104–112. [CrossRef]
9. Rakoff-Nahoum, S.; Paglino, J.; Eslami-Varzaneh, F.; Edberg, S.; Medzhitov, R. Recognition of commensal microflora by toll-like receptors is required for intestinal homeostasis. *Cell* **2004**, *118*, 229–241. [CrossRef] [PubMed]
10. Fukuda, S.; Toh, H.; Hase, K.; Oshima, K.; Nakanishi, Y.; Yoshimura, K.; Tobe, T.; Clarke, J.M.; Topping, D.L.; Suzuki, T.; et al. Bifidobacteria can protect from enteropathogenic infection through production of acetate. *Nature* **2011**, *469*, 543–549. [CrossRef] [PubMed]
11. Viaud, S.; Saccheri, F.; Mignot, G.; Yamazaki, T.; Daillre, R.; Hannani, D.; Enot, D.P.; Pfirschke, C.; Engblom, C.; Pittet, M.J.; et al. The intestinal microbiota modulates the anticancer immune effects of cyclophosphamide. *Science* **2013**, *342*, 971–976. [CrossRef]
12. Xu, J.; Gordon, J.I. Honor thy symbionts. *Proc. Natl. Acad. Sci. USA* **2003**, *100*, 10452–10459. [CrossRef]
13. Maruvada, P.; Leone, V.; Kaplan, L.M.; Chang, E.B. The Human microbiome and obesity: Moving beyond associations. *Cell Host Microbe* **2017**, *22*, 589–599. [CrossRef]
14. Beller, L.; Matthijnssens, J. What is (not) known about the dynamics of the human gut virome in health and disease. *Curr. Opin. Virol.* **2019**, *37*, 52–57. [CrossRef]
15. Sutton, T.D.S.; Hill, C. Gut bacteriophage: Current understanding and challenges. *Front. Endocrinol.* **2019**, *10*, 784. [CrossRef]

16. Nguyen, S.; Baker, K.; Padman, B.S.; Patwa, R.; Dunstan, R.A.; Weston, T.A.; Schlosser, K.; Bailey, B.; Lithgow, T.; Lazarou, M.; et al. Bacteriophage transcytosis provides a mechanism to cross epithelial cell layers. *mBio* **2017**, *8*. [CrossRef]
17. Gogokhia, L.; Buhrke, K.; Bell, R.; Hoffman, B.; Brown, D.G.; Hanke-Gogokhia, C.; Ajami, N.J.; Wong, M.C.; Ghazaryan, A.; Valentine, J.F.; et al. Expansion of bacteriophages is linked to aggravated intestinal inflammation and colitis. *Cell Host Microbe* **2019**, *25*, 285–299. [CrossRef] [PubMed]
18. Tetz, G.; Tetz, V. Bacteriophages as new human viral pathogens. *Microorganisms* **2018**, *6*, 54. [CrossRef] [PubMed]
19. Levin, B.R.; Stewart, F.M.; Chao, L. Resource-limited growth, competition, and predation: A model and experimental studies with bacteria and bacteriophage. *Math. Biosci.* **1977**, *111*, 3–24. [CrossRef]
20. Abedon, S.T.; Kuhl, S.J.; Blasdel, B.G.; Kutter, E.M. Phage treatment of human infections. *Bacteriophage* **2011**, *1*, 66–85. [CrossRef]
21. Barr, J.J.; Auro, R.; Furlan, M.; Whiteson, K.L.; Erb, M.L.; Pogliano, J.; Stotland, A.; Wolkowicz, R.; Cutting, A.S.; Doran, K.S.; et al. Bacteriophage adhering to mucus provide a non-host-derived immunity. *Proc. Natl. Acad. Sci. USA* **2013**, *110*, 10771–10776. [CrossRef]
22. Viertel, T.M.; Ritter, K.; Horz, H.-P. Viruses versus bacteria-novel approaches to phage therapy as a tool against multidrug-resistant pathogens. *J. Antimicrob. Chemother.* **2014**, *69*, 2326–2336. [CrossRef] [PubMed]
23. Shlezinger, M.; Khalifa, L.; Houri-Haddad, Y.; Coppenhagen-Glazer, S.; Resch, G.; Que, Y.-A.; Beyth, S.; Dorfman, E.; Hazan, R.; Beyth, N. Phage therapy: A new horizon in the antibacterial treatment of oral pathogens. *Curr. Top. Med. Chem.* **2017**, *17*, 1199–1211. [CrossRef] [PubMed]
24. Wernicki, A.; Nowaczek, A.; Urban-Chmiel, R. Bacteriophage therapy to combat bacterial infections in poultry. *Virol. J.* **2017**, *14*, 179. [CrossRef] [PubMed]
25. Chang, R.Y.K.; Wallin, M.; Lin, Y.; Leung, S.S.Y.; Wang, H.; Morales, S.; Chan, H.K. Phage therapy for respiratory infections. *Adv. Drug Deliv. Rev.* **2018**, *133*, 76–86. [CrossRef] [PubMed]
26. Gorski, A.; Midzybrodzki, R.; aczek, M.; Borysowski, J. Phages in the fight against COVID-19? *Future Microbiol.* **2020**, *15*, 1095–1100. [CrossRef]
27. Dabrowska, K.; Opolski, A.; Wietrzyk, J.; Gorski, A. Anticancer activity of bacteriophage T4 and its mutant HAP1 in mouse experimental tumour models. *Anticancer Res.* **2004**, *24*, 3991–3995.
28. Dabrowska, K.; Opolski, A.; Wietrzyk, J.; Switala-Jelen, K.; Boratynski, J.; Nasulewicz, A.; Lipinska, L.; Chybicka, A.; Kujawa, M.; Zabel, M.; et al. Antitumor activity of bacteriophages in murine experimental cancer models caused possibly by inhibition of beta3 integrin signaling pathway. *Acta Virol.* **2004**, *48*, 241–248.
29. Voreades, N.; Kozil, A.; Weir, T.L. Diet and the development of the human intestinal microbiome. *Front. Microbiol.* **2014**, *5*, 494. [CrossRef]
30. Leupold, J.H.; Yang, H.-S.; Colburn, N.H.; Asangani, I.; Post, S.; Allgayer, H. Tumor suppressor Pdcd4 inhibits invasion/intravasation and regulates urokinase receptor (u-PAR) gene expression via Sp-transcription factors. *Oncogene* **2007**, *26*, 4550–4562. [CrossRef]
31. Asangani, I.A.; Rasheed, S.A.K.; Nikolova, D.A.; Leupold, J.H.; Colburn, N.H.; Post, S.; Allgayer, H. MicroRNA-21 (miR-21) post-transcriptionally downregulates tumor suppressor Pdcd4 and stimulates invasion, intravasation and metastasis in colorectal cancer. *Oncogene* **2008**, *27*, 2128–2136. [CrossRef]
32. Rasheed, S.A.K.; Efferth, T.; Asangani, I.A.; Allgayer, H. First evidence that the antimalarial drug artesunate inhibits invasion and in vivo metastasis in lung cancer by targeting essential extracellular proteases. *Int. J. Cancer* **2010**, *127*, 1475–1485. [CrossRef]
33. Mudduluru, G.; George-William, J.N.; Muppala, S.; Asangani, I.A.; Kumarswamy, R.; Nelson, L.D.; Allgayer, H. Curcumin regulates miR-21 expression and inhibits invasion and metastasis in colorectal cancer. *Biosci. Rep.* **2011**, *31*, 185–197. [CrossRef] [PubMed]
34. Fischer, G.; Gardell, S.; Jorpes, E. On the chemical nature of acerin and the virucidal and antiviral effects of some vegetable tannins. *Experientia* **1954**, *10*, 329–330. [CrossRef] [PubMed]
35. Martinek, R.G.; Wolman, W. Xanthines, tannins, and sodium in coffee, tea, and cocoa. *J. Am. Med. Assoc.* **1955**, *158*, 1031–1051. [PubMed]
36. Friedman, M. Overview of antibacterial, antitoxin, antiviral, and antifungal activities of tea flavonoids and teas. *Mol. Nutr. Food Res.* **2007**, *51*, 116–134. [CrossRef]
37. Kon, K.V.; Rai, M.K. Plant essential oils and their constituents in coping with multidrug-resistant bacteria. *Expert Rev. Anti-Infect. Ther.* **2012**, *10*, 775–790. [CrossRef]
38. Tarr, P.I. *Escherichia coli* O157:H7: Overview of clinical and epidemiological issues. *J. Food Prot.* **1994**, *57*, 632–636. [CrossRef] [PubMed]
39. Su, C.; Brandt, L.J. *Escherichia coli* O157:H7 infection in humans. *Ann. Intern. Med.* **1995**, *123*, 698–714. [CrossRef]
40. Johnson, K.E.; Thorpe, C.M.; Sears, C.L. The emerging clinical importance of non-O157 Shiga toxin-producing *Escherichia coli*. *Clin. Infect. Dis.* **2006**, *43*, 1587–1595.
41. O'Brien, A.D.; Newland, J.W.; Miller, S.F.; Holmes, R.K.; Smith, H.W.; Formal, S.B. Shiga-like toxin-converting phages from *Escherichia coli* strains that cause hemorrhagic colitis or infantile diarrhea. *Science* **1984**, *226*, 694–696. [CrossRef] [PubMed]
42. Strockbine, N.A.; Marques, L.R.M.; Newland, J.W.; Smith, H.W.; Holmes, R.K.; O'Brien, A.D. Two toxin-converting phages from *Escherichia coli* O157:H7 strain 933 encode antigenically distinct toxins with similar biologic activities. *Infect. Immun.* **1986**, *53*, 135–140. [CrossRef]

43. Johansen, B.K.; Wasteson, Y.; Granum, P.E.; Brynestad, S. Mosaic structure of Shiga-toxin-2-encoding phages isolated from *Escherichia coli* O157:H7 indicates frequent gene exchange between lambdoid phage genomes. *Microbiology* **2001**, *147*, 1929–1936. [CrossRef] [PubMed]
44. Canchaya, C.; Fournous, G.; Chibani-Chennoufi, S.; Dillmann, M.L.; Brssow, H. Phage as agents of lateral gene transfer. *Curr. Opin. Microbiol.* **2003**, *6*, 417–424. [CrossRef]
45. Taieb, F.; Petit, C.; Nougayrde, J.-P.; Oswald, E. The enterobacterial genotoxins: Cytolethal distending toxin and colibactin. *EcoSal Plus* **2016**, *7*. [CrossRef]
46. Friedman, M.; Rasooly, R. Review of the inhibition of biological activities of food-related selected toxins by natural compounds. *Toxins* **2013**, *5*, 743–775. [CrossRef]
47. Oi, H.; Matsuura, D.; Miyake, M.; Ueno, M.; Takai, I.; Yamamoto, T.; Kubo, M.; Moss, J.; Noda, M. Identification in traditional herbal medications and confirmation by synthesis of factors that inhibit cholera toxin-induced fluid accumulation. *Proc. Natl. Acad. Sci. USA* **2002**, *99*, 3042–3046. [CrossRef] [PubMed]
48. Saito, T.; Miyake, M.; Toba, M.; Okamatsu, H.; Shimizu, S.; Noda, M. Inhibition by apple polyphenols of ADP-ribosyltransferase activity of cholera toxin and toxin-induced fluid accumulation in mice. *Microbiol. Immunol.* **2002**, *46*, 249–255. [CrossRef]
49. Morinaga, N.; Iwamaru, Y.; Yahiro, K.; Tagashira, M.; Moss, J.; Noda, M. Differential activities of plant polyphenols on the binding and internalization of cholera toxin in vero cells. *J. Biol. Chem.* **2005**, *280*, 23303–23309. [CrossRef] [PubMed]
50. Becker, P.M.; van der Meulen, J.; Jansman, A.J.M.; van Wikselaar, P.G. In vitro inhibition of ETEC K88 adhesion by pea hulls and of LT enterotoxin binding by faba bean hulls. *J. Anim. Physiol. Anim. Nutr.* **2012**, *96*, 1121–1126. [CrossRef]
51. D'Herelle, F. On an invisible microbe antagonistic toward dysenteric bacilli: Brief note by Mr. F. D'Herelle, presented by Mr. Roux. *Res. Microbiol.* **2007**, *158*, 553–554.
52. Chanishvili, N. Phage therapy-history from twort and d'herelle through soviet experience to current approaches. *Adv. Vir. Res.* **2012**, *83*, 3–40.
53. Salmond, G.P.C.; Fineran, P.C. A century of the phage: Past, present and future. *Nat. Rev. Microbiol.* **2015**, *13*, 777–786. [CrossRef] [PubMed]
54. Davies, E.V.; Winstanley, C.; Fothergill, J.L.; James, C.E. The role of temperate bacteriophages in bacterial infection. *FEMS Microbiol. Lett.* **2016**, *363*, 15. [CrossRef] [PubMed]
55. Erez, Z.; Steinberger-Levy, I.; Shamir, M.; Doron, S.; Stokar-Avihail, A.; Peleg, Y.; Melamed, S.; Leavitt, A.; Savidor, A.; Albeck, S.; et al. Communication between viruses guides lysis-lysogeny decisions. *Nature* **2017**, *541*, 488–493. [CrossRef]
56. Sharma, A.K.; Dhasmana, N.; Dubey, N.; Kumar, N.; Gangwal, A.; Gupta, M.; Singh, Y. Bacterial virulence factors: Secreted for survival. *Indian J. Microbiol.* **2017**, *57*, 1–10. [CrossRef] [PubMed]
57. Mogna, L.; Del Piano, M.; Deidda, F.; Nicola, S.; Soattini, L.; Debiaggi, R.; Sforza, F.; Strozzi, F.; Mogna, G. Assessment of the in vitro inhibitory activity of specific probiotic bacteria against different Escherichia coli strains. *J. Clin. Gastroenterol.* **2012**, *46*, S29–S32. [CrossRef]
58. Hsu, B.B.; Gibson, T.E.; Yeliseyev, V.; Liu, Q.; Lyon, L.; Bry, L.; Silver, P.A.; Gerber, G.K. Dynamic modulation of the gut microbiota and metabolome by bacteriophages in a mouse model. *Cell Host Microbe* **2019**, *25*, 803–814. [CrossRef] [PubMed]
59. Kakisu, E.; Abraham, A.G.; Farinati, C.T.; Ibarra, C.; De Antoni, G.L. Lactobacillus plantarum isolated from kefir protects vero cells from cytotoxicity by type-II shiga toxin from *Escherichia coli* O157:H7. *J. Dairy Res.* **2013**, *80*, 64–71. [CrossRef]
60. Barr, J.J. A bacteriophages journey through the human body. *Immunol. Rev.* **2017**, *279*, 106–122. [CrossRef]
61. Caldwell, J.A. Bacteriologic and bacteriophagic study of infected urines. *J. Infect. Dis.* **1928**, *43*, 353–362. [CrossRef]
62. Weber-Dabrowska, B.; Dabrowski, M.; Slopek, S. Studies on bacteriophage penetration in patients subjected to phage therapy. *Arch. Immunol. Ther. Exp.* **1987**, *35*, 563–568.
63. Moustafa, A.; Xie, C.; Kirkness, E.; Biggs, W.; Wong, E.; Turpaz, Y.; Bloom, K.; Delwart, E.; Nelson, K.E.; Venter, J.C.; et al. The blood DNA virome in 8,000 humans. *PLoS Pathog.* **2017**, *13*, 1–20. [CrossRef]
64. Ghose, C.; Ly, M.; Schwanemann, L.K.; Shin, J.H.; Atab, K.; Barr, J.J.; Little, M.; Schooley, R.T.; Chopyk, J.; Pride, D.T. The virome of cerebrospinal fluid: Viruses where we once thought there were none. *Front. Microbiol.* **2019**, *10*, 1–14. [CrossRef]
65. Gorski, A.; Wazna, E.; Dąbrowska, B.W.; Dąbrowska, K.; Świtała-Jeleń, K.; Międzybrodzki, R. Bacteriophage translocation. *FEMS Immunol. Med. Microbiol.* **2006**, *46*, 313–319. [CrossRef]
66. Heinemann, B.; Howard, A.J. Induction of lambda-bacteriophage in *Escherichia coli* as a screening test for potential antitumor agents. *Appl. Environ. Microbiol.* **1964**, *12*, 234–239. [CrossRef]
67. Chao, S.C.; Young, D.G.; Oberg, C.J. Screening for inhibitory activity of essential oils on selected bacteria, fungi and viruses. *J. Essent. Oil Res.* **2000**, *12*, 639–649. [CrossRef]
68. Boling, L.; Cuevas, D.A.; Grasis, J.A.; Kang, H.S.; Knowles, B.; Levi, K.; Maughan, H.; McNair, K.; Rojas, M.I.; Sanchez, S.E.; et al. Dietary prophage inducers and antimicrobials: Toward landscaping the human gut microbiome. *Gut Microbes* **2020**, *1*, 1–14. [CrossRef] [PubMed]
69. Goyal, S.K.; Samsher; Goyal, R.K. Stevia (*Stevia rebaudiana*) a bio-sweetener: A review. *Int. J. Food Sci. Nutr.* **2010**, *61*, 1–10. [CrossRef]
70. Durazzo, A.; Lucarini, M.; Souto, E.B.; Cicala, C.; Caiazzo, E.; Izzo, A.A.; Novellino, E.; Santini, A. Polyphenols: A concise overview on the chemistry, occurrence, and human health. *Phytother. Res.* **2019**, *33*, 2221–2243. [CrossRef]

71. Manach, C.; Scalbert, A.; Morand, C.; Rmsy, C.; Jimnez, L. Polyphenols: Food sources and bioavailability. *J. Clin. Nutr.* **2004**, *79*, 727–747. [CrossRef]
72. Kim, H.-S.; Quon, M.J.; Kim, J.-A. New insights into the mechanisms of polyphenols beyond antioxidant properties; lessons from the green tea polyphenol, epigallocatechin 3-gallate. *Redox Biol.* **2014**, *2*, 187–195. [CrossRef] [PubMed]
73. Nehlig, A.; Debry, G. Potential genotoxic, mutagenic and antimutagenic effects of coffee: A review. *Mutat. Res.* **1994**, *317*, 145–162. [CrossRef]
74. Setchell, K.D.R.; Welsh, M.B.; Lim, C.K. High-performance liquid chromatographic analysis of phytoestrogens in soy protein preparations with ultraviolet, electrochemical and thermospray mass spectrometric detection. *J. Chromatogr. A* **1987**, *386*, 315–323. [CrossRef]
75. Jiang, T.A. Health benefits of culinary herbs and spices. *J. AOAC Int.* **2019**, *102*, 395–411. [CrossRef] [PubMed]
76. Busch, C.; Burkard, M.; Leischner, C.; Lauer, U.M.; Frank, J.; Venturelli, S. Epigenetic activities of flavonoids in the prevention and treatment of cancer. *Clin. Epigenetics* **2015**, *7*, 64. [CrossRef]
77. Venturelli, S.; Burkard, M.; Biendl, M.; Lauer, U.M.; Frank, J.; Busch, C. Prenylated chalcones and flavonoids for the prevention and treatment of cancer. *Nutrition* **2016**, *32*, 1171–1178. [CrossRef] [PubMed]
78. Burkard, M.; Leischner, C.; Lauer, U.M.; Busch, C.; Venturelli, S.; Frank, J. Dietary flavonoids and modulation of natural killer cells: Implications in malignant and viral diseases. *J. Nutrit. Biochem.* **2017**, *46*, 1–12. [CrossRef]
79. Kosugi, A.; Nagao, M.; Suwa, Y.; Wakabayashi, K.; Sugimura, T. Roasting coffee beans produces compounds that induce prophage lambda in *E. coli* and are mutagenic in *E. coli* and *S. typhimurium*. *Mutat. Res.* **1983**, *116*, 179–184. [CrossRef]
80. Silva-Beltárn, N.P.; Ruiz-Cruz, S.; Chaidez, C.; Ornelas-Paz, J.D.J.; Lpez-Mata, M.A.; Mrquez-Ris, E.; Estrada, M.I. Chemical constitution and effect of extracts of tomato plants byproducts on the enteric viral surrogates. *Int. J. Environ. Health Res.* **2015**, *25*, 299–311. [CrossRef]
81. Lee, A.; Eschenbruch, R.; Waller, J. Effect of phenolic compounds, ethyl alcohol, and sodium metabisulphite on the lytic activity of phage PL-1 on a *Lactobacillus casei* S strain. *Can. J. Microbiol.* **1985**, *31*, 873–875. [CrossRef]
82. Su, X.; D'Souza, D.H. Inactivation of human norovirus surrogates by benzalkonium chloride, potassium peroxymonosulfate, tannic acid, and gallic acid. *Foodborne Pathog. Dis.* **2012**, *9*, 829–834. [CrossRef]
83. Khatibi, S.A.; Misaghi, A.; Moosavy, M.H. Effect of nanoliposomes containing Zataria multiflora Boiss. essential oil on gene expression of Shiga toxin 2 in *Escherichia coli* O157:H7. *J. Appl. Microbiol.* **2018**, *124*, 389–397. [CrossRef] [PubMed]
84. De Siqueira, R.S.; Dodd, C.E.R.; Rees, C.E.D. Evaluation of the natural virucidal activity of teas for use in the phage amplification assay. *Int. J. Food Microbiol.* **2006**, *111*, 259–262. [CrossRef]
85. Su, X.; Sangster, M.Y.; D'Souza, D.H. In vitro effects of pomegranate juice and pomegranate polyphenols on foodborne viral surrogates. *Foodborne Pathog. Dis.* **2010**, *7*, 1473–1479. [CrossRef] [PubMed]
86. Catel-Ferreira, M.; Tnani, H.; Hellio, C.; Cosette, P.; Lebrun, L. Antiviral effects of polyphenols: Development of bio-based cleaning wipes and filters. *J. Virol. Methods* **2015**, *212*, 1–7. [CrossRef]
87. Yang, J.; Tang, C.B.; Xiao, J.; Du, W.F.; Li, R. Influences of epigallocatechin gallate and citric acid on Escherichia coli O157:H7 toxin gene expression and virulence-associated stress response. *Lett. Appl. Microbiol.* **2018**, *67*, 435–441. [CrossRef] [PubMed]
88. Richter, H.E.; Loewen, P.C. Rapid inactivation of bacteriophage T7 by ascorbic acid is repairable. *BBA Gene Struct. Expr.* **1982**, *697*, 25–30. [CrossRef]
89. Yen, G.-C.; Lai, H.-H. Inhibitory effects of isoflavones on nitric oxide-or peroxynitrite-mediated DNA damage in RAW 264.7 cells and fX174 DNA. *Food Chem. Toxicol.* **2002**, *40*, 1433–1440. [CrossRef]
90. Su, X.; Howell, A.B.; D'Souza, D.H. The effect of cranberry juice and cranberry proanthocyanidins on the infectivity of human enteric viral surrogates. *Food Microbiol.* **2010**, *27*, 535–540. [CrossRef] [PubMed]
91. Su, X.; Howell, A.B.; D'Souza, D.H. Antiviral effects of cranberry juice and cranberry proanthocyanidins on foodborne viral surrogates—A time dependence study in vitro. *Food Microbiol.* **2010**, *27*, 985–991. [CrossRef]
92. Su, X.; Sangster, M.Y.; D'Souza, D.H. Time-dependent effects of pomegranate juice and pomegranate polyphenols on foodborne viral reduction. *Foodborne Pathog. Dis.* **2011**, *8*, 1177–1183. [CrossRef] [PubMed]
93. Su, X.; D'Souza, D.H. Grape seed extract for control of human enteric viruses. *Appl. Environ. Microbiol.* **2011**, *77*, 3982–3987. [CrossRef]
94. Sheng, L.; Rasco, B.; Zhu, M.J. Cinnamon oil inhibits Shiga toxin type 2 phage induction and Shiga toxin type 2 production in *Escherichia coli* O157:H7. *Appl. Environ. Microbiol.* **2016**, *82*, 6531–6540. [CrossRef] [PubMed]
95. Lipson, S.M.; Sethi, L.; Cohen, P.; Gordon, R.E.; Tan, I.P.; Burdowski, G.; Stotzky, G. Antiviral effects on bacteriophages and rotavirus by cranberry juice. *Phytomedicine* **2007**, *14*, 23–30. [CrossRef] [PubMed]
96. Silva-Beltrán, N.P. Antiviral effects of Brazilian green and red propolis extracts on Enterovirus surrogates. *Environ. Sci. Pollut. Res. Int.* **2020**, *23*, 28510–28517. [CrossRef] [PubMed]
97. Kim, Y.-G.; Lee, J.-H.; Kim, S.-I.; Baek, K.-H.; Lee, J. Cinnamon bark oil and its components inhibit biofilm formation and toxin production. *Int. J. Food Microbiol.* **2015**, *195*, 30–39. [CrossRef] [PubMed]
98. Davis, R.; Zivanovic, S. Enteric viral surrogate reduction by chitosan. *Food Environ. Virol.* **2015**, *7*, 359–365. [CrossRef]
99. Kochkina, Z.M.; Chirkov, S.N. Influence of Chitosan Derivatives on the Development of Phage Infection in the *Bacillus thuringiensis* Culture. *Mikrobiologiia* **2000**, *69*, 266–269.

100. Ly-Chatain, M.H.; Moussaoui, S.; Vera, A.; Rigobello, V.; Demarigny, Y. Antiviral effect of cationic compounds on bacteriophages. *Front. Microbiol.* **2013**, *4*, 46. [CrossRef]
101. Amorim, J.H.; Del Cogliano, M.E.; Fernandez-Brando, R.J.; Bilen, M.F.; Jesus, M.R.; Luiz, W.B.; Palermo, M.S.; Ferreira, R.C.; Servat, E.G.; Ghiringhelli, P.D.; et al. Role of bacteriophages in STEC infections: New implications for the design of prophylactic and treatment approaches. *F1000Research* **2014**, *3*, 74. [CrossRef]
102. Murata, A.; Oyadomari, R.; Ohashi, T.; Kitagawa, K. Mechanism of inactivation of bacteriophage deltaA containing single-stranded DNA by ascorbic acid. *J. Nutr. Sci. Vitaminol.* **1975**, *21*, 261–269. [CrossRef]
103. Kobayashi, S.; Ueda, K.; Morita, J.; Sakai, H.; Komano, T. DNA damage induced by ascorbate in the presence of Cu2+. *Biochim. Biophys. Acta* **1988**, *949*, 143–147. [CrossRef]
104. Cloos, J.; Gille, J.J.; Steen, I.; Lafleur, M.V.; Retèl, J.; Snow, G.B.; Braakhuis, B.J. Influence of the antioxidant N-acetylcysteine and its metabolites on damage induced by bleomycin in PM2 bacteriophage DNA. *Carcinogenesis* **1996**, *17*, 327–331. [CrossRef] [PubMed]
105. Gião, M.S.; Borges, A.B.; Guedes, C.J.; Hogg, T.A.; Pintado, M.E.; Malcata, F.X. Determination of antioxidant capacity using the biological system bacteriophage P22/bacterium Salmonella typhimurium. *J. Agric. Food Chem.* **2009**, *57*, 22–25. [CrossRef]
106. Kirtania, P.; Ghosh, S.; Bhawsinghka, N.; Chakladar, M.; Das Gupta, S.K. Vitamin C induced DevR-dependent synchronization of Mycobacterium smegmatis growth and its effect on the proliferation of mycobacteriophage D29. *FEMS Microbiol. Lett.* **2016**, *363*. [CrossRef]
107. Harding, A.S.; Schwab, K.J. Using limes and synthetic psoralens to enhance solar disinfection of water (SODIS): A laboratory evaluation with norovirus, *Escherichia coli*, and MS2. *Am. J. Trop. Med. Hyg.* **2012**, *86*, 566–572. [CrossRef]
108. Steiger, H.; Sinsheimer, R.L. Stimulation of phiX174 production in mitomycin C-treated Escherichia coli cells by caffeine. *J. Virol.* **1968**, *2*, 655. [CrossRef] [PubMed]
109. Harris, S.M.; Yue, W.F.; Olsen, S.A.; Hu, J.; Means, W.J.; McCormick, R.J.; Du, M.; Zhu, M.J. Salt at concentrations relevant to meat processing enhances Shiga toxin 2 production in Escherichia coli O157:H7. *Int. J. Food Microbiol.* **2012**, *159*, 186–192. [CrossRef]
110. Schons, M.; Inman, R.B. Caffeine-induced re-initiation of phage λ DNA replication. *J. Mol. Biol.* **1982**, *159*, 457–465. [CrossRef]
111. Camire, M.E.; Kubow, S.; Donnelly, D.J. Potatoes and human health. *Crit. Rev. Food Sci. Nutr.* **2009**, *49*, 823–840. [CrossRef]
112. Zaheer, K.; Akhtar, M.H. Potato Production, Usage, and Nutrition—A Review. *Crit. Rev. Food Sci. Nutr.* **2016**, *56*, 711–721. [CrossRef] [PubMed]
113. Silva-Beltrán, N.P.; Chaidez-Quiroz, C.; Lpez-Cuevas, O.; Ruiz-Cruz, S.; Lpez-Mata, M.A.; Del-Toro-snchez, C.L.; Marquez-Rios, E.; Ornelas-Paz, J.D.J. Phenolic compounds of potato peel extracts: Their antioxidant activity and protection against human enteric viruses. *J. Microbiol. Biotechnol.* **2017**, *27*, 234–241. [CrossRef] [PubMed]
114. Quiñones, B.; Massey, S.; Friedman, M.; Swimley, M.S.; Teter, K. Novel cell-based method to detect Shiga toxin 2 from *Escherichia coli* O157:H7 and inhibitors of toxin activity. *Appl. Environ. Microbiol.* **2009**, *75*, 1410–1416. [CrossRef]
115. Hadian, J.; Ebrahimi, S.N.; Mirjalili, M.H.; Azizi, A.; Ranjbar, H.; Friedt, W. Chemical and genetic diversity of zataria multi-florabiss. Accessions growing wild in Iran. *Chem. Biodivers.* **2011**, *8*, 176–188. [CrossRef]
116. Chavez, J.H.; Leal, P.C.; Yunes, R.A.; Nunes, R.J.; Barardi, C.R.M.; Pinto, A.R.; Simes, C.M.O.; Zanetti, C.R. Evaluation of antiviral activity of phenolic compounds and derivatives against rabies virus. *Vet. Microbiol.* **2006**, *116*, 53–59. [CrossRef] [PubMed]
117. Gil, M.I.; Tomas-Barberan, F.A.; Hess-Pierce, B.; Holcroft, D.M.; Kader, A.A. Antioxidant activity of pomegranate juice and its relationship with phenolic composition and processing. *J. Agric. Food Chem.* **2000**, *48*, 4581–4589. [CrossRef] [PubMed]
118. Haidari, M.; Ali, M. Pomegranate (*Punica granatum*) purified polyphenol extract inhibits influenza virus and has a synergistic effect with oseltamivir. *Phytomedicine* **2009**, *16*, 1127–1136. [CrossRef] [PubMed]
119. Sichel, G.; Corsaro, C.; Scalia, M. In vitro scavenger activity of some flavonoids and melanins against O2- dot. *Free Radic. Biol. Med.* **1991**, *11*, 1–8. [CrossRef]
120. Tyler, J.S.; Beeri, K.; Reynolds, J.L.; Alteri, C.J.; Skinner, K.G.; Friedman, J.H.; Eaton, K.A.; Friedman, D.I. Prophage induction is enhanced and required for renal disease and lethality in an EHEC mouse model. *PLoS Pathog.* **2013**, *9*, e1003236. [CrossRef]
121. Sugita-Konishi, Y.; Hara-Kudo, Y.; Amano, F.; Okubo, T.; Aoi, N.; Iwaki, M.; Kumagai, S. Epigallocatechin gallate and gallocatechin gallate in green tea catechins inhibit extracellular release of Vero toxin from enterohemorrhagic *Escherichia coli* O157:H7. *Biochim. Biophys. Acta* **1999**, *1472*, 42–50. [CrossRef]
122. Khan, N.S.; Ahmad, A.; Hadi, S.M. Anti-oxidant, pro-oxidant properties of tannic acid and its binding to DNA. *Chem.-Biol. Interact.* **2000**, *125*, 177–189. [CrossRef]
123. Kamimoto, M.; Nakai, Y.; Tsuji, T.; Shimamoto, T.; Shimamoto, T. Antiviral effects of persimmon extract on human norovirus and its surrogate, bacteriophage MS2. *J. Food Sci.* **2014**, *79*, M941–M946. [CrossRef] [PubMed]
124. Kameoka, S.; Leavitt, P.; Chang, C.; Kuo, S.M. Expression of antioxidant proteins in human intestinal Caco-2 cells treated with dietary flavonoids. *Cancer Lett.* **1999**, *146*, 161–167. [CrossRef]
125. Tsafa, E.; Al-Bahrani, M.; Bentayebi, K.; Przystal, J.; Suwan, K.; Hajitou, A. The natural dietary genistein boosts bacteriophage-mediated cancer cell killing by improving phage-targeted tumor cell transduction. *Oncotarget* **2016**, *7*, 52135–52149. [CrossRef]
126. Nogueira, M.C.L.; Oyarzbal, O.A.; Gombas, D.E. Inactivation of Escherichia coli O157:H7, Listeria monocytogenes, and Salmonella in cranberry, lemon, and lime juice concentrates. *J. Food Prot.* **2003**, *66*, 1637–1641. [CrossRef] [PubMed]
127. Horm, K.M.; Davidson, P.M.; Harte, F.M.; D'Souza, D.H. Survival and inactivation of human norovirus surrogates in blueberry juice by high-pressure homogenization. *Foodborne Pathog. Dis.* **2012**, *9*, 974–979. [CrossRef] [PubMed]

128. Sheng, L.; Olsen, S.A.; Hu, J.; Yue, W.; Means, W.J.; Zhu, M.J. Inhibitory effects of grape seed extract on growth, quorum sensing, and virulence factors of CDC top-six non-O157 Shiga toxin producing *E. coli*. *Int. J. Food Microbiol.* **2016**, *229*, 24–32. [CrossRef] [PubMed]
129. Rasooly, R.; Do, P.M.; Levin, C.E.; Friedman, M. Inhibition of Shiga toxin 2 (Stx2) in apple juices and its resistance to pasteurization. *J. Food Sci.* **2010**, *75*, M296–M301. [CrossRef]
130. Viuda-Martos, M.; Ruiz-Navajas, Y.; Fernndez-Lpez, J.; Prez-lvarez, J.A. Functional properties of honey, propolis, and royal jelly. *J. Food Sci.* **2008**, *73*, R117–R124. [CrossRef]
131. Rufatto, L.C.; Luchtenberg, P.; Garcia, C.; Thomassigny, C.; Bouttier, S.; Henriques, J.A.P.; Roesch-Ely, M.; Dumas, F.; Moura, S. Brazilian red propolis: Chemical composition and antibacterial activity determined using bioguided fractionation. *Microbiol. Res.* **2018**, *214*, 74–82. [CrossRef]
132. Iriti, M.; Varoni, E.M. Chitosan-induced antiviral activity and innate immunity in plants. *Environ. Sci. Pollut. Res.* **2015**, *22*, 2935–2944. [CrossRef]
133. Su, X.; Zivanovic, S.; D'Souza, D.H. Effect of chitosan on the infectivity of murine norovirus, feline calicivirus, and bacteriophage MS2. *J. Food Prot.* **2009**, *72*, 2623–2628. [CrossRef] [PubMed]
134. Davis, R.; Zivanovic, S.; D'Souza, D.H.; Davidson, P.M. Effectiveness of chitosan on the inactivation of enteric viral surrogates. *Food Microbiol.* **2012**, *32*, 57–62. [CrossRef] [PubMed]
135. Chirkov, S.N. The antiviral activity of chitosan (review). *Prikl. Biokhim. Mikrobiol.* **2002**, *38*, 1–8.
136. Liu, J.; Tian, S.; Meng, X.; Xu, Y. Effects of chitosan on control of postharvest diseases and physiological responses of tomato fruit. *Postharvest Biol. Technol.* **2007**, *44*, 300–306. [CrossRef]
137. Dragsted, L.O.; Daneshvar, B.; Vogel, U.; Autrup, H.N.; Wallin, H.; Risom, L.; Møller, P.; Mølck, A.M.; Hansen, M.; Poulsen, H.E.; et al. A sucrose-rich diet induces mutations in the rat colon. *Cancer Res.* **2002**, *62*, 4339–4345. [PubMed]
138. Duewel, H.S.; Daub, E.; Honek, J.F. Investigations of the interactions of saccharides with the lysozyme from bacteriophage lambda. *Biochim. Biophys. Acta* **1995**, *1247*, 149–158. [CrossRef]
139. Taylor, A.; Gorazdowska, M. Conversion of murein to non-reducing fragments by enzymes from phage lambda and Vi II lysates. *Biochim. Biophys. Acta* **1974**, *342*, 133–136. [CrossRef]
140. Aziz, M.; Karboune, S. Natural antimicrobial/antioxidant agents in meat and poultry products as well as fruits and vegetables: A review. *Crit. Rev. Food Sci. Nutr.* **2018**, *58*, 486–511. [CrossRef]
141. Du, W.-X.; Olsen, C.W.; Avena-Bustillos, R.J.; McHugh, T.H.; Levin, C.E.; Friedman, M. Effects of allspice, cinnamon, and clove bud essential oils in edible apple films on physical properties and antimicrobial activities. *J. Food Sci.* **2009**, *74*, M372–M378. [CrossRef] [PubMed]
142. Du, W.-X.; Olsen, C.W.; Avena-Bustillos, R.J.; McHugh, T.H.; Levin, C.E.; Mandrell, R.; Friedman, M. Antibacterial effects of allspice, garlic, and oregano essential oils in tomato films determined by overlay and vapor-phase methods. *J. Food Sci.* **2009**, *74*, M390–M397. [CrossRef] [PubMed]
143. Nowicki, D.; Bloch, S.; Nejman-Faleczyk, B.; Szalewska-Paasz, A.; Wgrzyn, A.; Wgrzyn, G. Defects in RNA polyadenylation impair both lysogenization by and lytic development of Shiga toxin-converting bacteriophages. *J. Gen. Virol.* **2015**, *96*, 1957–1968. [CrossRef] [PubMed]
144. Takemasa, N.; Ohnishi, S.; Tsuji, M.; Shikata, T.; Yokoigawa, K. Screening and analysis of spices with ability to suppress verocytotoxin production by *Escherichia coli* O157. *J. Food Sci.* **2009**, *74*, M461–M466. [CrossRef] [PubMed]
145. Morgan, A.R.; Cone, R.L.; Elgert, T.M. The mechanism of DNA strand breakage by vitamin C and superoxide and the protective roles of catalase and superoxide dismutase. *Nucleic Acids Res.* **1976**, *3*, 1139–1149. [CrossRef] [PubMed]
146. Morgan, W.A. DNA single-strand breakage in mammalian cells induced by redox cycling quinones in the absence of oxidative stress. *J. Biochem. Toxicol.* **1995**, *10*, 227–232. [CrossRef]
147. Schoenfeld, J.D.; Sibenaller, Z.A.; Mapuskar, K.A.; Wagner, B.A.; Cramer-Morales, K.L.; Furqan, M.; Sandhu, S.; Carlisle, T.L.; Smith, M.C.; Hejleh, T.A.; et al. O_2^- and H_2O_2-mediated disruption of Fe metabolism causes the differential susceptibility of NSCLC and GBM cancer cells to pharmacological ascorbate. *Cancer Cell* **2017**, *31*, 487–500. [CrossRef] [PubMed]
148. Yamamoto, N. Inactivation of T-group bacteriophages by ascorbic acid and some poly-phenol derivatives, and the catalytic effects of cupric ion and photo-excited riboflavin. *Biochim. Biophys. Acta* **1958**, *27*, 427–428. [CrossRef]
149. Gorgus, E.; Lohr, C.; Raquet, N.; Guth, S.; Schrenk, D. Limettin and furocoumarins in beverages containing citrus juices or extracts. *Food Chem. Toxicol.* **2010**, *48*, 93–98. [CrossRef]
150. Heckman, M.A.; Weil, J.; de Mejia, E.G. Caffeine (1, 3, 7-trimethylxanthine) in foods: A comprehensive review on consumption, functionality, safety, and regulatory matters. *J. Food Sci.* **2010**, *75*, R77–R87. [CrossRef]
151. Cui, W.Q.; Wang, S.T.; Pan, D.; Chang, B.; Sang, L.X. Caffeine and its main targets of colorectal cancer. *World J. Gastrointest. Oncol.* **2020**, *12*, 149–172. [CrossRef]
152. Moura, T.A.; Oliveira, L.; Rocha, M.S. Effects of caffeine on the structure and conformation of DNA: A force spectroscopy study. *Int. J. Biol. Macromol.* **2019**, *130*, 1018–1024. [CrossRef] [PubMed]
153. Zheng, D.-W.; Dong, X.; Pan, P.; Chen, K.-W.; Fan, J.-X.; Cheng, S.-X.; Zhang, X.-Z. Phage-guided modulation of the gut microbiota of mouse models of colorectal cancer augments their responses to chemotherapy. *Nat. Biomed. Eng.* **2019**, *3*, 717–728. [CrossRef] [PubMed]

154. Gelman, D.; Beyth, S.; Lerer, V.; Adler, K.; Poradosu-Cohen, R.; Coppenhagen-Glazer, S.; Hazan, R. Combined bacteriophages and antibiotics as an efficient therapy against VRE Enterococcus faecalis in a mouse model. *Res. Microbiol.* **2018**, *169*, 531–539. [CrossRef]
155. Mai, V.; Ukhanova, M.; Reinhard, M.K.; Li, M.; Sulakvelidze, A. Bacteriophage administration significantly reduces Shigella colonization and shedding by Shigella-challenged mice without deleterious side effects and distortions in the gut microbiota. *Bacteriophage* **2015**, *5*, e1088124. [CrossRef] [PubMed]
156. Mai, V.; Ukhanova, M.; Visone, L.; Abuladze, T.; Sulakvelidze, A. Bacteriophage administration reduces the concentration of listeria monocytogenes in the gastrointestinal tract and its translocation to spleen and liver in experimentally infected mice. *Int. J. Microbi.* **2010**, *2010*, 624234.
157. Draper, L.A.; Ryan, F.J.; Dalmasso, M.; Casey, P.G.; McCann, A.; Velayudhan, V.; Ross, R.P.; Hill, C. Autochthonous faecal viral transfer (FVT) impacts the murine microbiome after antibiotic perturbation. *BMC Biol.* **2020**, *18*, 173. [CrossRef]
158. Selle, K.; Fletcher, J.R.; Tuson, H.; Schmitt, D.S.; McMillan, L.; Vridhambal, G.S.; Rivera, A.J.; Montgomery, S.A.; Fortier, L.C.; Barrangou, R.; et al. In Vivo targeting of clostridioides difficile using phage-delivered CRISPR-Cas3 antimicrobials. *mBio* **2020**, *11*. [CrossRef]
159. Cheng, M.; Liang, J.; Zhang, Y.; Hu, L.; Gong, P.; Cai, R.; Zhang, L.; Zhang, H.; Ge, J.; Ji, Y.; et al. The Bacteriophage EF-P29 Efficiently Protects against Lethal Vancomycin-Resistant Enterococcus faecalis and Alleviates Gut Microbiota Imbalance in a Murine Bacteremia Model. *Front. Microbiol.* **2017**, *8*, 837. [CrossRef]
160. Galtier, M.; Sordi, L.D.; Sivignon, A.; De Vallée, A.; Maura, D.; Neut, C.; Rahmouni, O.; Wannerberger, K.; Darfeuille-Michaud, A.; Desreumaux, P.; et al. Bacteriophages Targeting adherent invasive escherichia coli strains as a promising new treatment for crohn's disease. *J. Crohn's Colitis* **2017**, *11*, 840–847. [CrossRef]
161. Duan, Y.; Llorente, C.; Lang, S.; Brandl, K.; Chu, H.; Jiang, L.; White, R.C.; Clarke, T.H.; Nguyen, K.; Torralba, M.; et al. Bacteriophage targeting of gut bacterium attenuates alcoholic liver disease. *Nature* **2019**, *575*, 505–511. [CrossRef] [PubMed]
162. Febvre, H.P.; Rao, S.; Gindin, M.; Goodwin, N.D.M.; Finer, E.; Vivanco, J.S.; Lu, S.; Manter, D.K.; Wallace, T.C.; Weir, T.L. PHAGE Study: Effects of supplemental bacteriophage intake on inflammation and gut microbiota in healthy adults. *Nutrients* **2019**, *11*, 666. [CrossRef] [PubMed]
163. Gindin, M.; Febvre, H.P.; Rao, S.; Wallace, T.C.; Weir, T.L. Bacteriophage for Gastrointestinal Health (PHAGE) study: Evaluating the safety and tolerability of supplemental bacteriophage consumption. *J. Am. Coll. Nutr.* **2019**, *38*, 68–75. [CrossRef]
164. Grubb, D.S.; Wrigley, S.D.; Freedman, K.E.; Wei, Y.; Vazquez, A.R.; Trotter, R.E.; Wallace, T.C.; Johnson, S.A.; Weir, T.L. PHAGE-2 Study: Supplemental Bacteriophages Extend Bifidobacterium animalis subsp. lactis BL04 Benefits on Gut Health and Microbiota in Healthy Adults. *Nutrients* **2020**, *12*, 2474. [CrossRef] [PubMed]
165. Cougnoux, A.; Dalmasso, G.; Martinez, R.; Buc, E.; Delmas, J.; Gibold, L.; Sauvanet, P.; Darcha, C.; Déchelotte, P.; Bonnet, M.; et al. Bacterial genotoxin colibactin promotes colon tumour growth by inducing a senescence-associated secretory phenotype. *Gut* **2014**, *63*, 1932–1942. [CrossRef] [PubMed]
166. Ishaque, N.; Abba, M.L.; Hauser, C.; Patil, N.; Paramasivam, N.; Huebschmann, D.; Leupold, J.H.; Balasubramanian, G.P.; Kleinheinz, K.; Toprak, U.H.; et al. Whole genome sequencing puts forward hypotheses on metastasis evolution and therapy in colorectal cancer. *Nat. Commun.* **2018**, *9*, 4782. [CrossRef] [PubMed]

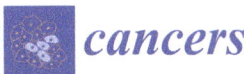

Article

The Immune Landscape of Colorectal Cancer

Artur Mezheyeuski [1,*], Patrick Micke [1], Alfonso Martín-Bernabé [2], Max Backman [1], Ina Hrynchyk [3], Klara Hammarström [1], Simon Ström [1], Joakim Ekström [1], Per-Henrik Edqvist [1], Magnus Sundström [1], Fredrik Ponten [1], Karin Leandersson [4], Bengt Glimelius [1] and Tobias Sjöblom [1]

[1] Department of Immunology, Genetics and Pathology, Uppsala University, 75185 Uppsala, Sweden; patrick.micke@igp.uu.se (P.M.); max.backman@igp.uu.se (M.B.); Klara.hammarstrom@igp.uu.se (K.H.); simonstrom96@gmail.com (S.S.); joakim.ekstrom@igp.uu.se (J.E.); per-henrik.edqvist@igp.uu.se (P.-H.E.); magnus.sundstrom@igp.uu.se (M.S.); fredrik.ponten@igp.uu.se (F.P.); bengt.glimelius@igp.uu.se (B.G.); tobias.sjoblom@igp.uu.se (T.S.)

[2] Department of Oncology-Pathology, Cancer Center Karolinska, Karolinska Institutet, 17164 Stockholm, Sweden; alfonso.martin.bernabe@ki.se

[3] City Clinical Pathologoanatomic Bureau, 220116 Minsk, Belarus; inahrinchyk@gmail.com

[4] Department of Translational Medicine, Lund University, 20502 Malmö, Sweden; karin.leandersson@med.lu.se

* Correspondence: artur.mezheyeuski@igp.uu.se

Simple Summary: We sought to provide a detailed overview of the immune landscape of colorectal cancer in the largest study to date in terms of patient numbers and analyzed immune cell types. We applied a multiplex in situ staining method in combination with an advanced scanning and image analysis pipeline akin to flow cytometry, and analyzed 5968 individual multi-layer images of tissue defining in a total of 39,078,450 cells. We considered the location of immune cells with respect to the stroma, and tumor cell compartment and tumor regions in the central part or the invasive margin. To the best of our knowledge, this study is the first comprehensive spatial description of the immune landscape in colorectal cancer using a large population-based cohort and a multiplex immune cell identification.

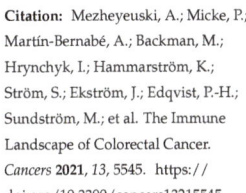

Citation: Mezheyeuski, A.; Micke, P.; Martín-Bernabé, A.; Backman, M.; Hrynchyk, I.; Hammarström, K.; Ström, S.; Ekström, J.; Edqvist, P.-H.; Sundström, M.; et al. The Immune Landscape of Colorectal Cancer. *Cancers* 2021, 13, 5545. https://doi.org/10.3390/cancers13215545

Academic Editor: Heike Allgayer

Received: 17 October 2021
Accepted: 2 November 2021
Published: 4 November 2021

Publisher's Note: MDPI stays neutral with regard to jurisdictional claims in published maps and institutional affiliations.

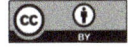

Copyright: © 2021 by the authors. Licensee MDPI, Basel, Switzerland. This article is an open access article distributed under the terms and conditions of the Creative Commons Attribution (CC BY) license (https://creativecommons.org/licenses/by/4.0/).

Abstract: While the clinical importance of CD8+ and CD3+ cells in colorectal cancer (CRC) is well established, the impact of other immune cell subsets is less well described. We sought to provide a detailed overview of the immune landscape of CRC in the largest study to date in terms of patient numbers and in situ analyzed immune cell types. Tissue microarrays from 536 patients were stained using multiplexed immunofluorescence panels, and fifteen immune cell subclasses, representing adaptive and innate immunity, were analyzed. Overall, therapy-naïve CRC patients clustered into an 'inflamed' and a 'desert' group. Most T cell subsets and M2 macrophages were enriched in the right colon (p-values 0.046–0.004), while pDC cells were in the rectum ($p = 0.008$). Elderly patients had higher infiltration of M2 macrophages ($p = 0.024$). CD8+ cells were linked to improved survival in colon cancer stages I-III ($q = 0.014$), while CD4+ cells had the strongest impact on overall survival in metastatic CRC ($q = 0.031$). Finally, we demonstrated repopulation of the immune infiltrate in rectal tumors post radiation, following an initial radiation-induced depletion. This study provides a detailed analysis of the in situ immune landscape of CRC paving the way for better diagnostics and providing hints to better target the immune microenvironment.

Keywords: colorectal cancer; multiplex; tumor immunology; immune landscape

1. Introduction

Cancer remains one of the leading causes of death worldwide and CRC is the third most common cancer type and the second most common cancer killer [1]. In addition to the traditional TNM classification system, molecular subgroups based on mutations and gene expression profiles are used to identify more homogeneous subgroups as CRC is intrinsically heterogeneous [2]. In particular, somatic mutations in driver genes, such as those of the RAS pathway, have major clinical implications for the response to specific therapies and molecular testing for such mutations is now a clinical standard in metastatic CRC (mCRC). During the past decade, a classification system based on the tumor immune environment has attracted attention. Galon et al. introduced an immune score that grouped CRCs with regard to the infiltration of T cells (CD3+ and CD8+ lymphocytes) in the tumor and the invasive margin [3]. The Immunoscore® provides independent prognostic information in addition to other clinical parameters including the TNM classification in CRC stage I–III [4,5]. Furthermore, not only the T cell lineage, but also the presence of other immune cell types including B cells and NK cells have been associated with better outcomes [6,7]. On the other hand, certain immune contexts of the primary tumor dominated by immune suppressive cells, like T regulatory cells or M2 type macrophages, were connected to tumor progression and poor prognosis [8]. These observations indicate an active involvement of the tumor immune environment in tumorigenesis and suggest a diagnostic, prognostic, and, potentially, also predictive value of a deeper immune classification of CRC.

The introduction of immune checkpoint inhibitors has demonstrated that cancer immunity can be modified, leading to immune-mediated long-lasting tumor regression in subsets of patients with several different solid tumor types [9]. Further, the pre-existing microenvironment seems of major relevance and high infiltration with immune cells is associated with better tumor response and long-term survival in patients treated with checkpoint inhibitors [10]. Transcriptomic analyses have revealed that these tumors also express inflammatory and effector cytokines, indicating a basic anti-tumor immune response, though not efficient enough to control tumor growth. This immune phenotype has been designated 'inflamed' or 'hot'. In contrast, tumors with less immune cell infiltrate were designated as 'desert' or 'cold' tumors [11,12]. In CRC, the 'inflamed' immune phenotype is often found in tumors with high microsatellite instability (MSI-H), most probably due to high tumor mutational load and the presentation of neoantigens leading to anti-cancer immunity [13,14]. The analysis of tumor exomes allows identification of such neoantigens. The number of mutations per exome ranges from ~100 in microsatellite stable (MSS) to ~1000 in MSI CRC [15–17]. Checkpoint inhibitor therapy is effective in these tumors [18,19] and is now approved for mCRC with MSI-H [18–21]. Taken together, there is evidence that the tumor immune microenvironment plays a major role in terms of CRC prognosis and, at the same time, indicates whether immune modulating treatment is beneficial.

Despite its obvious clinical relevance, knowledge of the immune microenvironment in CRC is fragmentary as most studies have focused on only a single cell type or a few subsets of immune cells. The most applied strategy is based on immunohistochemical analysis with semi-quantitative measurements, carrying a substantial risk of observer bias. Multiple markers may be analyzed in consecutive sections, but this has limited relevance when evaluating cell interactions [22]. Therefore, the focus of prior immunohistochemical studies was on the T cell lineage. More comprehensive studies rely on deconvolution of gene expression data, without spatial context of immune cells. This approach has disadvantages, as low abundance cell types are challenging to quantitate accurately in bulk mRNA profiles. Given these methodological difficulties, there are few comprehensive efforts towards in situ mapping of the tumor microenvironment [23]. However, novel immunofluorescence multiplex techniques in combination with advanced scanning and image analysis systems can tackle these obstacles to describe the immune response in cancer in a holistic and standardized manner [24].

The aim is to apply immunofluorescence multiplexing techniques to provide the first comprehensive overview of the immune landscape across a large population-based cohort of CRC patients. Relevant molecular and clinical subgroups are analyzed using antibody panels allowing in situ identification of 15 distinct subclasses of immune cells in association with clinical parameters and outcome. Finally, we compare the immune status in rectal tumors treated with different therapies and intervals prior to surgery to identify therapy-induced modulation of CRC immunity.

2. Materials and Methods

2.1. Study Cohort

The study cohort consists of prospectively collected CRC patients living in the Uppsala region of Sweden, most of which have been included in the Uppsala-Umeå Comprehensive Cancer Consortium (U-CAN) [25]. In total, 937 patients were diagnosed with CRC between 2010 and 2014 in the Uppsala region. Of them, 746 (80%) were included in tissue microarray (TMA). For the present study, only patients with TMA material from primary tumors were selected. After the staining procedures and quality control, 536 patients were available for analysis. The clinicopathological characteristics of the included patients and their tumors are presented in Table S1.

All patients received stage-stratified standard of care according to the Swedish national guidelines from 2008. According to the guidelines, colon tumors were recommended primary surgery and adjuvant chemotherapy if risk-factors for recurrence were present. If the colon tumor was considered inoperable, neoadjuvant chemotherapy was administered to shrink the tumor before surgery. Rectal tumors were grouped into three prognostic categories: early (low recurrence risk), intermediate (intermediate recurrence risk), and locally advanced (high recurrence risk) with recommendations of primary surgery or pre-operative radiotherapy or chemoradiotherapy with different time-intervals to surgery, dependent on group belonging. Formalin-fixed paraffin-embedded tissue blocks of primary tumors and distant metastases were used to construct TMAs. Each case was represented on the TMA with cores derived from the central part of the tumor and from the invasive margin. The study was approved by the regional ethical committee in Uppsala, Sweden (Dnr 2010/198 and Dnr 2015/419).

MSI status was evaluated in available cases by IHC analysis with antibodies against the two MMR proteins, PMS2 and MSH6. The tumor was denoted as MSI-H if at least one of these proteins was absent.

2.2. Multiplex Immunofluorescence Staining

For the multiplexed immunofluorescence staining, 4 µm thick sections were deparaffinized, rehydrated, and rinsed in distilled H_2O. Three staining protocols were established with three panels of antibodies: a lymphocyte panel, with CD4, CD8, CD20, FoxP3, CD45RO, and pan-cytokeratin (pan-CK) (as described in [26]); a NK/macrophage panel encompassing CD56, NKp46, CD3, CD68, CD163, and pan-CK; and a dendritic cell panel with CD3, CD1a, CD208, CD123, CD68, CD15, and pan-CK. The staining procedure was performed as described [27,28]. In total, 520 cases were evaluable for the lymphocyte panel, 508 cases for the NK/macrophage cell panel, and 498 cases for the dendritic cell panel (Table S1). Using a combination of immune markers, we quantified 15 immune cell subclasses (Figure 1a,b).

2.3. Imaging, Image Analysis, Thresholding and Immune Scores

The stained TMAs were imaged using the Vectra Polaris system (Akoya Biosciences, Marlborough, MA, USA) in a multispectral mode at a resolution of 2 pixels per µm. This resulted in 5968 individual multi-layer images, each representing a TMA core. Spectral deconvolution and initial image analysis were conducted in the inForm (2.4.6) software (Akoya Biosciences) (Figure S1). Each of the images was reviewed and manually curated by a pathologist to exclude artefacts, staining defects, and accumulation of immune cells in necrotic areas and intraglandular structures. The vendor-provided machine learning algorithm was trained and applied to split tissue into three categories: tumor compartment, stromal compartment, or blank areas as described [29]. Cell segmentation was performed using DAPI nuclear staining as described [27,28]. The perinuclear region at 3 µm (6 pixels) from the nuclear border was considered the cytoplasm area. The nuclear or cytoplasmic area was evaluated for the expression of nuclear or cytoplasmic/membrane markers, respectively. The cell phenotyping function of the inForm software was used to manually define cells positive to each of the markers. The intensity of the marker expression in selected cells was used to set the thresholds for marker positivity. The defined thresholds were then applied to the raw output data of the complete cohort outside the inForm pipeline. Every cell was characterized as positive or negative for each marker in the panel, and marker co-expression was used to define immune cell subtypes (Figure 1a,b). Immune cell infiltration was evaluated as the number of cells per analyzed tissue area, in the stromal compartment and tumor compartment. This algorithm was applied to quantify the 15 different immune cell subclasses in the stroma and tumor compartment in the center of the tumor and in the invasive margin, i.e., obtaining a cell quantification in four tissue regions. Immune scores were generated for each immune cell subclass. First, immune cell infiltration in each of the four localizations was dichotomized into 0 (low) and 1 (high), using the median as threshold. The sum of the values gives a score between 0 and 4 (Figure S1e).

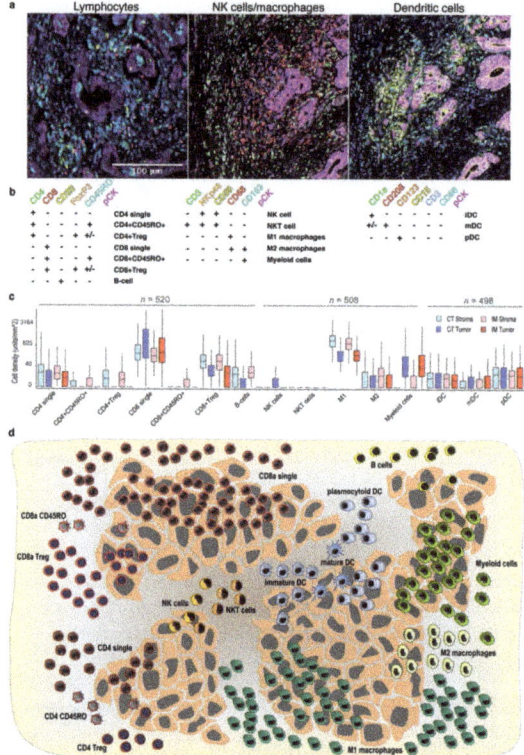

Figure 1. Characterization of immune cell subsets in the tumor and stroma compartments at the invasive margin and core of the tumor of primary CRC. (**a**) Representative images of the multiplex staining with three immune panels; (**b**) scheme of the immune marker combinations used to define the subgroups of immune cells; (**c**) immune cell densities in Tumor and Stroma compartments in Central Tumor (CT) and Invasive Margin (IM) (boxes show median values and interquartile range, and numbers represent cell counts per mm^2, cube root transformed); and (**d**) illustration of the mean immune cell infiltration in tumor center in tumor and stromal compartment.

2.4. Statistics

Statistical analyses were performed using R (version 3.5.1) and SPSS V20 (SPSS Inc., Chicago, IL, USA). In radically operated stage I–III patients, recurrence-free survival (RFS) was computed as the time from surgery to the first documented disease progression including local recurrence or distant metastases or death due to any reason, whichever occurred first [30]. Overall survival (OS) was the time from surgery to death due to any reason. To estimate relative hazards in both univariate and multivariable models, a Cox proportional hazards model was used. Hierarchical clustering analyses were conducted with the heatmap.plus package (version 1.3) in R. For the analyses of associations between MSS/MSI status and metastases type, the Chi-square test was used. The Ward algorithm was used for hierarchical clustering and $p < 0.05$ was considered statistically significant. The Benjamini–Hochberg procedure was used to adjust for multiple hypothesis testing, and adjusted q-values were reported.

3. Results

3.1. Identification and Quantification of Immune Cell Subclasses in CRC by Multiplex Staining

The successfully stained tissue microarray cores comprised of 536 surgically removed primary CRC cases with two cores from each tumor, representing the invasion margin and the central tumor area. Two thirds of the patients had colon cancer while one third rectal cancer, 54% of the patients were male and 35% were older than 70 years. In total, 59% of patients had stage III disease and 15% had metastatic disease at diagnosis. Most colon cancer patients (99%) were therapy-naïve at the time of surgery, while many rectal cancer patients had received pre-operative treatment (61%) (Table S1). The TMAs were stained with three different panels of immune markers along with pan-cytokeratin and DAPI as nuclear stain. Examples of multiplex immunofluorescent images are shown in Figure 1a and the analysis pipeline is illustrated in Figure S1. The expression of different immune markers was combined to assign each cell to one of 15 immune cell subtypes (Figure 1b), including different lymphocytes, macrophages, natural killer (NK) cells, dendritic cells (DCs), and myeloid cells (Figure 1b). The density of immune cell subtypes was annotated in the stroma and tumor compartments of the tumor center and at the invasive margin, resulting in four different metrics for each immune cell class. Overall, the most abundant cell types were CD8 single positive cells and M1 macrophages with median (mean) values of 314 (832) and 431 (685) cells per mm^2, respectively. NK cells and NKT cells demonstrated very low overall density with 77 and 81% of the cases being negative, respectively (Figure 1c,d). Taken together, the infiltration of immune cells was highly variable between tumors and immune cell subclasses, spanning from 0 to 11,994 cells/mm^2.

3.2. Spatial Distribution of Immune Cells in CRC

Next, we performed case-wise comparisons between the four tissue regions (stroma and tumor in the tumor center and stroma and tumor in the invasion margin). When comparing infiltration in stroma against tumor compartments (Figures 1d, S2 and S3), most immune cell subsets were more abundant in the stroma. Only CD8 single positive cells (see Figure 1B for immune cell sub-classification) and myeloid cells were more numerous in the tumor compartment ($q < 0.001$, Mann–Whitney U test with Benjamini–Hochberg correction). The distribution of immune cells between the center of the tumor and the invasive margin were similar, with a few notable exceptions. The most striking difference was observed for T cells, which were more abundant in the tumor center (Figure S4). In conclusion, there was greater enrichment of immune infiltrate in the stroma compared to the tumor cell compartment, but no significant differences between tumor center and invasive margin.

3.3. Interrelationship of Immune Cells and Immune Scores

We hypothesized that immune cells of the same lineage infiltrate tumor tissue in a coordinated fashion. Therefore, we correlated the abundance of all immune cell subtypes to each other in the four analyzed tumor regions (Figure S5). Indeed, the correlations for each specific immune subclass between the four tissue regions of the same tumor sample were in generally high. Due to this observation, we summarized the immune cell values in a single score for each immune cell subclass. These scores were generated in analogy to the original Immunoscore® [3] by summarizing the cell densities in all four regions into one score ranging from 0 to 4 (Figure S1e). Analysis using the immune scores revealed interrelations between different immune cells, with the highest correlations between lymphocyte subtypes, and between M1 macrophages and CD8+ lymphocytes. Interestingly, NK and NKT cells correlated negatively to mature dendritic cells and plasmacytoid dendritic cells (mDCs and pDCs). There was also a negative correlation of T cells to myeloid cells and M2 macrophages (Figure 2a). In conclusion, we identified distinct dominating immune infiltration patterns when a set of immune cell subclasses infiltrate tumor tissue coordinately.

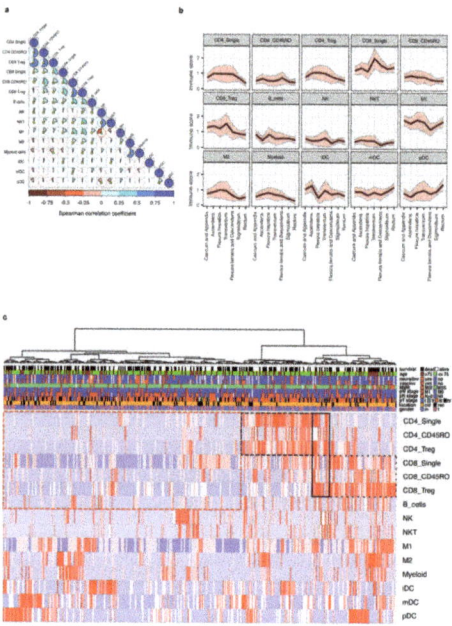

Figure 2. The immune scores interrelations, distribution across different clinical and pathological groups and unsupervised hierarchical clustering. (**a**) Graphical representation of Spearman's correlation matrix between immune scores. Pie charts and the intensity of shading represent the strength of correlation (Spearman correlation coefficient), blue color indicates direct while red color indicates inverse correlation. Asterisks indicate statistical significance ($p < 0.05$). (**b**) Immune scores mean levels (black line) and 95% confidence intervals (pink areas limited by gray lines) at specific primary tumor locations. For additional data, see Table S2. (**c**) Unsupervised hierarchical cluster analysis of immune scores. Cases were clustered based on the levels of immune scores. A total of 373 cases with complete immune score data from therapy-naïve patients were available. Clusters with enriched CD4 or CD8 cells are marked by dashed black line, while the cluster with low lymphocyte level is marked by dashed red line. For additional data, see Table S3.

3.4. Clustering of CRC Cases by Immune Cell Scores and Relation to Clinical Parameters

We next evaluated whether the immune scores were related to clinicopathological parameters. The findings largely replicated associations observed in region-restricted immune cell densities (Table S4). In line with published data [31,32], tumors of the right colon were characterized by higher immune scores for most T cell subclasses, M2 macrophages, and myeloid cells in comparison to the left colon and rectum, while pDC cells were enriched in the rectum. The most abundant immune infiltrates were seen in the tumors from flexura hepatica and colon transversum (Figure 2b and Table S2). Higher immune scores of CD8 single positive cells were observed in tumors with lower N stage. Most T cell subclasses, macrophages, and myeloid cells were enriched in MSI-H tumors. The M2 macrophages were associated with higher patient age.

To capture the dominating immune landscapes, we performed hierarchical clustering based on immune scores across all 373 therapy-naïve cases. The cluster analysis revealed two distinct groups (Figure 2c). The smaller cluster (n = 145) included tumors with high immune scores for T cells, reflecting an 'inflamed' phenotype. Interestingly, this cluster consisted of two distinct subgroups with high CD8 or CD4 scores. The second, larger cluster (n = 228), demonstrated low immune scores for T cells, representing the immune 'desert' phenotype. Within this cluster, several smaller subgroups were observed with either increased M2/myeloid cell scores, NK/NKT cell scores, immature dendritic cell (iDC) scores, or mDC/pDC scores. The 'inflamed' cluster was enriched with tumors (i) from the right colon, (ii) with high differentiation grade, (iii) without neural invasion, and (iv) with MSI. Other parameters, such as stage, sex, vascular engagement, local lymph node involvement, presence of distant metastases, or BRAF mutation status did not affect the distribution across the main clusters (Table S3). Interestingly, when we analyzed the impact on OS, the 'inflamed' and 'desert' immune clusters did not demonstrate significant differences. Taken together, tumors with an 'inflamed' or a 'desert' immune phenotype were clearly distinguishable, although, unexpectedly, not associated with improved or reduced survival.

3.5. Immune Scores and Survival

Clearly defined 'hot' and 'desert' tumors did not have significant survival differences. Therefore, we hypothesized that individual variations in different immune cell subsets may play more important roles in predicting patient survival and focused on the analyses of single immune scores. In a first set of survival analyses, we evaluated OS in all therapy naive patients (Figure 3a and Table S5); since preoperative treatment may influence the immune scores, these analyses were restricted to untreated patients. In line with previously published data [32], T cell immune scores had positive associations with improved survival, but only the immune score for CD8 single positive cells reached statistical significance (HR = 0.64, 95%CI [0.49–0.84], q = 0.014). In contrast, higher M2 macrophage scores were associated with shorter survival (HR = 1.50, 95%CI [1.20–2.00], q = 0.014). Due to the heterogeneity of CRC, both in terms of natural course of the disease and treatments, we investigated survival in specific patient subgroups with relevant endpoints. The same survival impact of CD8 cells and M2 macrophages was seen for radically operated stage I–III colon cancer patients, when disease-free survival (RFS) was analyzed. However, in the multivariable analysis, adjusted to clinicopathological factors, only single positive CD8 cells had a significant impact on prolonged RFS (HR = 0.64, 95%CI [0.41–0.98], p = 0.039) (Figure 3b and Tables S6 and S7). Subsequently, we evaluated stage IV patients separately. Immune scores for single positive CD4, single positive CD8 cells, and mDCs were associated with longer survival in the univariable analyses, although only the first retained statistical significance after adjustment for multiple testing (Figure 3c and Table S8). Thus, survival analysis in a therapy-naïve cohort and in colon cancer stage I–III confirmed previous findings indicating a major impact of CD8+ cells. In stage IV, single positive CD8+ were accompanied by mDCs and even stronger survival-predictive impact of single positive CD4+ cells.

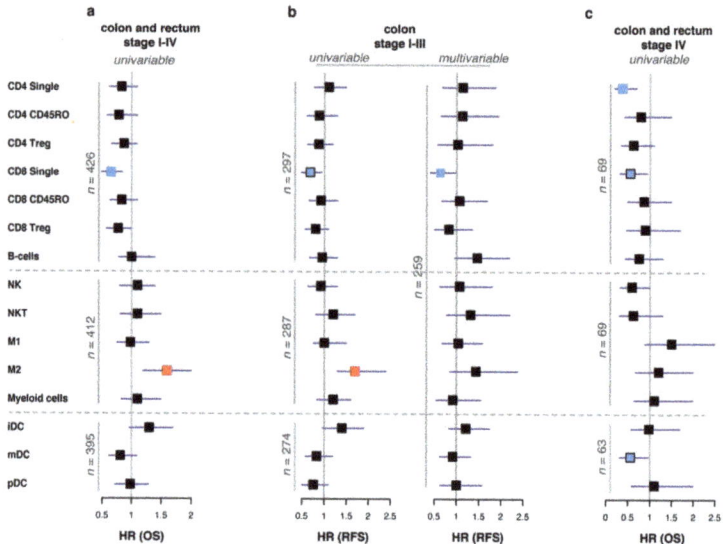

Figure 3. Immune scores predict patient survival. Forest plot of hazard ratios (HR) for immune scores in the univariable and multivariable Cox regression models. Filled squares indicate HR and whiskers represent 95% CI. Blue-colored squares indicate statistically significant ($p < 0.05$ and, where applicable, FDR q < 0.05) associations of the respective immune score with improved survival, while red squares represent association with reduced survival. Blue-colored squares with black contour indicate that the association was statistically significant in an individual test ($p < 0.05$) but lost statistical significance after adjustment for multiple testing (FDR q ≥ 0.05). (**a**) Univariable associations of immune scores with OS in a complete cohort of therapy-naïve patients. For detailed information see Table S5. (**b**) Association of immune scores with RFS in stage I–III colon cancer. Left panel illustrates the result of the univariable Cox regression models. Right panel illustrates the result of the multivariable Cox regression model, adjusted to clinicopathological parameters: pT, pN stages, tumor differentiation, patient age, surgery type (elective or acute), and adjuvant treatment. For detailed information see Supplementary Tables S6 and S7. (**c**) Univariable associations of immune scores with OS in stage IV therapy-naïve colorectal cancer patients. For detailed information, see Table S8.

3.6. Rectal Cancer

Rectal and colon cancer are often considered separate diseases [33]. This is also reflected by the different immune phenotype observed with lower numbers of CD4 single positive cells, CD4 Treg cells, and higher mDC, pDC, NKT cells in therapy-naïve rectal cancer compared to colon cancer (Table S2, Figure 4a), suggesting a lower level of natural immune activation in rectal cancer patients. Since most rectal cancer patients receive neoadjuvant radiotherapy or chemoradiotherapy (RT/CRT), we analyzed samples from 78 patients treated with RT/CRT. These patients were dichotomized regarding neoadjuvant treatment type, that was either (i) short-course RT (5 × 5 Gy in one week) followed by immediate surgery or (ii) short-course RT with delayed surgery (later than three weeks), CRT with delayed surgery, or short-course RT and chemotherapy in the interval to surgery. The analyses revealed that many immune cell counts decreased in the group that received RT/CRT therapy and was operated soon after the treatment and increased again in the delayed surgery group (Figure 4b), with the most characteristic profile seen for CD4+CD45RO+, CD8+CD45RO+, CD8 regulatory cells, M2 macrophages, iDCs, and pDCs. Interesting, CD4 and CD8 single cells, as well as B cells, showed quite a stable level of infiltration independent from neoadjuvant treatment type. None of the immune cell subclasses showed statistically significant differences when comparing tumors from primary surgery and those from the delayed surgery group, with the exception of M1 macrophages which demonstrated lower densities in the pretreated delayed surgery group. Taken together, the immune profiles differ between rectal and colon cancers in several aspects. In rectal cancer, the pattern reflects repopulation of the immune infiltrate in tumor tissue post radiation, following an initial radiation-induced depletion.

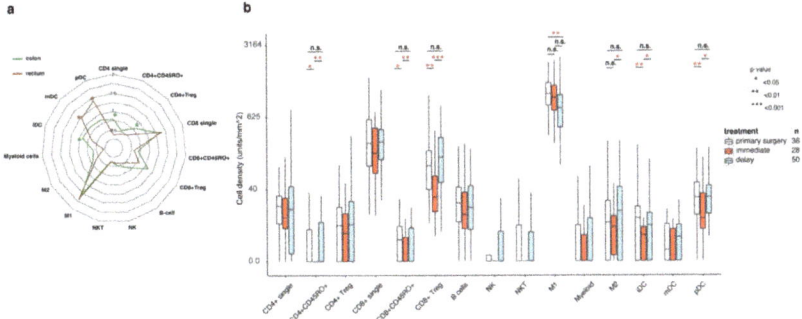

Figure 4. Immune infiltration in rectal cancers is restored after RT/CRT pre-treatment and delayed surgery, while vasculature is changed. (**a**) Radar plots of immune scores in therapy-naïve colon cancer patients (green) and rectal cancer patients (brown). (**b**) Immune infiltrate levels for patients who had primary surgery (white), radiation therapy followed by immediate surgery (<21 days), or delayed surgery after (chemo)radiotherapy. Numbers represent cell counts per mm^2, cube root transformed. Boxes show median values and interquartile range of the ratios, whiskers represent 1.5 IQR. Wilcoxon signed-rank test with Pratt method assuming asymptotic distribution was used for statistical analysis. Statistically significant differences: * $p < 0.05$, ** $p < 0.01$ and *** $p < 0.001$; not statistically significant differences: n.s.

4. Discussion

Tumors are composed of malignant cells and host elements of the tumor microenvironment which can support or suppress tumor progression and influence anti-cancer treatment. Although T cells have been considered as the most important anti-tumoral immune cells, detailed analysis of T cell subtypes and of other immune cells classes has been limited due to methodological difficulties. The functions of different immune cells can vary dramatically, depending on their activation and differentiation status. These differences are reflected in unique protein expression profiles, requiring techniques for multiplex in situ analysis to enable quantification of immune cell classes in clinical samples [34]. This study describes the immune cell microenvironment of CRC with 15 subgroups of immune cells at a hitherto unrivaled resolution. We applied a multiplex in situ staining method in combination with an advanced scanning and image analysis pipeline, akin to flow cytometry in situ, and analyzed 5968 individual multi-layer images of tissue defining a total of 39,078,450 cells. Each image was reviewed and thoroughly curated by a pathologist to exclude artefacts, staining defects, and necrotic areas. Furthermore, we considered the location of immune cells with respect to the stroma and tumor cell compartment as well as tumor regions in the central part or the invasion margin. To the best of our knowledge, this study is the first comprehensive spatial description of the immune landscape in CRC using a large population-based cohort and a multiplex immune cell identification.

In addition to commonly analyzed immune cells, like CD4 and CD8 cells, or FoxP3+ cells, we could accurately discriminate additional subsets of T lymphocytes. This increased the depth of cell sub-classification and, at the same time, improved the purity of each cell class. For instance, in conventional immunohistochemical analysis, FoxP3 positive cells have usually been considered regulatory T cells. Our approach refined cell counting by excluding FoxP3+ cells of non-lymphocyte or unknown origin, e.g., cancer cells or immune cells negative for other markers [28,35]. Furthermore, we found that a large proportion of the FoxP3+ cells are of the CD8+ lineage. CD8+FoxP3+ T cells have previously been suggested to be immunosuppressive CD8+ Tregs [36], although conflicting data exist showing that FoxP3 may be induced upon CD8+ T cell activation [37]. The unexpected high abundance of the specific cell type observed here should be the subject of further investigations.

We could clearly identify two distinct immune phenotypes: immune 'inflamed', characterized by high infiltration of lymphocytes, and immune 'desert' tumors. Interestingly, the 'inflamed' cluster in our analysis consisted of two subgroups with tumors with either CD4+ or CD8+ infiltration, and with only a small group of cases with concurrent high CD4 and CD8 levels. One may speculate that this finding might explain the general resistance of CRC to immune checkpoint inhibitors, considering that the presence of both immune cell linages is necessary for effective cancer cell elimination. Finally, the presence of dendritic cells, cells of the myeloid lineage, and NK cells define further subgroups within the immune desert background. Taken together our analyses refine the immune classification of CRC.

Despite being expectedly associated with dMMR/MSI-H cases, immune 'inflamed' tumors did not demonstrate a statistically significant association with improved patient survival. We next extended our analysis of individual immune cells in the context of clinical outcome. In an objective and unbiased analysis, previously reported relations were confirmed, but we could also uncover new information about the prognostic impact of further immune cell subclasses. Thus, Immunoscore®, which considers amount and localization of CD3 and CD8 cells showed an independent prognostic impact in a large multicenter prospective study [5]. Our CD8 immune score, although generated slightly differently from the Immunoscore®, had prognostic value in this cohort. Another immune cell subclass which emerged as a potent prognostic biomarker was the M2 macrophages. These cells have a broad and not yet fully understood role, but can be considered as protumoral elements and hallmarks of an immunosuppressive microenvironment [38]. Our findings suggest that the adverse effect of M2 macrophages should be considered in efforts to improve the prognostic accuracy of immune scoring systems.

Finally, we evaluated changes in the immune microenvironment of primary rectal cancer tissue subjected to preoperative RT/CRT. Our results demonstrated immune deprivation in tumor tissue undergoing resection directly after irradiation. The local immunosuppressive effect of irradiation is well established, and diverse radio-sensitivity of different immune cell types has been reported (reviewed in [39]). In agreement with these reports, we observed lower cell counts for all evaluated cell types. While there are several studies describing the immediate effect of RT/CRT on the tumor microenvironment, data about delayed effects, after weeks or months, are largely missing. Here, tumors resected after a delay following RT or CRT were characterized by an immune microenvironment largely similar to non-irradiated tumors. Accordingly, the immune suppressive effect of therapy should be considered when combinations of immune and conventional therapy are planned and may give a rationale for the sequencing of different therapy modalities in clinical trials. However, this simplistic explanation is complicated by the fact that the tumors that received or did not receive neoadjuvant treatment were not randomized, but rather selected according to stage and other characteristics on magnetic resonance imaging and type and intensity of therapy varied. The patients of the three analyzed groups, i.e., primary surgery, preoperative RT followed by immediate surgery, and preoperative RT/CRT followed by delayed surgery, are not comparable with regards to clinicopathological characteristics. With this caveat, the causes for the reported observations may be more elaborate than a direct link between RT/CRT and immune cell count. Overall, early (or so called 'good') rectal tumors [40] were operated immediately and had lower stages and few other risk factors (like extramural vascular invasion) than intermediate or 'bad' tumors subjected to RT and immediate surgery. Further, the group of locally advanced tumors receiving preoperative RT/CRT and delayed surgery (so called 'ugly' tumors) usually represent even more advanced tumor forms: stage cT4a/b or cT3 tumors with threatened/involved mesorectal fascia. Taking this together, the immune characteristics can not only be compared between neoadjuvant treatment groups, but also need to be normalized to their non-pretreated counterparts, with respective T and N-stages. With this background, using data presented in Table S4 as reference, one could expect 'ugly' tumors to have lower levels of immune infiltration. However, our data demonstrate that 'ugly' tumors after RT/CRT were immunologically comparable with non-pretreated 'good' tumors for most of the immune cells (except M1 macrophages). Therefore, we hypothesize that RT/CRT may convert 'ugly' tumors into immunologically 'good' ones. Although intriguing, this interpretation should be considered with caution because the number of cases is relatively small and due to the absence of proper non-treated reference tissue for RT/CRT cases. Further studies, involving patients randomized with regards to pre-operative treatment (in terms of the type of treatment and of the timing prior surgery) are therefore warranted. Ideally, such studies should include sampling before the neoadjuvant treatment.

5. Conclusions

In conclusion, to the best of our knowledge this study is the largest in terms of patient numbers and analyzed immune cell subclasses in CRC. We provide a detailed un-biased overview of the in situ immune landscape of CRC and were able to confirm but also extend the concept of cancer immunity. Many of the observations may have clinical relevance for CRC patients by paving the way for better cancer diagnostics or by providing hints to better target the immune microenvironment therapeutically. The applied multiplex technique and the analysis pipeline are applicable on common diagnostic tissue samples; therefore, it is possible that a comprehensive analysis of the immune microenvironment will become a part of the future clinical routine in the era of immunotherapy.

Supplementary Materials: The following are available online at https://www.mdpi.com/article/10.3390/cancers13215545/s1. Figure S1: flow chart illustrating the analytical pipeline: (a) original multispectral image 'mixed' channels; (b) multispectral multilayer image with separated channels; (c) schematic illustration of the image processing related to compartment segmentation. The Tumor (brown), Stroma (green) and Non-tissue (yellow) compartments are segmented, based on machine-learning image analysis approach. Areas of necrosis and artefacts were marked for exclusion from further analysis (gray). Immune cell infiltrates were analyzed or in Tumor and Stroma compartment separately. (d) Individual cell segmentation. (e) Generation of immune scores for each of 15 immune cell subclasses. Figure S2: pairwise comparison of immune cell densities in Tumor and Stroma compartments. Figure S3: illustration of the mean immune cell infiltration in invasive margin in tumor and stroma compartment. Numbers represent cell counts per mm^2, cube root transformed. Figure S4: pairwise comparison of immune cell densities in CT and IM. Figure S5: cross-correlation between the abundance of immune cells. (a) Graphical representation of the Spearman's correlation matrix of the abundance of immune cell subclasses. Circle size represents the strength of correlation, blue color indicates direct while red color indicates inversed correlation. (b, c, d, e) Graphical representation of the Spearman's correlation matrix of the abundance of immune cell subclasses only in: (b) stroma compartment in invasive margin; (c) tumor compartment in invasive margin; (d) stroma compartment in tumor center; (e) tumor compartment in tumor center, Table S1: baseline clinicopathological characteristics. Values are the number (percentage) unless indicated otherwise. Percentages may not add to 100% due to rounding. Table S2: immune scores in tumors with different clinical and pathological characteristics. Chi-square test was used for statistical analysis. Table S3: distribution of clinicopathological parameters in tumors within 'inflamed' and 'Immune desert' clusters. See also Figure 2c. Table S4: differences in immune cell distribution across cancer samples from patients with different clinicopathological characteristics. The direction of the association is illustrated by the location of the asterisks. *-$p < 0.05$; **-$p < 0.01$; ***-$p < 0.001$. Table S5: univariable associations of immune scores with OS in a complete cohort of therapy-naïve patients. See also Figure 3a. Table S6: association of immune scores with RFS in stage I–III colon cancer, univariable Cox regression models. See also Figure 3b, left panel. Table S7: association of immune scores with RFS in stage I–III colon cancer, multivariable Cox regression model, adjusted to clinicopathological parameters. See also Figure 3b, right panel. Table S8: univariable associations of immune scores with OS in stage VI therapy-naïve colon cancer patients. See also Figure 3c.

Author Contributions: Conceptualization, A.M., P.M., B.G. and T.S.; methodology, A.M.; software, A.M.; formal analysis, AM, A.M.-B., M.S., K.H., S.S. and P.-H.E.; resources, A.M., P.M., F.P., B.G. and T.S.; data curation, A.M., M.B. and I.H.; writing—original draft preparation, A.M. and P.M.; writing—review and editing, A.M., P.M., F.P., K.L., B.G. and T.S.; visualization, A.M. and J.E.; supervision, P.M, K.L., B.G. and T.S.; project administration, A.M. and P.-H.E.; funding acquisition, A.M., P.M., B.G. and T.S. All authors have read and agreed to the published version of the manuscript.

Funding: This study was supported by a postdoctoral grant from the Swedish Cancer Society to A.M. (CAN 2017/1066) and project grants from the Swedish Cancer Society to T.S. (CAN 2018/772), B.G. (CAN 2019/0382), and P.M. (CAN 2018/816); the Lions Cancer Foundation Uppsala to P.M.; and the Selanders foundation and P.O. Zetterling Foundation to A.M. U-CAN is supported by the Swedish Government (SRA CancerUU) and locally by Uppsala University and Region Uppsala.

Institutional Review Board Statement: The study was approved by the regional ethical committee in Uppsala, Sweden (Dnr 2010/198 and Dnr 2015/419).

Informed Consent Statement: Informed consent was obtained from all subjects involved in the study.

Data Availability Statement: Data regarding methodology, image analysis, curation and data processing, and raw data of stroma fraction are available from the corresponding author.

Conflicts of Interest: The authors declare no conflict of interest.

References

1. Sung, H.; Ferlay, J.; Siegel, R.L.; Laversanne, M.; Soerjomataram, I.; Jemal, A.; Bray, F. Global Cancer Statistics 2020: GLOBOCAN Estimates of Incidence and Mortality Worldwide for 36 Cancers in 185 Countries. *CA Cancer J. Clin.* **2021**, *71*, 209–249. [CrossRef]
2. Guinney, J.; Dienstmann, R.; Wang, X.; De Reynies, A.; Schlicker, A.; Soneson, C.; Marisa, L.; Roepman, P.; Nyamundanda, G.; Angelino, P.; et al. The consensus molecular subtypes of colorectal cancer. *Nat. Med.* **2015**, *21*, 1350–1356. [CrossRef] [PubMed]
3. Galon, J.; Fridman, W.H.; Pages, F. The adaptive immunologic microenvironment in colorectal cancer: A novel perspective. *Cancer Res.* **2007**, *67*, 1883–1886. [CrossRef] [PubMed]
4. Mlecnik, B.; Tosolini, M.; Kirilovsky, A.; Berger, A.; Bindea, G.; Meatchi, T.; Bruneval, P.; Trajanoski, Z.; Fridman, W.H.; Pages, F.; et al. Histopathologic-based prognostic factors of colorectal cancers are associated with the state of the local immune reaction. *J. Clin. Oncol.* **2011**, *29*, 610–618. [CrossRef]
5. Pages, F.; Mlecnik, B.; Marliot, F.; Bindea, G.; Ou, F.S.; Bifulco, C.; Lugli, A.; Zlobec, I.; Rau, T.T.; Berger, M.D.; et al. International validation of the consensus Immunoscore for the classification of colon cancer: A prognostic and accuracy study. *Lancet* **2018**, *391*, 2128–2139. [CrossRef]
6. Edin, S.; Kaprio, T.; Hagstrom, J.; Larsson, P.; Mustonen, H.; Bockelman, C.; Strigard, K.; Gunnarsson, U.; Haglund, C.; Palmqvist, R. The Prognostic Importance of CD20($^+$) B lymphocytes in Colorectal Cancer and the Relation to Other Immune Cell subsets. *Sci. Rep.* **2019**, *9*, 19997. [CrossRef]
7. Coppola, A.; Arriga, R.; Lauro, D.; Del Principe, M.I.; Buccisano, F.; Maurillo, L.; Palomba, P.; Venditti, A.; Sconocchia, G. NK Cell Inflammation in the Clinical Outcome of Colorectal Carcinoma. *Front. Med.* **2015**, *2*, 33. [CrossRef]
8. Schreiber, R.D.; Old, L.J.; Smyth, M.J. Cancer immunoediting: Integrating immunity's roles in cancer suppression and promotion. *Science* **2011**, *331*, 1565–1570. [CrossRef]
9. Couzin-Frankel, J. Breakthrough of the year 2013. Cancer immunotherapy. *Science* **2013**, *342*, 1432–1433. [CrossRef]
10. Havel, J.J.; Chowell, D.; Chan, T.A. The evolving landscape of biomarkers for checkpoint inhibitor immunotherapy. *Nat. Rev. Cancer* **2019**, *19*, 133–150. [CrossRef]
11. Joyce, J.A.; Fearon, D.T. T cell exclusion, immune privilege, and the tumor microenvironment. *Science* **2015**, *348*, 74–80. [CrossRef] [PubMed]
12. Chen, D.S.; Mellman, I. Elements of cancer immunity and the cancer-immune set point. *Nature* **2017**, *541*, 321–330. [CrossRef]
13. Smyrk, T.C.; Watson, P.; Kaul, K.; Lynch, H.T. Tumor-infiltrating lymphocytes are a marker for microsatellite instability in colorectal carcinoma. *Cancer* **2001**, *91*, 2417–2422. [CrossRef]
14. Dolcetti, R.; Viel, A.; Doglioni, C.; Russo, A.; Guidoboni, M.; Capozzi, E.; Vecchiato, N.; Macri, E.; Fornasarig, M.; Boiocchi, M. High prevalence of activated intraepithelial cytotoxic T lymphocytes and increased neoplastic cell apoptosis in colorectal carcinomas with microsatellite instability. *Am. J. Pathol.* **1999**, *154*, 1805–1813. [CrossRef]
15. Sjoblom, T.; Jones, S.; Wood, L.D.; Parsons, D.W.; Lin, J.; Barber, T.D.; Mandelker, D.; Leary, R.J.; Ptak, J.; Silliman, N.; et al. The consensus coding sequences of human breast and colorectal cancers. *Science* **2006**, *314*, 268–274. [CrossRef] [PubMed]
16. Lu, Y.C.; Robbins, P.F. Cancer immunotherapy targeting neoantigens. *Semin. Immunol.* **2016**, *28*, 22–27. [CrossRef]
17. Heemskerk, B.; Kvistborg, P.; Schumacher, T.N. The cancer antigenome. *EMBO J.* **2013**, *32*, 194–203. [CrossRef]
18. Le, D.T.; Uram, J.N.; Wang, H.; Bartlett, B.R.; Kemberling, H.; Eyring, A.D.; Skora, A.D.; Luber, B.S.; Azad, N.S.; Laheru, D.; et al. PD-1 Blockade in Tumors with Mismatch-Repair Deficiency. *N. Engl. J. Med.* **2015**, *372*, 2509–2520. [CrossRef]

19. Overman, M.J.; McDermott, R.; Leach, J.L.; Lonardi, S.; Lenz, H.J.; Morse, M.A.; Desai, J.; Hill, A.; Axelson, M.; Moss, R.A.; et al. Nivolumab in patients with metastatic DNA mismatch repair-deficient or microsatellite instability-high colorectal cancer (CheckMate 142): An open-label, multicentre, phase 2 study. *Lancet Oncol.* **2017**, *18*, 1182–1191. [CrossRef]
20. Overman, M.J.; Lonardi, S.; Wong, K.Y.M.; Lenz, H.J.; Gelsomino, F.; Aglietta, M.; Morse, M.A.; Van Cutsem, E.; McDermott, R.; Hill, A.; et al. Durable Clinical Benefit with Nivolumab Plus Ipilimumab in DNA Mismatch Repair-Deficient/Microsatellite Instability-High Metastatic Colorectal Cancer. *J. Clin. Oncol.* **2018**, *36*, 773–779. [CrossRef]
21. Marmorino, F.; Boccaccino, A.; Germani, M.M.; Falcone, A.; Cremolini, C. Immune Checkpoint Inhibitors in pMMR Metastatic Colorectal Cancer: A Tough Challenge. *Cancers* **2020**, *12*, 2317. [CrossRef] [PubMed]
22. Bindea, G.; Mlecnik, B.; Tosolini, M.; Kirilovsky, A.; Waldner, M.; Obenauf, A.C.; Angell, H.; Fredriksen, T.; Lafontaine, L.; Berger, A.; et al. Spatiotemporal dynamics of intratumoral immune cells reveal the immune landscape in human cancer. *Immunity* **2013**, *39*, 782–795. [CrossRef] [PubMed]
23. Kather, J.N.; Suarez-Carmona, M.; Charoentong, P.; Weis, C.A.; Hirsch, D.; Bankhead, P.; Horning, M.; Ferber, D.; Kel, I.; Herpel, E.; et al. Topography of cancer-associated immune cells in human solid tumors. *eLife* **2018**, *7*, e36967. [CrossRef] [PubMed]
24. Berry, S.; Giraldo, N.A.; Green, B.F.; Cottrell, T.R.; Stein, J.E.; Engle, E.L.; Xu, H.; Ogurtsova, A.; Roberts, C.; Wang, D.; et al. Analysis of multispectral imaging with the AstroPath platform informs efficacy of PD-1 blockade. *Science* **2021**, *372*, 2609. [CrossRef] [PubMed]
25. Glimelius, B.; Melin, B.; Enblad, G.; Alafuzoff, I.; Beskow, A.; Ahlstrom, H.; Bill-Axelson, A.; Birgisson, H.; Bjor, O.; Edqvist, P.H.; et al. U-CAN: A prospective longitudinal collection of biomaterials and clinical information from adult cancer patients in Sweden. *Acta Oncol.* **2018**, *57*, 187–194. [CrossRef] [PubMed]
26. Herrera, M.; Mezheyeuski, A.; Villabona, L.; Corvigno, S.; Strell, C.; Klein, C.; Holzlwimmer, G.; Glimelius, B.; Masucci, G.; Sjoblom, T.; et al. Prognostic Interactions between FAP$^+$ Fibroblasts and CD8a$^+$ T Cells in Colon Cancer. *Cancers* **2020**, *12*, 3238. [CrossRef]
27. Mezheyeuski, A.; Bergsland, C.H.; Backman, M.; Djureinovic, D.; Sjoblom, T.; Bruun, J.; Micke, P. Multispectral imaging for quantitative and compartment-specific immune infiltrates reveals distinct immune profiles that classify lung cancer patients. *J. Pathol.* **2018**, *244*, 421–431. [CrossRef]
28. Lundgren, S.; Elebro, J.; Heby, M.; Nodin, B.; Leandersson, K.; Micke, P.; Jirstrom, K.; Mezheyeuski, A. Quantitative, qualitative and spatial analysis of lymphocyte infiltration in periampullary and pancreatic adenocarcinoma. *Int. J. Cancer* **2020**, *146*, 3461–3473. [CrossRef]
29. Micke, P.; Strell, C.; Mattsson, J.; Martin-Bernabe, A.; Brunnstrom, H.; Huvila, J.; Sund, M.; Warnberg, F.; Ponten, F.; Glimelius, B.; et al. The prognostic impact of the tumour stroma fraction: A machine learning-based analysis in 16 human solid tumour types. *EBioMedicine* **2021**, *65*, 103269. [CrossRef]
30. Punt, C.J.; Buyse, M.; Kohne, C.H.; Hohenberger, P.; Labianca, R.; Schmoll, H.J.; Pahlman, L.; Sobrero, A.; Douillard, J.Y. Endpoints in adjuvant treatment trials: A systematic review of the literature in colon cancer and proposed definitions for future trials. *J. Natl. Cancer Inst.* **2007**, *99*, 998–1003. [CrossRef]
31. Ogino, S.; Nosho, K.; Irahara, N.; Meyerhardt, J.A.; Baba, Y.; Shima, K.; Glickman, J.N.; Ferrone, C.R.; Mino-Kenudson, M.; Tanaka, N.; et al. Lymphocytic reaction to colorectal cancer is associated with longer survival, independent of lymph node count, microsatellite instability, and CpG island methylator phenotype. *Clin. Cancer Res.* **2009**, *15*, 6412–6420. [CrossRef]
32. Galon, J.; Costes, A.; Sanchez-Cabo, F.; Kirilovsky, A.; Mlecnik, B.; Lagorce-Pages, C.; Tosolini, M.; Camus, M.; Berger, A.; Wind, P.; et al. Type, density, and location of immune cells within human colorectal tumors predict clinical outcome. *Science* **2006**, *313*, 1960–1964. [CrossRef]
33. Hong, T.S.; Clark, J.W.; Haigis, K.M. Cancers of the colon and rectum: Identical or fraternal twins? *Cancer Discov.* **2012**, *2*, 117–121. [CrossRef] [PubMed]
34. Taube, J.M.; Akturk, G.; Angelo, M.; Engle, E.L.; Gnjatic, S.; Greenbaum, S.; Greenwald, N.F.; Hedvat, C.V.; Hollmann, T.J.; Juco, J.; et al. The Society for Immunotherapy of Cancer statement on best practices for multiplex immunohistochemistry (IHC) and immunofluorescence (IF) staining and validation. *J. Immunother. Cancer* **2020**, *8*, e000155. [CrossRef]
35. Karanikas, V.; Speletas, M.; Zamanakou, M.; Kalala, F.; Loules, G.; Kerenidi, T.; Barda, A.K.; Gourgoulianis, K.I.; Germenis, A.E. Foxp3 expression in human cancer cells. *J. Transl. Med.* **2008**, *6*, 19. [CrossRef] [PubMed]
36. Yu, Y.; Ma, X.; Gong, R.; Zhu, J.; Wei, L.; Yao, J. Recent advances in CD8($^+$) regulatory T cell research. *Oncol. Lett.* **2018**, *15*, 8187–8194. [CrossRef] [PubMed]
37. Kmieciak, M.; Gowda, M.; Graham, L.; Godder, K.; Bear, H.D.; Marincola, F.M.; Manjili, M.H. Human T cells express CD25 and Foxp3 upon activation and exhibit effector/memory phenotypes without any regulatory/suppressor function. *J. Transl. Med.* **2009**, *7*, 89. [CrossRef]
38. Yu, T.; Gan, S.; Zhu, Q.; Dai, D.; Li, N.; Wang, H.; Chen, X.; Hou, D.; Wang, Y.; Pan, Q.; et al. Modulation of M2 macrophage polarization by the crosstalk between Stat6 and Trim24. *Nat. Commun.* **2019**, *10*, 4353. [CrossRef]
39. Jarosz-Biej, M.; Smolarczyk, R.; Cichon, T.; Kulach, N. Tumor Microenvironment as A "Game Changer" in Cancer Radiotherapy. *Int. J. Mol. Sci.* **2019**, *20*, 3212. [CrossRef]
40. Blomqvist, L.; Glimelius, B. The 'good', the 'bad', and the 'ugly' rectal cancers. *Acta Oncol.* **2008**, *47*, 5–8. [CrossRef]

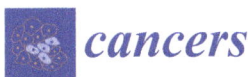

Article

Changes in Methylation across Structural and MicroRNA Genes Relevant for Progression and Metastasis in Colorectal Cancer

Nitin Patil [1,†], Mohammed L. Abba [1,†], Chan Zhou [1], Shujian Chang [1], Timo Gaiser [2], Jörg H. Leupold [1] and Heike Allgayer [1,*]

[1] Department of Experimental Surgery—Cancer Metastasis, Mannheim Medical Faculty, Ruprecht Karls University of Heidelberg, 68167 Mannheim, Germany; Nitin.Patil@medma.uni-heidelberg.de (N.P.); Mohammed.Abba@medma.uni-heidelberg.de (M.L.A.); chan.zhou@medma.uni-heidelberg.de (C.Z.); xdw@jiangnan.edu.cn (S.C.); joerg.leupold@medma.uni-heidelberg.de (J.H.L.)

[2] Institute of Pathology, Mannheim Medical Faculty, Ruprecht Karls University of Heidelberg, Theodor Kutzer Ufer 1-3, 68167 Mannheim, Germany; Timo.Gaiser@umm.de

* Correspondence: heike.allgayer@medma.uni-heidelberg.de; Tel.: +49-(0)621-383-71630 or +49-(0)621-383-71635; Fax: +49-(0)621-383-71631

† Shared first authors and equal contributions.

Citation: Patil, N.; Abba, M.L.; Zhou, C.; Chang, S.; Gaiser, T.; Leupold, J.H.; Allgayer, H. Changes in Methylation across Structural and MicroRNA Genes Relevant for Progression and Metastasis in Colorectal Cancer. *Cancers* **2021**, *13*, 5951. https://doi.org/10.3390/cancers13235951

Academic Editor: David Wong

Received: 10 November 2021
Accepted: 24 November 2021
Published: 26 November 2021

Publisher's Note: MDPI stays neutral with regard to jurisdictional claims in published maps and institutional affiliations.

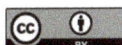

Copyright: © 2021 by the authors. Licensee MDPI, Basel, Switzerland. This article is an open access article distributed under the terms and conditions of the Creative Commons Attribution (CC BY) license (https://creativecommons.org/licenses/by/4.0/).

Simple Summary: Changes in the expression of key molecules such as microRNAs (miRs) can drive or suppress carcinogenesis and metastasis. A number of established transcriptional and genetic mechanisms regulate miR gene expression, but methylation/epigenetics have been analyzed less. Here, we systematically evaluated genome-wide methylation changes, focusing on miR, downstream targets, and further genes relevant for metastasis in colorectal cancers (CRC), including CpG islands, open seas, and north and south shore regions. A number of miRs deregulated during CRC progression/metastasis were significantly affected by methylation changes, especially within CpG islands and open seas. Several of these miRs cooperate in cancer- and metastasis-related pathways, while methylation changes otherwise primarily affect protein-coding genes. Our results highlight alternative routes to the transcriptional and genetic control of miR and further gene expression relevant for CRC progression and metastasis by changes in gene methylation. They also bear important therapeutic implications since drugs that alter methylation states are now in clinical use.

Abstract: MiRs are important players in cancer and primarily genetic/transcriptional means of regulating their gene expression are known. However, epigenetic changes modify gene expression significantly. Here, we evaluated genome-wide methylation changes focusing on miR genes from primary CRC and corresponding normal tissues. Differentially methylated CpGs spanning CpG islands, open seas, and north and south shore regions were evaluated, with the largest number of changes observed within open seas and islands. Kyoto Encyclopedia of Genes and Genomes (KEGG) pathway enrichment analysis revealed several of these miRs to act in important cancer-related pathways, including phosphatidylinositol 3-kinase (PI3K)–protein kinase B (Akt) and mitogen-activated protein kinase (MAPK) pathways. We found 18 miR genes to be significantly differentially methylated, with MIR124-2, MIR124-3, MIR129-2, MIR137, MIR34B, MIR34C, MIR548G, MIR762, and MIR9-3 hypermethylated and MIR1204, MIR17, MIR17HG, MIR18A, MIR19A, MIR19B1, MIR20A, MIR548F5, and MIR548I4 hypomethylated in CRC tumor compared with normal tissue, most of these miRs having been shown to regulate steps of metastasis. Generally, methylation changes were distributed evenly across all chromosomes with predominance for chromosomes 1/2 and protein-coding genes. Interestingly, chromosomes abundantly affected by methylation changes globally were rarely affected by methylation changes within miR genes. Our findings support additional mechanisms of methylation changes affecting (miR) genes that orchestrate CRC progression and metastasis.

Keywords: genome-wide methylation array; colorectal cancer; methylation; miRNA; metastasis

1. Introduction

CRC is presently the second leading cause of cancer deaths and third most commonly diagnosed cancer worldwide [1]. The mortality associated with CRC is largely due to its ability to establish distant metastases, with the 5-year survival rate for metastatic CRC being approximately 10% without treatment [2].

The successive acquisition of genetic and epigenetic alterations has been shown to drive the initiation and progression of adenomas to carcinomas in CRC. These mediate the transformation of a normal colorectal epithelium to a benign adenoma, and the accumulation of further multiple genetic and epigenetic changes in particular clones can result in an invasive and metastatic phenotype [3–5]. A multitude of research efforts have sought to identify and investigate the key molecules involved in the initiation and progression of CRC. A large number of molecular drivers have been identified, of which molecules such as adenomatous polyposis coli (APC), tumor protein P53 (TP53), kirsten rat sarcoma virus (KRAS), and catenin beta-1 (CTNNB1) appear to play crucial roles [4].

Almost three decades ago, a group of small non-coding RNAs was identified, which renders important mediators of post-transcriptional gene regulation. This group of molecules, also called miRs, represents small endogenous RNA molecules (18–22 nt) that repress the expression of protein-coding genes [6,7], the predominant function of miRs being RNA silencing and the negative regulation of gene expression at the post-transcriptional level [8]. The interaction of miR seed sequences with sequences in the 3′ untranslated region (UTR) of their target mRNAs leads to translational repression. Interestingly, miR binding sites have also been identified in other mRNA regions, including the 5′ UTR and coding sequence as well as within promoter regions [9,10]. The analyses of large patient datasets of diverse cancer entities identified over 10,000 miR–mRNA interactions to be associated with cancer progression. Almost 40% of these interactions exhibited a high fidelity of miR function [11]. The aberrational regulation of miRs has been shown to interfere with several important signaling cascades including epidermal growth factor receptor (EGFR), kirsten rat sarcoma virus (KRAS), PI3K, Wingless and Int-1 (Wnt), myelocytomatosis (Myc), HIPO and Notch pathways, amongst others, which are vital to tumor progression and metastasis [12]. In addition, an accumulating number of studies, including our own, make it clear that miRs are important players in different steps of metastasis in multiple cancer types, including CRC [5,13–17]. The means of regulation of miR gene expression in this context can be different; however, most studies so far have investigated, and demonstrated, changes in transcription as major mechanisms of regulating miR expression during metastasis [17,18].

Epigenetic modifications have emerged as a major mechanistic hallmark that drives malignant diseases, with the most prominent epigenetic changes comprising the methylation of CpG islands, the methylation of histone proteins, and deacetylation [19]. It is now well established that aberrant epigenetic modifications play a critical role in cancer progression and metastasis irrespective of genetic lesions [20]. Comparatively, malignant cells have been described to be typically hypermethylated at CpG islands [21].

In this study of colorectal carcinomas, we explored genome-wide methylation changes, specifically focusing on miRs genes due to the important role they play in cancer progression and metastasis. Toward this end, we selected all miR gene regions that were affected by methylation including the gene body, islands, shelves, shores, and open seas. KEGG pathway enrichment analysis revealed that the mRNAs these miRs regulate play important roles in cancer progression and metastasis. Using a two-fold (up or down) differential methylation difference between tumor and normal samples, we found 18 miRs to be differentially methylated in tumor samples, nine of them being hypomethylated and nine hypermethylated as compared to normal colorectal tissue. In line with the literature and own previous studies, these miRs, and their deregulated expression in CRC, have been identified to play potent roles in cancer progression and metastasis. Our findings support additional mechanisms orchestrating CRC progression and metastasis by affecting gene and miR regulation via methylation.

2. Material and Methods

2.1. Tissue Material and Ethical Consent

In general, all of the samples were analyzed completely anonymized, retrospectively, and without the possibility to track back any results to the individual patient. The study was approved by the local board of ethics (Medical Ethics Committee II, University of Heidelberg), ethics approval: 2012-608R-MA, to T.G. Information regarding UICC staging and pathological grading were collected in line with the stipulated international formats [22,23]. Tissue specimens from tumor and corresponding normal mucosa distant from the tumor site were collected after macroscopic verification by a pathologist, and frozen immediately in liquid nitrogen. In total, samples of 24 patients were analyzed in the study (24 tumor and 24 matched normal samples). All patients were of Caucasian descent.

2.2. Genomic DNA Isolation

Genomic DNA was isolated from resected tumor and corresponding normal samples using the QIAamp DNA mini kit (Qiagen GmbH, Hilden Germany) according to the manufacturer's instructions. DNA concentration was measured with the Nanodrop spectrophotometer and 500–1000 ng of DNA/sample were used in later experiments.

2.3. Methylation Profiling

DNA samples were submitted to the Genomics and Proteomics core facility of the German Cancer Research Center (DKFZ), Heidelberg Germany for methylation profiling using the Illumina Infinium 450 K Methylation Array according to the standard protocol. In summary, DNA samples were bisulfite converted using the Zymo EZ DNA Methylation Kit. Then, the bisulfite converted DNA was denatured and further amplified. Afterwards, the DNA were fragmented using enzymatic digestion with FMS fragmentation solution and then precipitated. Then, the re-suspended DNA fragments were hybridized to the BeadChip. After an overnight incubation step, the un-hybridized probes were washed away, and the BeadChip was stained and scanned with the Illumina iScan system.

2.4. Bioinformatics Analysis

The level of methylation was determined at each locus by the intensity of the two possible fluorescent signals from the C (methylated) and T (unmethylated) alleles. Pre-processing was done in two steps, using the R package "minfi" [24]. Background subtraction was followed by normalizing to internal controls that were applied to the Meth and Unmeth intensities separately. Filtering was done according to Sturm et al. [25] by the removal of probes targeting the X and Y chromosomes, the removal of probes containing a single-nucleotide polymorphism (dbSNP132 Common) within five base pairs, by including the targeted CpG site, and probes not mapping uniquely to the human reference genome (hg19), allowing for one mismatch. In total, 438,370 probes were subjected to analysis. For analysis, the relative level of methylation was calculated as the ratio of the methylated probe signal to total locus signal intensity (beta value).

Pairwise comparisons were performed using the Wilcoxon signed-rank test. For multiple testing, the step-down maxT testing procedure was applied to provide strong control of the family-wise type I error rate [26]. Genome annotation was based on the University of California Santa Cruz (UCSC) Genome Browser (http://genome.ucsc.edu, accessed on 20 September 2021; UCSC Genome Bioinformatics, Santa Cruz, CA, USA), whereas miR annotation was from miRBase (http://www.mirbase.org, accessed on 20 September 2021) Release 22.

2.5. Data Availability

All methylation data discussed in the manuscript have been deposited in the NCBI Gene Expression Omnibus and can be accessed using the GEO Series accession number GSE184494 (https://www.ncbi.nlm.nih.gov/geo/query/acc.cgi?acc=GSE184494, accessed on 20 September 2021).

2.6. KEGG Analysis

All potential mRNA targets of all miR genes were individually identified using the Targetscan and miRDB online tools. Then, the common gene signatures of the individual miRs were imported into the DAVID online tool (david.abcc.ncifcrf.gov, accessed on 29 September 2021), and all functional KEGG pathways were identified [27]. All significant pathways were considered ($p < 0.05$), and the most frequently delineated pathways were used in the final analysis. The generated pathways that were irrelevant to cancer in general or CRC specifically were manually curated. Then, the resulting list of pathways was used to generate a heat map in Microsoft Excel based on the frequency of occurrence of the given miRs. Furthermore, canonical pathways that interacted with the highest number of miRs as well as miRs that individually interacted with the most pathways were delineated.

2.7. Ingenuity Pathway Analysis (IPA)

The IPA pathway tool from QIAGEN Germany was used for the analysis. All predicted targets of mature miRs encoded by hyper and hypomethylated mRNA genes were imported into the ingenuity pathway core analysis pipeline using the default settings with the exception of following changes. Node types were limited to canonical pathways, disease, function, fusion gene product, G-protein coupled receptor, mature miR, miR, and others. Species was limited only to humans. Tissues and cell filters were limited to cancer or colorectal disease. The mutation filter was set to functional effect and translational impact. From the resulting pathways, only the top hit pathways with oncogenic relevance were selected.

3. Results

3.1. Methylation Array and Associated Bioinformatics: General Distribution of Differentially Methylated Sites between Coding, Non-Coding, and Intergenic Regions

Tissue samples from 24 matched primary CRC and corresponding normal colorectal tissue pairs were profiled on the Infinium 450 K Bead Array. The analyzed samples were completely anonymized, without the possibility to track back any results to the individual patient. The median age of the patients at diagnosis was 65 years; 38% were females, and 62% were males. There was no evidence of a familiar hereditary background in all cases. Only 4% of the patients had pT1 stages, while 21% had pT2, 58% had pT3, and 17% had pT4 stages, this being comparable to the distribution of stages within other, also larger western CRC cohorts [1,28]. Half (50%) of the patients had pN0 and 50% had pN1-2 stage. As far as clinical information was available, five patients showed clinically diagnosed metastasis (M1) to the liver (Supplementary Table S1).

The output of differentially methylated genes between colorectal tumor and corresponding normal tissues comprised both protein and non-protein coding genes. For each methylated CpG site, the median tumor and normal beta values, together with p-values, were analyzed using the Wilcoxon Signed-Rank test. For all genes that were significantly differentially methylated ($p \leq 0.05$), the median difference beta values were calculated to determine if the genes were hyper- or hypomethylated with respect to the normal colorectal samples. The methylated sites for the genes were also mapped to correspond to CpG islands, north and south shores, north and south shelves, as well as open seas. We took the CpG island definition of a 200 bp region of DNA with a GC content higher than 50% and an observed CpG versus expected CpG ratio greater or equal to 0.6. We considered methylation sites up to 2 kb upstream/downstream of CpG islands as north and south shores, respectively, and shelves as −4 kb upstream/downstream of CpG islands. Open seas represented isolated CpGs within the genome >4 kb from CGIs. Moreover, the transcriptional start site (TSS) TSS200 and TSS1500 regions represent sites that are located up to −200 and −1500 bp upstream of the transcriptional start site, respectively. The definitions of north and south shores, north and south shelves, and open seas were applied as previously published [29].

Globally, 34.8% of differentially methylated CpGs occurred in islands, 18.2% occurred in shores, 7.6% occurred in shelves, and 39.4% occurred in open seas (Figure 1A). Specifically, 18% of the methylated regions were found within the TSS1500, 11% were found in the TSS200 site, respectively; 16% were found within 5′ UTRs, 9% were found within the 1st exons of genes, 42% were found in the gene body, and 4% were found in the 3′ UTR regions, respectively (Figure 1B). Regions neighboring the gene body at both the 5′ and 3′ flanking regions also showed significant methylation differences, with 5′ UTRs accounting for 4657 and the 3′ UTRs with 1045 differentially methylated sites, respectively (Figure 1B). More than half (65%) of the aberrant DNA methylation sites were associated with protein-coding genes, 31% were associated with genes for non-coding RNAs (including miR genes, long non-coding RNAs (lncRNA) genes, etc.), and 4% were located in intergenic regions (Figure 1C).

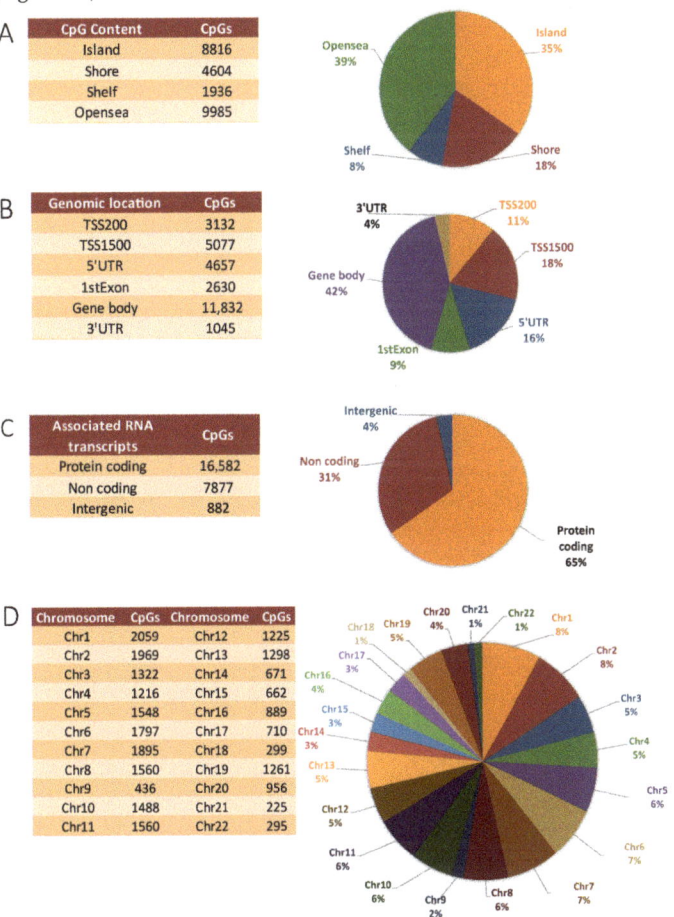

Figure 1. DNA methylation landscape in CRC tissues. (**A**) Genomic distribution of CpG sites in relation to CpG islands and neighboring shores, shelves, and open seas. (**B**) Functional genomic and neighborhood location and distribution of methylated CpG sites. (**C**) Distribution of CpGs in relation to coding, non-coding, and intergenic regions, respectively. (**D**) Chromosome distribution of the differential methylated sites.

As shown in Figure 1D, the overall changes in DNA methylation were mainly seen within chromosome 1 (8.13%), followed by chromosomes 2 (7.77%) and chromosome 7 (7.48%). The least affected chromosomes were chromosome 9 (1.7%), chromosome 18 and

22 (both 1.1%), and chromosome 21 (0.88%). The global methylation pattern across all chromosomes, including the proportions of both hyper- and hypomethylated CpGs in tumor versus corresponding normal tissue, and their relations to the specific genomic features (islands, shelves, shores, and open seas) is represented in Table 1. Our global analysis shows that methylation changes predominantly affected protein-coding genes. Methylation preferentially occurred within gene bodies, and the chromosomal distribution was relatively proportional to chromosome size, with a few exceptions. The majority of methylation changes were seen on chromosomes 1, 2, 7, 6, 11, 8, 5, 10, 3, 13, 19, 12, and 4, respectively, in decreasing order of magnitude. The other autosomes were less affected, with chromosomes 21, 22, 18, and 9 showing the least changes in their methylation pattern in tumor as compared to normal tissue (Figure 1D).

Table 1. Overview of genome-wide methylation burden across all chromosomes. The number of hypermethylation and hypomethylation events in relation to CpG islands and neighborhood regions are given.

Chromosome (Chr)	Status	OpenSea	Island	Shelf	Shore
Chr1	Hypomethylated	786	39	142	179
	Hypermethylated	57	636	10	210
Chr2	Hypomethylated	861	40	137	168
	Hypermethylated	36	568	5	154
Chr3	Hypomethylated	532	17	73	70
	Hypermethylated	30	430	15	155
Chr4	Hypomethylated	442	5	83	85
	Hypermethylated	12	462	7	120
Chr5	Hypomethylated	588	28	91	118
	Hypermethylated	62	541	4	116
Chr6	Hypomethylated	781	13	96	111
	Hypermethylated	75	503	17	201
Chr7	Hypomethylated	728	55	151	195
	Hypermethylated	50	533	21	162
Chr8	Hypomethylated	597	29	93	142
	Hypermethylated	26	502	7	164
Chr9	Hypomethylated	106	13	26	69
	Hypermethylated	12	177	5	28
Chr10	Hypomethylated	506	26	101	121
	Hypermethylated	40	573	5	116
Chr11	Hypomethylated	686	19	84	131
	Hypermethylated	41	448	4	147
Chr12	Hypomethylated	485	18	78	115
	Hypermethylated	43	357	20	109
Chr13	Hypomethylated	517	17	85	97
	Hypermethylated	29	372	11	170
Chr14	Hypomethylated	253	9	39	58
	Hypermethylated	13	220	5	74
Chr15	Hypomethylated	313	9	35	39
	Hypermethylated	9	219	4	34
Chr16	Hypomethylated	267	29	68	121
	Hypermethylated	35	295	15	59
Chr17	Hypomethylated	242	7	75	80
	Hypermethylated	27	229	4	46
Chr18	Hypomethylated	37	14	33	27
	Hypermethylated	1	161	4	22
Chr19	Hypomethylated	262	40	114	119
	Hypermethylated	37	524	18	147
Chr20	Hypomethylated	223	41	88	127
	Hypermethylated	2	385	5	85
Chr21	Hypomethylated	67	4	18	23
	Hypermethylated	5	88	0	20
Chr22	Hypomethylated	63	23	37	49
	Hypermethylated	1	98	3	21

3.2. Hypermethylated and Hypomethylated CpG Areas across Genomic Features

Next, we evaluated the location of all of the differentially methylated CpGs in relation to functional genomic regions and genomic features. Altogether, 11,513 (45%) sites were hypermethylated and 13,828 (55%) sites were hypomethylated in the tumor as compared to normal colorectal tissue (Figure 2A). Moreover, we found that open seas harbored the largest number of differentially methylated sites, with the greater majority of sites being hypomethylated (9342 sites) as opposed to only 643 being hypermethylated in the tumor as compared to corresponding normal tissues. The next most abundantly affected genomic feature was CpG islands comprising 8816 sites, of which the majority was hypermethylated (8321 as compared to 495 hypomethylated sites) in tumor tissue. In the case of shelves, we also observed a predominant hypomethylation of CpGs (1747) as compared to 189 hypermethylated sites in the tumor tissues. No significant difference in number was observed between hypermethylated (2360) and hypomethylated (2244) sites in shores (Figure 2B).

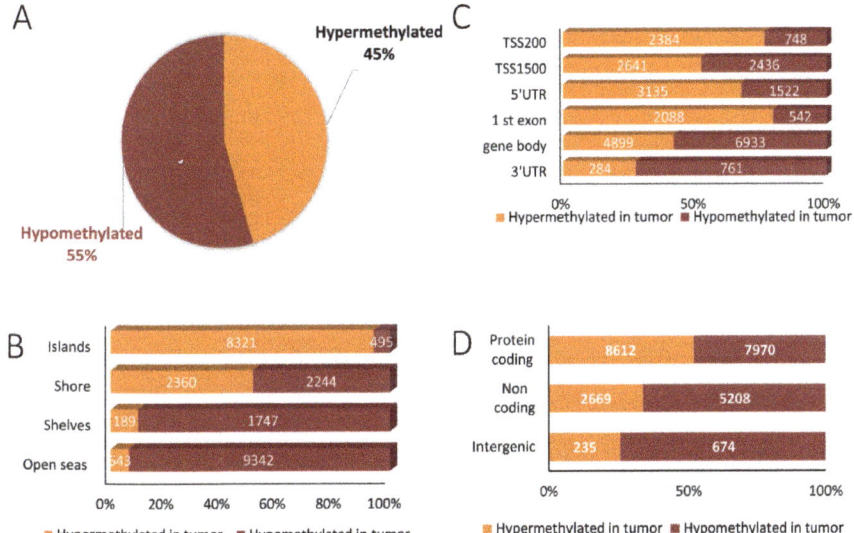

Figure 2. The methylation landscape of all genes across genomic features relative to hypermethylated and hypomethylated states. (**A**) Relative contribution of unique hypermethylated and hypomethylated CpG sites. (**B**) Percentages of CpG hypermethylation and hypomethylation events according to their CpG content and neighborhood context. (**C**) The distribution of hypermethylated and hypomethylated CpGs examined in different functional genomic regions. (**D**) The differentially methylated sites within protein-coding genes, non-coding genes, and intergenic regions.

In a separate analysis, functional genomic regions were evaluated with a total of 28,373 differentially methylated sites. Here, methylation changes within the gene body were the most abundant (11,832 affected sites). Of these, 4899 were hypermethylated and 6933 hypomethylated in tumor as compared to normal colorectal tissues. Promoter regions within 200 and up to 1500 bp relative to the transcriptional start sites were the next most abundantly differentially methylated regions with 8209 sites. Of these, 5025 sites were hypermethylated and 3184 sites hypomethylated in tumor as compared to corresponding normal tissues (Figure 2C). These findings are in line with the overall observation that most of the methylation changes were observed in protein-coding regions (16,582 methylation sites) as opposed to 7877 sites for non-coding regions (Figure 2D).

3.3. Methylation-Specific Patterns across miR Genes

The methylation pattern in miR genes across all chromosomes, including the contribution of both hypermethylated and hypomethylated CpGs, and their context to specific genomic features (islands, shelves shores, and open seas) is represented in Table 2. Interestingly, for miR genes, methylation changes occurred predominantly in promoter regions located within 1500 bp from transcription start sites. In addition, chromosomes 14, 20, and 19 accounted for over 43% of the methylation changes observed for miR genes in tumor versus normal tissue. An interesting observation was that chromosomes that were abundantly affected by methylation changes within the global gene profile were largely unaffected by methylation changes within miR genes. Of note, the chromosomes 4, 12, 17, 18, and 21 showed no methylation changes within miR genes (Table 2).

Table 2. Overview of miR-specific methylation changes across all chromosomes. The number of CpG hypermethylation and hypomethylation events in tumor as compared to normal tissue is shown, according to their neighborhood context.

Chromosome	Status	OpenSea	Island	Shelf	Shore
Chr1	Hypomethylated	5	0	0	0
	Hypermethylated	0	1	0	2
Chr2	Hypomethylated	1	0	0	0
	Hypermethylated	0	0	0	0
Chr3	Hypomethylated	6	0	0	0
	Hypermethylated	1	1	0	0
Chr4	Hypomethylated	0	0	0	0
	Hypermethylated	0	0	0	0
Chr5	Hypomethylated	1	0	0	0
	Hypermethylated	0	0	0	0
Chr6	Hypomethylated	5	0	0	0
	Hypermethylated	0	0	0	0
Chr7	Hypomethylated	12	0	0	0
	Hypermethylated	0	0	0	0
Chr8	Hypomethylated	1	0	0	1
	Hypermethylated	0	3	0	7
Chr9	Hypomethylated	1	0	0	0
	Hypermethylated	0	0	0	0
Chr10	Hypomethylated	0	1	3	2
	Hypermethylated	0	0	0	0
Chr11	Hypomethylated	2	0	0	0
	Hypermethylated	2	12	0	0
Chr12	Hypomethylated	0	0	0	0
	Hypermethylated	0	0	0	0
Chr13	Hypomethylated	12	0	3	1
	Hypermethylated	0	0	0	0
Chr14	Hypomethylated	25	1	1	2
	Hypermethylated	0	0	0	0
Chr15	Hypomethylated	1	1	0	1
	Hypermethylated	0	5	0	0
Chr16	Hypomethylated	1	0	0	0
	Hypermethylated	0	0	0	1
Chr17	Hypomethylated	0	0	0	0
	Hypermethylated	0	0	0	0
Chr18	Hypomethylated	0	0	0	0
	Hypermethylated	0	0	0	0
Chr19	Hypomethylated	20	0	0	0
	Hypermethylated	0	0	0	0
Chr20	Hypomethylated	5	0	0	0
	Hypermethylated	0	18	0	1
Chr21	Hypomethylated	0	0	0	0
	Hypermethylated	0	0	0	0
Chr22	Hypomethylated	0	0	0	0
	Hypermethylated	1	0	0	0

Overall, similar trends were observed for the miR genes as with the whole genome profile. When we specifically focused on miR genes, we found 170 unique sites that were differentially methylated, with 115 being hypomethylated and 55 being hypermethylated in the tumors. Regarding their location within functional genomic regions, the highest number of differentially methylated sites was observed in open seas (103 sites), of which

99 were hypomethylated and only four were hypermethylated in tumor tissues. Overall, in the case of CpG islands, 42 differentially methylated sites were identified from which a total of 40 sites were hypermethylated and only two were hypomethylated in tumor tissues when compared to corresponding normal tissues. Within shores, a total of 21 differentially methylated sites were identified of which 10 sites were hypomethylated and 11 were hypermethylated in tumor as compared to normal tissue. Only four sites were hypomethylated within sea shelves; none were found here that were hypermethylated (Figure 3A). A more focused evaluation of the miR genes interestingly showed promoter regions to be more abundantly hit by methylation changes as opposed to the gene body, as shown in Figure 3B. The 5′ and 3′ UTR regions were minimally affected by methylation changes in the miR genes (Figure 3B). Interestingly, aberrantly methylated miR sites were found only in 17 autosomal chromosomes. Chromosomes 4, 12, 17, 18, 21, and sex chromosomes were devoid of miR methylation sites (Figure 3C).

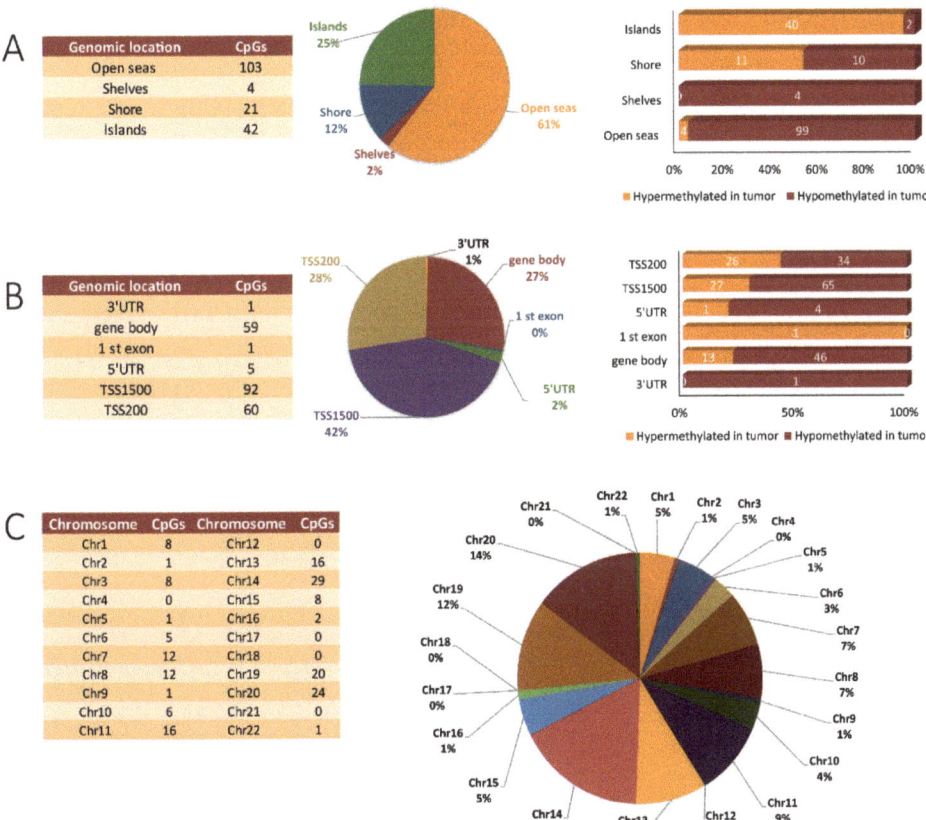

Figure 3. MiR gene methylation profiling in CRC tissues. (**A**) Genomic distribution of differentially methylated CpG sites in miR genes in relation to CpG islands, shores, shelves, and open sea regions. (**B**) The number and percentage of hypermethylated and hypomethylated CpG sites of miR genes ordered according to their functional genomic distribution. (**C**) Chromosome location of the differentially methylated sites of miR genes.

3.4. Identification of Significant Differentially Methylated miRs

In total, 170 unique CpG sites were affected by methylation changes across miR genes. These sites concerned 107 distinct miR genes. In order to ascertain the most significant differentially methylated candidates, we selected all miR genes with a fold change methylation difference between tumor and normal tissue of two and above (hypomethylated and hypermethylated). This analysis revealed 37 distinct CpG sites within miR genes to be significantly hit by methylation changes. These sites represented 18 unique miR genes (Figure 4). Of these miR genes, MIR124-3 was the most hypermethylated in the tumor samples (16-fold methylation difference). The MIR1204 gene was the most hypomethylated in tumor samples when compared with corresponding normal resected tissues (−2.9-fold methylation difference). The regions responsible for these methylation changes were most visible within CpG islands and mostly affected TSS regions up to 1500 bp, as described in Figure 3B. These 18 unique miR genes were further analyzed for their reported impact on colorectal carcinogenesis and tumor progression.

Status	UCSC_RefGene_Name	Fold change	Relation_to_Island	UCSC_RefGene_Group
Hypomethylated	MIR1204;PVT1		S_Shore	TSS200;Body
Hypomethylated	MIR548F9;NBEA;MA821L1		N_Shore	Body;Body;TSS1500
Hypomethylated	MIR19A;MIR17HG;MIR17HG;MIR20A;MIR17;MIR19B1;MIR18A		S_Shore	TSS1500;Body;Body;TSS1500;TSS1500;TSS1500;TSS1500
Hypomethylated	MIR19A;MIR17HG;MIR17HG;MIR17;MIR18A		S_Shore	TSS1500;Body;Body;TSS1500;TSS1500
Hypomethylated	MIR548F5;DCLK1		OpenSea	Body;Body
Hypomethylated	MIR548I4;CNTNAP2		OpenSea	TSS1500;Body
Hypermethylated	MIR129-2		Island	Body
Hypermethylated	MIR548G;C3orf26;C3orf26		Island	Body;1stExon;5'UTR
Hypermethylated	MIR124-3		Island	TSS1500
Hypermethylated	MIR762;BCL7C		N_Shore	TSS1500;Body
Hypermethylated	MIR124-3		Island	TSS200
Hypermethylated	MIR137		Island	Body
Hypermethylated	MIR137		S_Shore	TSS200
Hypermethylated	MIR9-3		Island	TSS1500
Hypermethylated	MIR34B;BTG4;MIR34C		Island	TSS200;TSS1500;TSS1500
Hypermethylated	MIR124-2		S_Shore	TSS1500
Hypermethylated	MIR124-3		Island	Body
Hypermethylated	MIR124-3		Island	TSS1500
Hypermethylated	MIR9-3		Island	TSS1500
Hypermethylated	MIR129-2		Island	TSS200
Hypermethylated	MIR124-3		Island	TSS200
Hypermethylated	MIR124-2		S_Shore	TSS200
Hypermethylated	MIR548G;COL8A1;COL8A1		OpenSea	Body;TSS200;TSS200
Hypermethylated	MIR129-2		Island	TSS200
Hypermethylated	MIR129-2		Island	TSS200
Hypermethylated	MIR34B;BTG4;MIR34C		Island	Body;TSS1500;TSS1500
Hypermethylated	MIR124-3		Island	TSS200
Hypermethylated	MIR9-3		Island	TSS1500
Hypermethylated	MIR129-2		Island	TSS200
Hypermethylated	MIR124-3		Island	TSS200
Hypermethylated	MIR137		S_Shore	TSS200
Hypermethylated	MIR124-3		Island	TSS1500
Hypermethylated	MIR34B;BTG4;MIR34C		Island	TSS200;TSS1500;TSS1500
Hypermethylated	MIR124-3		Island	Body
Hypermethylated	MIR34B;BTG4;MIR34C		Island	TSS200;TSS1500;TSS1500
Hypermethylated	MIR34B;BTG4;MIR34C		Island	TSS200;TSS1500;TSS1500
Hypermethylated	MIR124-3		Island	TSS1500

Figure 4. Heat map of differentially methylated miR genes. The heat map showcases all >2-fold differentially methylated CpG sites within miR genes between tumor and normal colorectal samples. A total of 37 unique sites covering 18 miR genes were identified (nine hypermethylated and nine hypomethylated). The color in each small box represents the relative methylation level of the individual positions within genes in colorectal carcinomas as compared to normal colorectal tissue. The light green color to red color represents a low to high relative methylation status of the individual site, respectively. For the sake of completeness, genes with overlapping open reading frames sharing similar genomic locations are also shown.

Toward this end, we compared these microRNA genes that were affected by methylation changes with recent literature (Table 3) to see whether the observed methylation pattern correlated with current miR gene expression and functional data. In line with our findings, we saw most of our hypermethylated miRs described as downregulated in several tumor types including CRC, and to play a role as potential tumor and/or metastasis suppressors. Similarly, in case of hypomethylated miR genes found in this study, most studies supported an oncogenic and/or pro-metastatic role while being more highly expressed in diverse solid cancers, including CRC.

Table 3. Methylation status of 16 of the miR genes found in this this study and supporting expression and functional data from the current literature on the respective miRs. For two miRs found in this study, supporting literature is not yet available to the best of our knowledge.

Hypermethylated miRs Found in Our Study	miR Expression in Cancer	Regulation	Role	Cancer Types	Target Genes	References
hsa-miR-124-2	Downregulated	Hypermethylated	Tumor suppressor	Cervical cancer	IGFBP7	[30]
hsa-miR-124-3	Downregulated	Hypermethylated	Tumor suppressor	Prostate cancer, Cervical cancer, HCC, Bladder cancer, CRC	IGFBP7, CRKL, Sp1, EDNRB, CCL20, DNMT3B, STAT3	[30–37]
hsa-miR-129-2	Downregulated	Hypermethylated	Tumor suppressor	Esophageal carcinoma, Breast cancer, CRC	SOX4, BCL2L2, BCL2	[38–40]
hsa-miR-137	Downregulated	Hypermethylated	Tumor suppressor	Endometrial cancer, CRC, Pancreatic cancer	EZH2, LSD1, TCF4, LSD1, KLF12, KDM4A	[14,41–45]
hsa-miR-34B	Downregulated	Hypermethylated	Tumor suppressor	Cervical cancer, Lung adenocarcinoma, Breast cancer, Oropharyngeal (oral) cancer, NSCLC	TGF-β1, BMF, Cyclin D1, JAG1	[46–51]
hsa-miR-34C	Downregulated	Hyper-methylated	Tumor suppressor	Nasopharyngeal carcinoma, Prostate cancer	MET	[52,53]
hsa-miR-34b/c	Downregulated	Hypermethylated	Tumor suppressor	CRC	-	[54]
hsa-miR-762	Upregulated	-	Tumor promoter	Breast cancer	IRF7	[55]
hsa-miR-9-3	Downregulated	Hypermethylated	Tumor suppressor	Hodgkin's lymphoma, Gastric cancer	ITGB1	[56,57]
Hypomethylated miRs Found in Our Study	miR Expression in Cancer	Regulation	Role	Cancer Types	Target Genes	References
hsa-miR-1204	Upregulated	-	Tumor promoter	Breast cancer, Glioblastoma	VDR, CREB-1	[58,59]
hsa-miR-17	Upregulated	-	Tumor promoter	CRC	-	[60]
hsa-miR-18A	Upregulated	-	Tumor promoter	Prostate cancer, Breast cancers, Osteosarcoma, Nasopharyngeal carcinoma, CRC	STK4, IRF2, Dicer1	[14,61–64]
hsa-miR-19A	Upregulated	-	Tumor promoter	CRC, Gastric cancer, HCC	TIA1, MXD1, PTEN	[14,65–68]
hsa-miR-19B1	Upregulated	-	Tumor promoter	Gastric cancer	MXD1	[67]
hsa-miR-20A	Upregulated	-	Tumor promoter	CRC	WTX	[69]
hsa-miR-548F5	-	Hyper-methylated		Schwannomas	-	[70]

Abbreviations: B-cell lymphoma 2 (BCL2), BCL2-like 2 (BCL2L2), Bcl-2-modifying factor (BMF), CAMP responsive element binding protein 1 (CREB-1), Chemokine (C-C motif) ligand-20 (CCL20), CRK-like proto-oncogene, adaptor protein (CRKL), DNA methyl-transferase (DNMT3B), Enoyl coenzyme A hydratase short-chain 1 mitochondrial (ECHS1), Hepatocellular carcinoma (HCC), Histone-lysine N-methyltransferase (EZH2), Insulin-like growth factor-binding protein 7 (IGFBP7), Integrin Subunit Beta 1 (ITGB1), integrin αV endothelin receptor type B (EDNRB), Interferon regulatory factor 7 (IRF7), Interferon regulatory factor (IRF)2, Jagged1 (JAG1), Kruppel-like factor 12 (KLF12), Lysine demethylase (KDM4A), Lysine-specific demethylase 1 (LSD1), Lysine-specific histone demethylase 1A (LSD1), Max dimerization protein 1 (MXD1), MET proto-oncogene, receptor tyrosine kinase (MET), Non-small cell lung cancer (NSCLC), Phosphatase and tensin homolog (PTEN), Serine/threonine-protein kinase 4 (STK4), Signal transducer and activator of transcription 3 (STAT3), Specificity protein 1 (Sp1), SRY-related HMG-box (SOX4), T-cell intracellular antigen 1 (TIA1), Transcription factor 4 (TCF4), Transforming growth factor beta 1 (TGF-β1), Vitamin D receptor (VDR), Wilms tumor gene on the X chromosome (WTX).

3.5. Pathway Enrichment Analysis of Differentially Methylated miR Genes

To further explore the potential functions of differentially methylated sites affecting miRs, we identified all putative targets of the selected 18 miR genes, using the Targetscan and miRDB online tools. All miR targets were individually uploaded into the DAVID

Ease online platform. Next, we carried out the KEGG enrichment analysis by using the DAVID bioinformatics resource. Here, we performed a functional and pathway enrichment analysis to map the differentially methylated genes to various types of molecular networks. All pathways with p-values < 0.05 for individual miRs were compiled and only pathways known to have a published impact on cancer development were considered. The lists of the pathways for each miR were analyzed together, and pathways that were common to all miRs were followed further. In total, 17 cancer-relevant pathways were identified for all of these miRs differentially methylated in their genes in our study, including the MAPK, EGFR, ras-proximate-1 or ras-related protein 1 (Rap1), mammalian target of rapamycin (mTOR), and Ras signaling pathway, the Hippo signaling pathway, the PI3K–Akt signaling pathways, and an implication of events leading to chromosomal instability (CIN) and microsatellite instability (MSI). The latter comprise several cellular pathways leading to the development of CRC (Figure 5A). The most recurrent pathways for all miRs implicated to be differentially methylated in CRC in our study were selected for further evaluation and are summarized in Figure 5. Additionally, we performed two further independent analyses, as shown in Figure 5B,C, respectively, to evaluate which of the individual pathways were targeted by the majority of the miRs we identified to be differentially methylated in their genes and vice versa. Our analysis showed that hsa-miR-762, hsa-miR-18a-3p, hsa-miR-17-5p, hsa-miR-20a-5p, hsa-miR-20a-3p, hsa-miR-548f-3p, hsa-miR-17-3p, hsa-miR-19a-3p, hsa-miR-19b-3p, hsa-miR-34b-5p, and hsa-miR-548g-3p targeted eleven or more of the pathways identified in the network (Figure 5B). All of these miRs have been implicated previously, by us and others, to be critical molecular players in the regulation of metastasis and/or CRC progression [54,55,58,71,72].

Furthermore, we evaluated the most recurring pathways targeted by all of these miRs together. Toward this end, the MAPK, ErbB, Rap1, mTOR, Ras signaling pathways as well as the Hippo and PI3K–Akt signaling pathways were regulated by all of these miRs, implicating changes in the methylation of the corresponding miR genes as a crucial event in the mediation of CRC progression and metastasis (Figure 5C). The identification of this network of important signaling pathways as targets of the differentially methylated miRs shown here further validates the vital role that these miRs play in CRC. To corroborate the DAVID analysis, pathways specific for gene targets of hypermethylated and hypomethylated miRs were evaluated using the IPA tool. For the hypermethylated miR targets, CRC metastasis signaling, WNT/β-catenin, and TGF-β signaling were the most significant pathways targeted (Figure 5D). For the hypomethylated miRs, molecular mechanisms of cancer, TGF-β signaling, and WNT/β-catenin were most visible as the targeted pathway groups in this tool (Figure 5E). Taken together, the pathway analyses from DAVID Ease and IPA analysis had very similar outcomes.

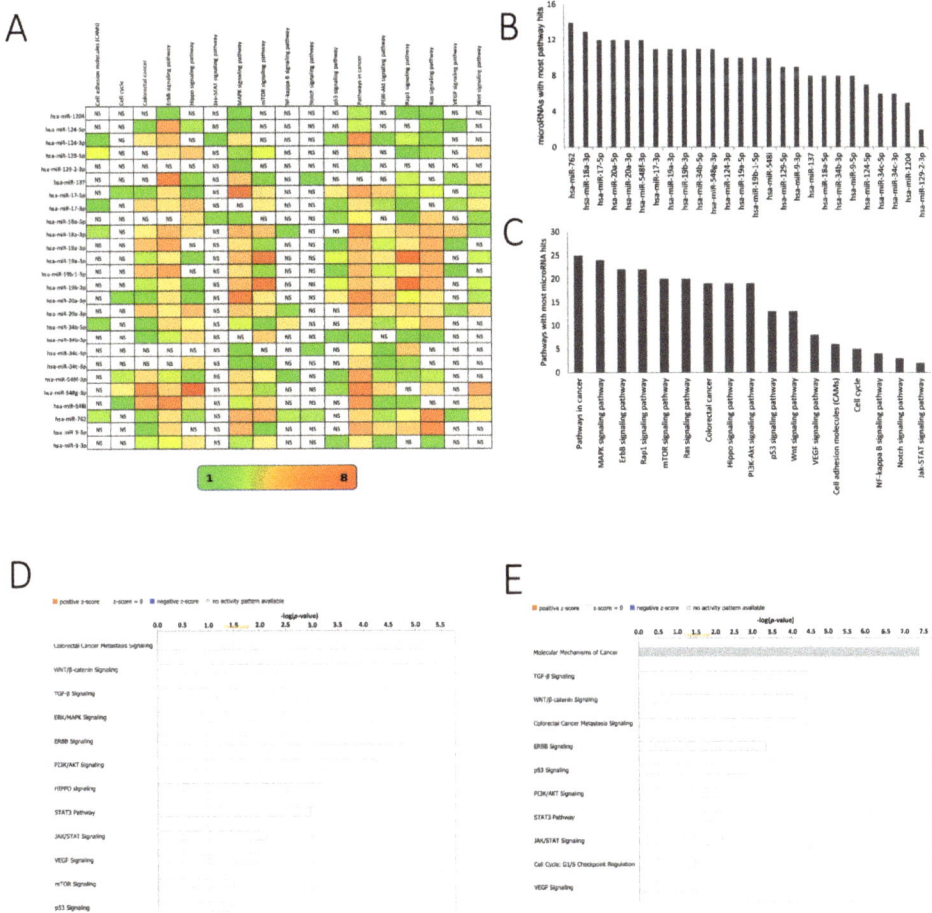

Figure 5. KEGG pathway enrichment analysis by using DAVID Ease. (**A**) Number of genes related to the enriched KEGG pathway. The color of the bar corresponds to log10 (*p*-value). (**B**) Bar diagram showcasing miRs regulating the highest number of canonical pathways in descending order. (**C**) Bar diagram showcasing canonical pathways regulated by the largest number of miRs from the differential methylation list (see Figure 4) in descending order. (**D**) Ingenuity pathway analysis of targets of hypermethylated miR genes. The threshold line is equivalent to a −log *p* value of 0.05. (**E**) Ingenuity pathway analysis of targets of hypomethylated miR genes. The threshold line is equivalent to a −log *p* value of 0.05.

4. Discussion

The significant role played by miRs in the mediation of colorectal carcinogenesis, progression, and metastasis is well established. Depending on the genes targeted, miRs could have both oncogenic or tumor-suppressor functions. This is evident from several studies in CRC as well as in other solid carcinoma [14,15,17,36,39,58,60,71,73]. Importantly, the expression of any miR is only one factor to define its netto influence on its target genes; other parameters are, e.g., the specificity of interaction of the miR with its target mRNA (seed) sequence, the accessibility of the target mRNA for the microRNA by, for example, intracellular compartmentalization, and others [7,9,74]. The abundance of miR expression is being regulated at a number of levels, of which especially genetically acting ones have been abundantly studied so far, especially the transcriptional regulation of gene expression but also copy number changes; however, of course, epigenetics and especially the methylation of CpG sites could play a role as in other genes as well [5,8,19]. Interestingly, very few studies have investigated the impact of methylation on global miR gene expression so far. Moreover, most of these studies have been limited to studying methylation changes within the gene promoters only [29,75,76].

However, in our present study, we performed a genome-wide methylation analysis, covering 99% of all RefSeq genes and also comprising low CpG island density, which could remain undetected using other capture methods [29,77]. Furthermore, our evaluation of methylation changes was not only limited to promoter regions but also included shelves, shores, and open sea regions. A total of 25,341 CpG sites were found to be differentially methylated between colorectal tumor and corresponding normal samples ($p < 0.05$, Wilcoxon Signed-Rank test). Furthermore, most of the changes were observed within CpG island (35%) and open seas (39%). Interestingly, a greater proportion of differentially methylated sites were found in the gene body, which was followed by promoter regions up to 1500 base pairs from transcriptional start sites. Expectedly, most methylation changes occurred in the promoter region of coding genes. These findings are in line with published data that the methylation of promoters, especially those of tumor-suppressor genes, leads to a disruption of functional protein expression, which plays a critical role in cancer progression and other important functional processes [78,79].

The distribution of methylation changes across the different chromosomes was relatively proportional to chromosome size, with chromosomes 1, 2, 7, and 6 accounting for the most changes. These findings mirror those of other studies that have investigated chromosome and genome-wide methylation profiles [80,81]. Although both hypermethylation and hypomethylation events are common in cancer, the literature indicates that hypomethylation events are slightly more common [82]. Similarly, in our study, we also found both hypermethylation and hypomethylation events in the tumor as compared to normal tissues, with hypomethylation being slightly more predominant, with 55% hypomethylated as compared to 45% hypermethylated sites globally. Interestingly, hypomethylation and hypermethylation events were not evenly spread across genomic features or regions. Over 90% of the hypermethylation changes observed in tumor tissues were located within CpG islands, whereas the exact opposite was evident in open seas. Across all genomic regions, hypomethylation was more predominant with the exception of 3′ UTR and 1st exon regions.

Interestingly, hypermethylation was more evident in protein-coding genes, but the reverse was the case in non-coding regions, leading to the hypothesis that epigenetic alterations in coding and non-coding sequences might cooperate in human tumorigenesis. In line with the objectives of our study, we proceeded to specifically evaluate miR genes, many of which have been shown to regulate CRC progression and metastasis [14,36,37,40,42,43,54,60,65,66,68,69,83]. For miR genes, differential methylation was observed predominantly in the open seas and CpG islands. Functionally, these methylation events were more visible in the regions of −200 to 1500 base pairs relative to the transcription start sites. As mentioned above, over 95% of methylation events in open seas were hypomethylated, and those in CpG islands were hypermethylated. Surprisingly, the abundantly methylated chromosomes seen globally were not the same for the miR genes, with chromosomes 14, 20, 19, 13, and 11 mostly hit by methylation events within miR genes in contrast to the overall methylation pattern. A previous compilation by Ghorai and Ghosh identified chromosomes 1, 14, and 19 to harbor the largest number of cancer-associated miRs in the human genome [84]. These chromosomes with the highest number of miR genes overlap with the chromosomes hit by miR-gene specific methylation changes in our study. This underscores an implication that methylation is a potential key event in regulating tumor-associated miR expression, in addition to further mechanisms already shown to be essential, such as the transcriptional regulation of miRs, copy number changes, or changes in subcellular localization such as cytosolic, nuclear, or a concentration in exosomes to guide miR activity toward certain compartments in cancer [5,9,14,18,82]. To further focus on the most significant differentially methylated miR genes, we chose all sites that showed at least a two-fold methylation difference between tumor and corresponding normal samples. Using this selection criterion, we found 37 unique miR-related CpG sites. The majority of these significant differentially methylated sites were located in CpG islands, most of these occurring within 1500 base pairs from the transcriptional start site. The 37 unique CpG sites were located within a total of 18 distinct miR genes. Of these 18 miRs genes, nine genes were hypomethylated and nine genes were hypermethylated. Many of these miRs we found significantly differentially methylated in CRC also already have been shown to take functional roles in diverse further cancer entities besides CRC, which were in part related to changes in the methylation of their genes. For example, a tumor-suppressor function has been ascribed to all three loci encoding mature hsa-miR-124 (hsa-miR-124-1/-2/-3), which has been shown to be hypermethylated in cervical tumors [30], prostate cancer [31], nasopharyngeal carcinoma [85], HCC [32,33], bladder cancer [34], and CRC [35–37]. Likewise, mature miR-129-2 miR has been shown to be a tumor suppressor in esophageal cancer [38], breast cancer [39], and CRC [40]. The hypermethylation of miR-137 was observed in endometrial cancer [41], CRC [42,43], and pancreatic cancer [44,45].

MiR miR-34 family members have been well described as tumor suppressors by our own group in CRC [71] and by others in different kinds of carcinomas including cervical cancer [46], lung adenocarcinoma [47,48], breast cancer [49], oropharyngeal cancer [50], NSCLC [51], nasopharyngeal carcinoma [52], and prostate cancer [53]. Moreover, Toyota et al. demonstrated the downregulation of miR-34b/c expression in a panel of colorectal tumor tissues, again confirming these miRs as tumor suppressors in CRC [54]. These results also mirror our own findings. Other hypermethylated miR genes in our present study include miR-548G and the miR-9 family, which comprises tumor-suppressor miRs seen in Hodgkin's lymphoma [56] and gastric cancer [57] so far.

Significantly hypomethylated miR genes in our present study included miR-1204 with established roles in breast cancer [58] and glioblastoma [59]. The mir-17-92 polycistron encodes six individual miR transcripts comprising miR-17, 18a, 19a, 20, 19b, and 92a. From our analysis, several members of this polycistron were hypomethylated, including MIR17HG, a known promoter of tumorigenesis and metastasis in CRC [60], miR-18a (miR-18a) having been shown to be important in prostate cancer [61], breast cancers [62], osteosarcoma [63], and nasopharyngeal carcinoma [64]. Additionally, miR-19a with documented roles to promote proliferation and migration in CRC [65,66], gastric cancer [67], and HCC [68] was hypomethylated in our analysis. Likewise, miR-20a has been shown to have a tumor-promoting activity in CRC [69]. Taken together, it is an established notion that the miRs we found as significantly changed in the methylation of their genes in colorectal carcinomas, as opposed to normal tissues, are highly relevant molecules that contribute to diverse aspects of (CRC) carcinogenesis, tumor progression, and metastasis.

This is further underlined by our evaluation of the canonical pathways that were attributable to the mRNA molecular targets of these particular miRs. We discovered that several of the miRs might act as a network regulating essential (CRC) cancer-associated pathways, e.g., the EGFR, MAPK, Ras, or the mTOR signaling pathway, amongst others. These strongly enriched canonical pathways, in addition to others, contributed to a generalized and significant enrichment of pathways in cancer in our study. Our findings are supported by the work of Sanchez-Vega et al. who, using 9125 samples from 33 cancer types, found similar pathways to be equally important. Interestingly, this study included DNA methylation changes in addition to mutations, copy number changes, mRNA expression, and gene fusion data to decode these pathway signatures [12]. With our own studies, using our data from miR expression analysis and whole genome sequencing, we were also able to postulate important contributions from a number of these differentially methylated miRs to CRC metastasis as a result of alterations in the pathways mentioned above [5,13,14].

Certainly, our study does have limitations, some of them being the small sample size and the non-availability of corresponding expression data from the same patients. Moreover, a sample triplet comprising tumor, normal, and metastatic tissues from the same patients would have provided a more significant inference in the context of cancer progression and metastasis; however, as the scientific community is well aware, metastasis samples are extremely rare to receive for any experimental analysis. In addition, due to the completely anonymized design of our study we, unfortunately, are unable to associate particular methylation changes to specific tumor stages of the cohort. Still, due to the fact that we studied a mixed population containing patients with some early, but, as a majority of cases, late cancer stages (e.g., 75% pT3 and pT4 stages, 50% pN1/2 stages, 5% M1), it is more likely that the methylation signature we identified is more representative of advanced tumor stages, possibly including features that support metastasis. Along these lines, we consider it interesting to speculate that the priming of certain genes/pathways that initiate or promote progression and/or metastatic steps by changes in methylation might already be visible in primary tumor samples.

Taken together, our present study, which is one of the few to perform genome-wide methylation analysis with a focus on microRNA genes, covering 99% of all RefSeq genes and also comprising low CpG island density, suggests it to be very likely that, besides other means of (genetic) deregulation, changes in methylation already at the primary tumor stage might contribute to the deregulation of expression of miRs and other (associated) genes, which contribute to advanced stages and metastasis development in CRC. Certainly, a definitive causal impact of our observed methylation changes can only be established with further experimental studies.

5. Conclusions

Taken together, our comprehensive analysis of differential miR gene methylation strongly implicates DNA methylation to have an important role in the regulation of a number of important miRs that regulate key cancer pathways in CRC, its progression, and its metastasis. It is interesting to speculate that methylation might have not only an equally important function in regulating miR gene expression in this and other cancer entities as compared to other means of regulation, such as transcription, mutations, or other genetic alterations, but that it might be more powerful by superimposing itself to modulate suchlike other means epigenetically. As a result, the modulation of methylation using clinically available therapeutic agents might be able to modulate essential miR-regulated molecular networks in CRC, and particular methylation events could be studied further as biomarkers in the risk classification of CRC.

Supplementary Materials: The following are available online at https://www.mdpi.com/article/10.3390/cancers13235951/s1, Table S1: Clinical pathological characteristics of the tumour samples used for the methylation analysis. pT, pN, M stipulates the tumour node metastasis classification of the UICC, G reflects the tumour's grade of differentiation. All tumours were microsatellite stable.

Author Contributions: Conceptualization of the project: H.A., M.L.A.; Methodology: samples, and tissue preparation: M.L.A., N.P., C.Z., S.C., J.H.L., T.G.; Data generation and analysis M.L.A., N.P., J.H.L.; Writing—original draft and editing: N.P., M.L.A., J.H.L., H.A.; Writing—final drafting and approval of manuscript: M.L.A., N.P., C.Z., S.C., J.H.L., T.G., H.A.; Funding acquisition: H.A.; Supervision of the project: M.L.A., H.A. All authors have read and agreed to the published version of the manuscript.

Funding: H.A. was supported by the Alfried Krupp von Bohlen und Halbach Foundation, Essen, the Deutsche Krebshilfe, Bonn (70112168), the Deutsche Forschungsgemeinschaft (DFG, grant number AL 465/9-1), the HEiKA Initiative (Karlsruhe Institute of Technology/University of Heidelberg collaborative effort), Hella-Buehler-Foundation, Heidelberg, and the DKFZ-MOST Cooperation, Heidelberg (grant number CA149), M.L.A. was supported by the Deutsche Krebshilfe, Bonn (70112168) and the Medical Faculty Mannheim of the University of Heidelberg (MEAMEDMA).

Institutional Review Board Statement: The study was conducted according to the guidelines of the Declaration of Helsinki and approved by the institutional review board of ethics (Medical Ethics Committee II, University of Heidelberg), ethics approval: 2012-608R-MA, to T.G.

Informed Consent Statement: Patient consent was waived due to the completely anonymized, retrospective nature of the study.

Data Availability Statement: The array data have been deposited in the NCBI Gene Expression Omnibus and can be accessed using the GEO Series accession number GSE184494 (https://www.ncbi.nlm.nih.gov/geo/query/acc.cgi?acc=GSE184494, accessed on 20 September 2021).

Acknowledgments: The paper contains parts of the thesis performed by Chan Zhou in partial fulfilment of the requirements for the "med." at Mannheim Medical Faculty, University of Heidelberg. HA was supported by the Alfried Krupp von Bohlen und Halbach Foundation, Essen, the Deutsche Krebshilfe, Bonn (70112168), the Deutsche Forschungsgemeinschaft (DFG, grant number AL 465/9-1), the HEiKA Initiative (Karlsruhe Institute of Technology/University of Heidelberg collaborative effort), Hella-Buehler-Foundation, Heidelberg, and the DKFZ-MOST Cooperation, Heidelberg (grant number CA149), MLA was supported by the Deutsche Krebshilfe, Bonn (70112168) and the Medical Faculty Mannheim of the University of Heidelberg (MEAMEDMA).

Conflicts of Interest: The authors declare no conflict of interest.

References

1. Sung, H.; Ferlay, J.; Siegel, R.L.; Laversanne, M.; Soerjomataram, I.; Jemal, A.; Bray, F. Global cancer statistics 2020: Globocan estimates of incidence and mortality worldwide for 36 cancers in 185 countries. *CA Cancer J. Clin.* **2021**, *71*, 209–249. [CrossRef]
2. Rawla, P.; Sunkara, T.; Barsouk, A. Epidemiology of colorectal cancer: Incidence, mortality, survival, and risk factors. *Prz. Gastroenterol.* **2019**, *14*, 89–103. [CrossRef]
3. Hanahan, D.; Weinberg, R.A. Hallmarks of cancer: The next generation. *Cell* **2011**, *144*, 646–674. [CrossRef]
4. Fearon, E.R.; Vogelstein, B. A genetic model for colorectal tumorigenesis. *Cell* **1990**, *61*, 759–767. [CrossRef]
5. Ishaque, N.; Abba, M.L.; Hauser, C.; Patil, N.; Paramasivam, N.; Huebschmann, D.; Leupold, J.H.; Balasubramanian, G.P.; Kleinheinz, K.; Toprak, U.H.; et al. Whole genome sequencing puts forward hypotheses on metastasis evolution and therapy in colorectal cancer. *Nat. Commun.* **2018**, *9*, 4782–4795. [CrossRef]
6. Zhang, B.; Wang, Q.; Pan, X. Micrornas and their regulatory roles in animals and plants. *J. Cell. Physiol.* **2007**, *210*, 279–289. [CrossRef] [PubMed]
7. Bartel, D.P. Micrornas: Genomics, biogenesis, mechanism, and function. *Cell* **2004**, *116*, 281–297. [CrossRef]
8. Chen, K.; Rajewsky, N. The evolution of gene regulation by transcription factors and micrornas. *Nat. Rev. Genet.* **2007**, *8*, 93–103. [CrossRef]
9. Lang, F.; Contreras-Gerenas, M.F.; Gelléri, M.; Neumann, J.; Kröger, O.; Sadlo, F.; Berniak, K.; Marx, A.; Cremer, C.; Wagenknecht, H.-A.; et al. Tackling tumour cell heterogeneity at the super-resolution level in human colorectal cancer tissue. *Cancers* **2021**, *13*, 3692–3713. [CrossRef]
10. Reinhart, B.J.; Slack, F.J.; Basson, M.; Pasquinelli, A.E.; Bettinger, J.C.; Rougvie, A.E.; Horvitz, H.R.; Ruvkun, G. The 21-nucleotide let-7 rna regulates developmental timing in caenorhabditis elegans. *Nature* **2000**, *403*, 901–906. [CrossRef] [PubMed]
11. Shu, J.; Silva, B.; Gao, T.; Xu, Z.; Cui, J. Dynamic and modularized microrna regulation and its implication in human cancers. *Sci. Rep.* **2017**, *7*, 13356–13372. [CrossRef]
12. Sanchez-Vega, F.; Mina, M.; Armenia, J.; Chatila, W.K.; Luna, A.; La, K.C.; Dimitriadoy, S.; Liu, D.L.; Kantheti, H.S.; Saghafinia, S.; et al. Oncogenic signaling pathways in the cancer genome atlas. *Cell* **2018**, *173*, 321–337.e10. [CrossRef]
13. Allgayer, H.; Leupold, J.H.; Patil, N. Defining the "metastasome": Perspectives from the genome and molecular landscape in colorectal cancer for metastasis evolution and clinical consequences. *Semin. Cancer Biol.* **2020**, *60*, 1–13. [CrossRef] [PubMed]
14. Mudduluru, G.; Abba, M.; Batliner, J.; Patil, N.; Scharp, M.; Lunavat, T.R.; Leupold, J.H.; Oleksiuk, O.; Juraeva, D.; Thiele, W.; et al. A systematic approach to defining the microrna landscape in metastasis. *Cancer Res.* **2015**, *75*, 3010–3019. [CrossRef] [PubMed]
15. Asangani, I.A.; Rasheed, S.A.; Nikolova, D.A.; Leupold, J.H.; Colburn, N.H.; Post, S.; Allgayer, H. Microrna-21 (mir-21) post-transcriptionally downregulates tumor suppressor pdcd4 and stimulates invasion, intravasation and metastasis in colorectal cancer. *Oncogene* **2008**, *27*, 2128–2136. [CrossRef]
16. Abba, M.; Benner, A.; Patil, N.; Heil, O.; Allgayer, H. Differentially expressed micrornas in colorectal cancer metastasis. *Genom. Data* **2015**, *6*, 33–35. [CrossRef]
17. Peng, Y.; Croce, C.M. The role of micrornas in human cancer. *Signal Transduct. Target. Ther.* **2016**, *1*, 15004–15012. [CrossRef]
18. Kunej, T.; Godnic, I.; Horvat, S.; Zorc, M.; Calin, G.A. Cross talk between microrna and coding cancer genes. *Cancer J.* **2012**, *18*, 223–231. [CrossRef]
19. Darwiche, N. Epigenetic mechanisms and the hallmarks of cancer: An intimate affair. *Am. J. Cancer Res.* **2020**, *10*, 1954–1978.
20. Kanwal, R.; Gupta, S. Epigenetic modifications in cancer. *Clin. Genet.* **2012**, *81*, 303–311. [CrossRef]
21. Goh, L.; Murphy, S.K.; Muhkerjee, S.; Furey, T.S. Genomic sweeping for hypermethylated genes. *Bioinformatics* **2007**, *23*, 281–288. [CrossRef] [PubMed]
22. Fleming, M.; Ravula, S.; Tatishchev, S.F.; Wang, H.L. Colorectal carcinoma: Pathologic aspects. *J. Gastrointest. Oncol.* **2012**, *3*, 153–173. [PubMed]

23. Amin, M.B.; Edge, S.B.; American Joint Committee of Cancer. *AJCC Cancer Staging Manual*; Springer: Cham, Switzerland, 2017.
24. Aryee, M.J.; Jaffe, A.E.; Corrada-Bravo, H.; Ladd-Acosta, C.; Feinberg, A.P.; Hansen, K.D.; Irizarry, R.A. Minfi: A flexible and comprehensive bioconductor package for the analysis of infinium DNA methylation microarrays. *Bioinformatics* **2014**, *30*, 1363–1369. [CrossRef] [PubMed]
25. Sturm, D.; Witt, H.; Hovestadt, V.; Khuong-Quang, D.A.; Jones, D.T.; Konermann, C.; Pfaff, E.; Tonjes, M.; Sill, M.; Bender, S.; et al. Hotspot mutations in h3f3a and idh1 define distinct epigenetic and biological subgroups of glioblastoma. *Cancer Cell* **2012**, *22*, 425–437. [CrossRef]
26. Westfall, P.H.; Stanley, Y.S. *Resampling-Based Multiple Testing: Examples and Methods for p-Value Adjustment*, Wiley Series in Probability and Statistics ed.; John Wiley & Sons Inc.: New York, NY, USA, 1993.
27. Dennis, G., Jr.; Sherman, B.T.; Hosack, D.A.; Yang, J.; Gao, W.; Lane, H.C.; Lempicki, R.A. David: Database for annotation, visualization, and integrated discovery. *Genome Biol.* **2003**, *4*, P3. [CrossRef]
28. Siegel, R.L.; Miller, K.D.; Goding Sauer, A.; Fedewa, S.A.; Butterly, L.F.; Anderson, J.C.; Cercek, A.; Smith, R.A.; Jemal, A. Colorectal cancer statistics, 2020. *CA Cancer J. Clin.* **2020**, *70*, 145–164. [CrossRef]
29. Bibikova, M.; Barnes, B.; Tsan, C.; Ho, V.; Klotzle, B.; Le, J.M.; Delano, D.; Zhang, L.; Schroth, G.P.; Gunderson, K.L.; et al. High density DNA methylation array with single cpg site resolution. *Genomics* **2011**, *98*, 288–295. [CrossRef]
30. Wilting, S.M.; van Boerdonk, R.A.A.; Henken, F.E.; Meijer, C.J.L.M.; Diosdado, B.; Meijer, G.A.; le Sage, C.; Agami, R.; Snijders, P.J.F.; Steenbergen, R.D.M. Methylation-mediated silencing and tumour suppressive function of hsa-mir-124 in cervical cancer. *Mol. Cancer* **2010**, *9*, 167–180. [CrossRef]
31. Chu, M.; Chang, Y.; Guo, Y.; Wang, N.; Cui, J.; Gao, W.-Q. Regulation and methylation of tumor suppressor mir-124 by androgen receptor in prostate cancer cells. *PLoS ONE* **2015**, *10*, e0116197. [CrossRef]
32. Majid, A.; Wang, J.; Nawaz, M.; Abdul, S.; Ayesha, M.; Guo, C.; Liu, Q.; Liu, S.; Sun, M.-Z. Mir-124-3p suppresses the invasiveness and metastasis of hepatocarcinoma cells via targeting crkl. *Front. Mol. Biosci.* **2020**, *7*, 223–237. [CrossRef]
33. Cai, Q.Q.; Dong, Y.W.; Wang, R.; Qi, B.; Guo, J.X.; Pan, J.; Liu, Y.Y.; Zhang, C.Y.; Wu, X.Z. Mir-124 inhibits the migration and invasion of human hepatocellular carcinoma cells by suppressing integrin αv expression. *Sci. Rep.* **2017**, *7*, 40733–40742. [CrossRef]
34. Fu, W.; Wu, X.; Yang, Z.; Mi, H. The effect of mir-124-3p on cell proliferation and apoptosis in bladder cancer by targeting ednrb. *Arch. Med Sci.* **2019**, *15*, 1154–1162. [CrossRef]
35. Lu, M.L.; Zhang, Y.; Li, J.; Fu, Y.; Li, W.H.; Zhao, G.F.; Li, X.H.; Wei, L.; Liu, G.B.; Huang, H. Microrna-124 inhibits colorectal cancer cell proliferation and suppresses tumor growth by interacting with plcb1 and regulating wnt/β-catenin signaling pathway. *Eur. Rev. Med Pharmacol. Sci.* **2019**, *23*, 121–136. [PubMed]
36. Shahmohamadnejad, S.; Nouri Ghonbalani, Z.; Tahbazlahafi, B.; Panahi, G.; Meshkani, R.; Emami Razavi, A.; Shokri Afra, H.; Khalili, E. Aberrant methylation of mir-124 upregulates dnmt3b in colorectal cancer to accelerate invasion and migration. *Arch. Physiol. Biochem.* **2020**, 1–7. [CrossRef]
37. Zhang, J.; Lu, Y.; Yue, X.; Li, H.; Luo, X.; Wang, Y.; Wang, K.; Wan, J. Mir-124 suppresses growth of human colorectal cancer by inhibiting stat3. *PLoS ONE* **2013**, *8*, e70300–e70310. [CrossRef]
38. Kang, M.; Li, Y.; Liu, W.; Wang, R.; Tang, A.; Hao, H.; Liu, Z.; Ou, H. Mir-129-2 suppresses proliferation and migration of esophageal carcinoma cells through downregulation of sox4 expression. *Int. J. Mol. Med.* **2013**, *32*, 51–58. [CrossRef]
39. Tang, X.; Tang, J.; Liu, X.; Zeng, L.; Cheng, C.; Luo, Y.; Li, L.; Qin, S.-L.; Sang, Y.; Deng, L.-M.; et al. Downregulation of mir-129-2 by promoter hypermethylation regulates breast cancer cell proliferation and apoptosis. *Oncol. Rep.* **2016**, *35*, 2963–2969. [CrossRef] [PubMed]
40. Karaayvaz, M.; Zhai, H.; Ju, J. Mir-129 promotes apoptosis and enhances chemosensitivity to 5-fluorouracil in colorectal cancer. *Cell Death Dis.* **2013**, *4*, e659–e667. [CrossRef] [PubMed]
41. Zhang, W.; Chen, J.-H.; Shan, T.; Aguilera-Barrantes, I.; Wang, L.-S.; Huang, T.H.-M.; Rader, J.S.; Sheng, X.; Huang, Y.-W. Mir-137 is a tumor suppressor in endometrial cancer and is repressed by DNA hypermethylation. *Lab. Investig.* **2018**, *98*, 1397–1407. [CrossRef]
42. Bi, W.P.; Xia, M.; Wang, X.J. Mir-137 suppresses proliferation, migration and invasion of colon cancer cell lines by targeting tcf4. *Oncol. Lett.* **2018**, *15*, 8744–8748. [CrossRef]
43. Ding, X.; Zhang, J.; Feng, Z.; Tang, Q.; Zhou, X. Mir-137-3p inhibits colorectal cancer cell migration by regulating a kdm1a-dependent epithelial–mesenchymal transition. *Dig. Dis. Sci.* **2021**, *66*, 2272–2282. [CrossRef] [PubMed]
44. He, Z.; Guo, X.; Tian, S.; Zhu, C.; Chen, S.; Yu, C.; Jiang, J.; Sun, C. Microrna-137 reduces stemness features of pancreatic cancer cells by targeting klf12. *J. Exp. Clin. Cancer Res.* **2019**, *38*, 126–141. [CrossRef]
45. Neault, M.; Mallette, F.A.; Richard, S. Mir-137 modulates a tumor suppressor network-inducing senescence in pancreatic cancer cells. *Cell Rep.* **2016**, *14*, 1966–1978. [CrossRef] [PubMed]
46. Cao, Z.; Zhang, G.; Xie, C.; Zhou, Y. Mir-34b regulates cervical cancer cell proliferation and apoptosis. *Artif. Cells Nanomed. Biotechnol.* **2019**, *47*, 2042–2047. [CrossRef] [PubMed]
47. Catuogno, S.; Cerchia, L.; Romano, G.; Pognonec, P.; Condorelli, G.; de Franciscis, V. Mir-34c may protect lung cancer cells from paclitaxel-induced apoptosis. *Oncogene* **2013**, *32*, 341–351. [CrossRef]
48. Kim, J.S.; Kim, E.J.; Lee, S.; Tan, X.; Liu, X.; Park, S.; Kang, K.; Yoon, J.-S.; Ko, Y.H.; Kurie, J.M.; et al. Mir-34a and mir-34b/c have distinct effects on the suppression of lung adenocarcinomas. *Exp. Mol. Med.* **2019**, *51*, 1–10. [CrossRef]

49. Lee, Y.-M.; Lee, J.-Y.; Ho, C.-C.; Hong, Q.-S.; Yu, S.-L.; Tzeng, C.-R.; Yang, P.-C.; Chen, H.-W. Mirna-34b as a tumor suppressor in estrogen-dependent growth of breast cancer cells. *Breast Cancer Res.* **2011**, *13*, R116–R131. [CrossRef]
50. Hsieh, M.-J.; Lin, C.-W.; Su, S.-C.; Reiter, R.J.; Chen, A.W.-G.; Chen, M.-K.; Yang, S.-F. Effects of mir-34b/mir-892a upregulation and inhibition of abcb1/abcb4 on melatonin-induced apoptosis in vcr-resistant oral cancer cells. *Mol. Ther. Nucleic Acids* **2020**, *19*, 877–889. [CrossRef]
51. Wang, L.-G.; Ni, Y.; Su, B.-H.; Mu, X.-R.; Shen, H.-C.; Du, J.-J. Microrna-34b functions as a tumor suppressor and acts as a nodal point in the feedback loop with met. *Int. J. Oncol.* **2013**, *42*, 957–962. [CrossRef]
52. Li, Y.Q.; Ren, X.Y.; He, Q.M.; Xu, Y.F.; Tang, X.R.; Sun, Y.; Zeng, M.S.; Kang, T.B.; Liu, N.; Ma, J. Mir-34c suppresses tumor growth and metastasis in nasopharyngeal carcinoma by targeting met. *Cell Death Dis.* **2015**, *6*, e1618. [CrossRef]
53. Hagman, Z.; Haflidadottir, B.S.; Ansari, M.; Persson, M.; Bjartell, A.; Edsjö, A.; Ceder, Y. The tumour suppressor mir-34c targets met in prostate cancer cells. *Br. J. Cancer* **2013**, *109*, 1271–1278. [CrossRef] [PubMed]
54. Toyota, M.; Suzuki, H.; Sasaki, Y.; Maruyama, R.; Imai, K.; Shinomura, Y.; Tokino, T. Epigenetic silencing of microrna-34b/c and b-cell translocation gene 4 is associated with cpg island methylation in colorectal cancer. *Cancer Res.* **2008**, *68*, 4123–4132. [CrossRef]
55. Li, Y.; Huang, R.; Wang, L.; Hao, J.; Zhang, Q.; Ling, R.; Yun, J. Microrna-762 promotes breast cancer cell proliferation and invasion by targeting irf7 expression. *Cell Prolif.* **2015**, *48*, 643–649. [CrossRef] [PubMed]
56. Ben Dhiab, M.; Ziadi, S.; Louhichi, T.; Ben Gacem, R.; Ksiaa, F.; Trimeche, M. Investigation of mir9-1, mir9-2 and mir9-3 methylation in hodgkin lymphoma. *Pathobiology* **2015**, *82*, 195–202. [CrossRef]
57. Meng, Q.; Xiang, L.; Fu, J.; Chu, X.; Wang, C.; Yan, B. Transcriptome profiling reveals mir-9-3p as a novel tumor suppressor in gastric cancer. *Oncotarget* **2017**, *8*, 37321–37331. [CrossRef]
58. Liu, X.; Bi, L.; Wang, Q.; Wen, M.; Li, C.; Ren, Y.; Jiao, Q.; Mao, J.-H.; Wang, C.; Wei, G.; et al. Mir-1204 targets vdr to promotes epithelial-mesenchymal transition and metastasis in breast cancer. *Oncogene* **2018**, *37*, 3426–3439. [CrossRef]
59. Zhao, X.; Shen, F.; Ma, J.; Zhao, S.; Meng, L.; Wang, X.; Liang, S.; Liang, J.; Hu, C.; Zhang, X. Creb1-induced mir-1204 promoted malignant phenotype of glioblastoma through targeting nr3c2. *Cancer Cell Int.* **2020**, *20*, 111–120. [CrossRef]
60. Xu, J.; Meng, Q.; Li, X.; Yang, H.; Xu, J.; Gao, N.; Sun, H.; Wu, S.; Familiari, G.; Relucenti, M.; et al. Long noncoding rna mir17hg promotes colorectal cancer progression via mir-17-5p. *Cancer Res.* **2019**, *79*, 4882–4895. [CrossRef]
61. Hsu, T.I.; Hsu, C.H.; Lee, K.H.; Lin, J.T.; Chen, C.S.; Chang, K.C.; Su, C.Y.; Hsiao, M.; Lu, P.J. Microrna-18a is elevated in prostate cancer and promotes tumorigenesis through suppressing stk4 in vitro and in vivo. *Oncogenesis* **2014**, *3*, e99. [CrossRef] [PubMed]
62. Egeland, N.G.; Jonsdottir, K.; Aure, M.R.; Sahlberg, K.; Kristensen, V.N.; Cronin-Fenton, D.; Skaland, I.; Gudlaugsson, E.; Baak, J.P.A.; Janssen, E.A.M. Mir-18a and mir-18b are expressed in the stroma of oestrogen receptor alpha negative breast cancers. *BMC Cancer* **2020**, *20*, 377–390. [CrossRef]
63. Lu, C.; Peng, K.; Guo, H.; Ren, X.; Hu, S.; Cai, Y.; Han, Y.; Ma, L.; Xu, P. Mir-18a-5p promotes cell invasion and migration of osteosarcoma by directly targeting irf2. *Oncol. Lett.* **2018**, *16*, 3150–3156. [CrossRef] [PubMed]
64. Luo, Z.; Dai, Y.; Zhang, L.; Jiang, C.; Li, Z.; Yang, J.; McCarthy, J.B.; She, X.; Zhang, W.; Ma, J.; et al. Mir-18a promotes malignant progression by impairing microrna biogenesis in nasopharyngeal carcinoma. *Carcinogenesis* **2013**, *34*, 415–425. [CrossRef] [PubMed]
65. Huang, L.; Wang, X.; Wen, C.; Yang, X.; Song, M.; Chen, J.; Wang, C.; Zhang, B.; Wang, L.; Iwamoto, A.; et al. Hsa-mir-19a is associated with lymph metastasis and mediates the tnf-α induced epithelial-to-mesenchymal transition in colorectal cancer. *Sci. Rep.* **2015**, *5*, 13350–13361. [CrossRef]
66. Liu, Y.; Liu, R.; Yang, F.; Cheng, R.; Chen, X.; Cui, S.; Gu, Y.; Sun, W.; You, C.; Liu, Z.; et al. Mir-19a promotes colorectal cancer proliferation and migration by targeting tia1. *Mol. Cancer* **2017**, *16*, 53–69. [CrossRef] [PubMed]
67. Wu, Q.; Yang, Z.; An, Y.; Hu, H.; Yin, J.; Zhang, P.; Nie, Y.; Wu, K.; Shi, Y.; Fan, D. Mir-19a/b modulate the metastasis of gastric cancer cells by targeting the tumour suppressor mxd1. *Cell Death Dis.* **2014**, *5*, e1144–e1154. [CrossRef]
68. Jiang, X.-M.; Yu, X.-N.; Liu, T.-T.; Zhu, H.-R.; Shi, X.; Bilegsaikhan, E.; Guo, H.-Y.; Song, G.-Q.; Weng, S.-Q.; Huang, X.-X.; et al. Microrna-19a-3p promotes tumor metastasis and chemoresistance through the pten/akt pathway in hepatocellular carcinoma. *Biomed. Pharmacother.* **2018**, *105*, 1147–1154. [CrossRef]
69. Zhu, G.-F.; Xu, Y.-W.; Li, J.; Niu, H.-L.; Ma, W.-X.; Xu, J.; Zhou, P.-R.; Liu, X.; Ye, D.-L.; Liu, X.-R.; et al. Mir20a/106a-wtx axis regulates rhogdia/cdc42 signaling and colon cancer progression. *Nat. Commun.* **2019**, *10*, 112–125. [CrossRef]
70. Torres-Martin, M.; Lassaletta, L.; de Campos, J.M.; Isla, A.; Pinto, G.R.; Burbano, R.R.; Melendez, B.; Castresana, J.S.; Rey, J.A. Genome-wide methylation analysis in vestibular schwannomas shows putative mechanisms of gene expression modulation and global hypomethylation at the hox gene cluster. *Genes Chromosomes Cancer* **2015**, *54*, 197–209. [CrossRef]
71. Mudduluru, G.; Ceppi, P.; Kumarswamy, R.; Scagliotti, G.V.; Papotti, M.; Allgayer, H. Regulation of axl receptor tyrosine kinase expression by mir-34a and mir-199a/b in solid cancer. *Oncogene* **2011**, *30*, 2888–2899. [CrossRef]
72. Shi, Y.; Qiu, M.; Wu, Y.; Hai, L. Mir-548-3p functions as an anti-oncogenic regulator in breast cancer. *Biomed. Pharmacother. Biomed. Pharmacother.* **2015**, *75*, 111–116. [CrossRef]
73. Laudato, S.; Patil, N.; Abba, M.L.; Leupold, J.H.; Benner, A.; Gaiser, T.; Marx, A.; Allgayer, H. P53-induced mir-30e-5p inhibits colorectal cancer invasion and metastasis by targeting itga6 and itgb1. *Int. J. Cancer* **2017**, *141*, 1879–1890. [CrossRef]
74. Bentwich, I. Prediction and validation of micrornas and their targets. *FEBS Lett.* **2005**, *579*, 5904–5910. [CrossRef]
75. Sproul, D.; Kitchen, R.R.; Nestor, C.E.; Dixon, J.M.; Sims, A.H.; Harrison, D.J.; Ramsahoye, B.H.; Meehan, R.R. Tissue of origin determines cancer-associated cpg island promoter hypermethylation patterns. *Genome Biol.* **2012**, *13*, R84–R99. [CrossRef]

76. Bandres, E.; Agirre, X.; Bitarte, N.; Ramirez, N.; Zarate, R.; Roman-Gomez, J.; Prosper, F.; Garcia-Foncillas, J. Epigenetic regulation of microrna expression in colorectal cancer. *Int. J. Cancer* **2009**, *125*, 2737–2743. [CrossRef] [PubMed]
77. Kurdyukov, S.; Bullock, M. DNA methylation analysis: Choosing the right method. *Biology* **2016**, *5*, 3–23. [CrossRef] [PubMed]
78. Pfeifer, G.P. Defining driver DNA methylation changes in human cancer. *Int. J. Mol. Sci.* **2018**, *19*, 1166. [CrossRef] [PubMed]
79. Wajed, S.A.; Laird, P.W.; DeMeester, T.R. DNA methylation: An alternative pathway to cancer. *Ann. Surg.* **2001**, *234*, 10–20. [CrossRef] [PubMed]
80. Eckhardt, F.; Lewin, J.; Cortese, R.; Rakyan, V.K.; Attwood, J.; Burger, M.; Burton, J.; Cox, T.V.; Davies, R.; Down, T.A.; et al. DNA methylation profiling of human chromosomes 6, 20 and 22. *Nat. Genet.* **2006**, *38*, 1378–1385. [CrossRef]
81. Hernando-Herraez, I.; Garcia-Perez, R.; Sharp, A.J.; Marques-Bonet, T. DNA methylation: Insights into human evolution. *PLoS Genet.* **2015**, *11*, e1005661–e1005672. [CrossRef]
82. Ehrlich, M. DNA hypomethylation in cancer cells. *Epigenomics* **2009**, *1*, 239–259. [CrossRef]
83. Li, J.; Zhong, Y.; Cai, S.; Zhou, P.; Yao, L. Microrna expression profiling in the colorectal normal-adenoma-carcinoma transition. *Oncol. Lett.* **2019**, *18*, 2013–2018. [CrossRef] [PubMed]
84. Ghorai, A.; Ghosh, U. Mirna gene counts in chromosomes vary widely in a species and biogenesis of mirna largely depends on transcription or post-transcriptional processing of coding genes. *Front. Genet.* **2014**, *5*, 100–110. [CrossRef] [PubMed]
85. Peng, X.H.; Huang, H.R.; Lu, J.; Liu, X.; Zhao, F.P.; Zhang, B.; Lin, S.X.; Wang, L.; Chen, H.H.; Xu, X.; et al. Mir-124 suppresses tumor growth and metastasis by targeting foxq1 in nasopharyngeal carcinoma. *Mol. Cancer* **2014**, *13*, 186–198. [CrossRef] [PubMed]

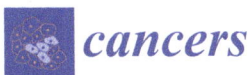

Article

Combination of Wnt/β-Catenin Targets S100A4 and DKK1 Improves Prognosis of Human Colorectal Cancer

Mathias Dahlmann [1], Anne Monks [2], Erik D. Harris [2], Dennis Kobelt [1], Marc Osterland [1], Fadi Khaireddine [1], Pia Herrmann [1], Wolfgang Kemmner [1], Susen Burock [3], Wolfgang Walther [1], Robert H. Shoemaker [4,†] and Ulrike Stein [1,5,*]

[1] Experimental and Clinical Research Center, a Cooperation between the Charité—Universitätsmedizin Berlin and the Max-Delbrück-Center for Molecular Medicine in the Helmholtz Association, Lindenberger Weg 80, 13125 Berlin, Germany; mathias.dahlmann@mdc-berlin.de (M.D.); dennis.kobelt@charite.de (D.K.); marc.osterland@fu-berlin.de (M.O.); fadykhaireddine@hotmail.com (F.K.); pia.herrmann@charite.de (P.H.); wolfgang.kemmner@charite.de (W.K.); wowalt@mdc-berlin.de (W.W.)

[2] Molecular Pharmacology Laboratory, Leidos Biomedical Research, Inc., FNLCR, Frederick, MD 21702, USA; annemonks25@gmail.com (A.M.); erik.harris@nih.gov (E.D.H.)

[3] Charité Comprehensive Cancer Center, Charité—Universitätsmedizin Berlin, Corporate Member of Freie Universität Berlin and Humboldt—Universität zu Berlin, Invalidenstraße 80, 10117 Berlin, Germany; susen.burock@charite.de

[4] Screening Technologies Branch, Developmental Therapeutics Program, Division of Cancer Treatment and Diagnosis, National Cancer Institute-Frederick, Building 440, Frederick, MD 21702, USA; shoemakr@mail.nih.gov

[5] German Cancer Consortium, 69121 Heidelberg, Germany

* Correspondence: ustein@mdc-berlin.de

† Present address: Chemopreventive Agent Development Research Group, Division of Cancer Prevention, National Cancer Institute, 9609 Medical Center Drive, Bethesda, MD 20892, USA.

Citation: Dahlmann, M.; Monks, A.; Harris, E.D.; Kobelt, D.; Osterland, M.; Khaireddine, F.; Herrmann, P.; Kemmner, W.; Burock, S.; Walther, W.; et al. Combination of Wnt/β-Catenin Targets S100A4 and DKK1 Improves Prognosis of Human Colorectal Cancer. *Cancers* 2022, 14, 37. https://doi.org/10.3390/cancers14010037

Academic Editors: Heike Allgayer and Sandra J. van Vliet

Received: 7 October 2021
Accepted: 8 December 2021
Published: 22 December 2021

Publisher's Note: MDPI stays neutral with regard to jurisdictional claims in published maps and institutional affiliations.

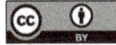

Copyright: © 2021 by the authors. Licensee MDPI, Basel, Switzerland. This article is an open access article distributed under the terms and conditions of the Creative Commons Attribution (CC BY) license (https://creativecommons.org/licenses/by/4.0/).

Simple Summary: Aberrant Wnt/β-catenin signaling contributes to the development, progression, and metastasis of CRC, by altering target gene expression connected to cancer cell proliferation and motility. S100A4 is a Wnt/β-catenin target gene, which strongly enhances migration and invasion of CRC cells and thus CRC metastasis. Here, we report the transcriptional cross-regulation of S100A4 and the Wnt antagonist DKK1, in which the expression of S100A4 down-regulates DKK1 expression, sustaining activated Wnt signaling. S100A4 is an established prognostic biomarker for CRC patient survival, and the combination of S100A4 and DKK1 can be used to improve the prognosis of overall and metastasis-free survival.

Abstract: Metastasis is directly linked to colorectal cancer (CRC) patient survival. Wnt signaling through β-catenin plays a key role. Metastasis-inducing S100A4 is a Wnt/β-catenin target gene and a prognostic biomarker for CRC and other cancer types. We aimed to identify S100A4-dependent expression alterations to better understand CRC progression and metastasis for improved patient survival. S100A4-induced transcriptome arrays, confirmatory studies in isogenic CRC cell lines with defined β-catenin genotypes, and functional metastasis studies were performed. S100A4-regulated transcriptome examination revealed the transcriptional cross-regulation of metastasis-inducing S100A4 with Wnt pathway antagonist Dickkopf-1 (DKK1). S100A4 overexpression down-regulated DKK1, S100A4 knock-down increased DKK1. Recombinant DKK1 reduced S100A4 expression and S100A4-mediated cell migration. In xenografted mice, systemic S100A4-shRNA application increased intratumoral DKK1. The inverse correlation of S100A4 and DKK1 was confirmed in five independent publicly available CRC expression datasets. Combinatorial analysis of S100A4 and DKK1 in two additional independent CRC patient cohorts improved prognosis of overall and metastasis-free survival. The newly discovered transcriptional cross-regulation of Wnt target S100A4 and Wnt antagonist DKK1 is predominated by an S100A4-induced Wnt signaling feedback loop, increasing cell motility and metastasis risk. S100A4 and DKK1 combination improves the identification of CRC patients at high risk.

Keywords: S100A4; DKK1; Wnt signaling; colorectal cancer; patient survival

1. Introduction

Colorectal cancer (CRC) is a major cause of cancer death worldwide and particularly in Western countries [1]. Turning healthy epithelial colon cells into CRC cells is frequently caused by increased Wnt signaling [2–5]. In sporadic CRC, somatic mutations in the *Adenomatous Polyposis Coli* (APC) are found in 70–80% of patients [6]. APC truncation distinctly reduces the degradation of β-catenin, which subsequently accumulates in the nucleus and triggers Wnt/β-catenin target gene expression even without upstream activation of the signaling pathway [7,8]. Similarly, aberrantly activated Wnt/β-catenin signaling is mediated by gain-of-function mutations in β-catenin itself, which occur in almost 50% of CRC tumors without APC mutations [9]. The majority of gain-of-function mutations (amino acid substitutions or in-frame deletions) within β-catenin occur in exon 3 at a regulatory region (aa32-aa45) for protein phosphorylation and binding of the E3 ubiquitin-protein ligase β-TrCP, which triggers the subsequent proteasomal degradation of β-catenin, resulting in a stabilization of mutated β-catenin in these cells [10].

One of the Wnt signaling target genes in CRC is the metastasis-inducing small Ca^{2+} binding protein S100A4 [11,12]. Its high abundance in tumor tissue, both intracellular and in the interstitial fluid, increases the metastatic potential of CRC cells and decreases overall survival (OS) and metastasis-free survival (MFS) of patients [13,14]. Therapeutic approaches to reduce S100A4 expression, and thereby restrict cancer progression and metastasis, including RNA interference (RNAi) [15–17] and small molecules for intervention strategies in the Wnt pathway [18–21].

Wnt/β-catenin signaling also regulates the expression of Dickkopf-1 (DKK1) [22]. DKK1 itself is an established Wnt antagonist, which competes to recruit Wnt co-receptors, such as LRP5/6, and is thus preventing the activation of Wnt signaling [23,24]. Elevated DKK1 expression in multiple myeloma and prostate cancer leads to enhanced bone metastasis [25–27], and the expression level of DKK1 affects the organotropism of breast cancer metastasis [28,29]. As an inhibitor of proliferative Wnt signaling, DKK1 has also been reported as a mediator to metastatic latency, where quiescent metastatic cells evade immune surveillance for later sporadic outgrowth [30]. Although DKK1 expression is associated with poor survival in many solid cancers, it is often found down-regulated in CRC and reports of its prognostic value in CRC metastasis are controversial [31–33].

In this study, we aimed to explore S100A4-induced transcriptome alterations in CRC cells. We discovered a so far undescribed feedback loop within the Wnt pathway. S100A4, the expression of which is induced by active Wnt/β-catenin signaling, suppresses the expression of DKK1. We analyzed this transcriptional cross-regulation of metastasis-inducing S100A4 and the Wnt antagonist DKK1 in CRC in cell culture and confirmed it in CRC xenografted mice. In addition, we found the activating transcription factor 5 (ATF5) involved in the expression regulation of DKK1 in CRC cells with restored low Wnt/β-catenin pathway activity. Combinatorial analysis of inverse S100A4 and DKK1 expression in human CRC patient specimens improved prognostication for patient survival.

2. Materials and Methods

2.1. Cell Lines, Culture Conditions, and Treatment

The CRC cell line HCT116 (heterozygous gain-of-function Δ45-β-catenin), and the single allele derivatives HAB68 (Δ45-β-catenin) and HAB92 (wild-type β-catenin), were kindly provided by Todd Waldman (Georgetown University, Washington, DC, USA). Plasmid transfection was performed with FugeneHD (Promega, Madison, WI, USA), according to the manufacturer's instructions. Transfection of HAB92 and HCT116 cells with pcDNA3.1 or pcDNA3.1/S100A4 resulted in the control cell lines HAB92/vector and HCT116/vector, and in the S100A4 overexpressing cell lines HAB92/S100A4 and HCT116/S100A4, respectively. Transfection of HCT116 cells with S100A4-specific (shS100A4) or unspecific control shRNA-plasmids (shCtrl) resulted in HCT116/shS100A4 and HCT116/shCtrl cells, respectively. HAB92/shDKK1 and HAB92/shCtrl cells were generated by transfecting DKK1-specific (shDKK1) or unspecific (shCtrl) shRNA-plasmids (all SABiosciences, Frederick, MD, USA). Generated cell lines with modulated target gene expression were generated from clonal expansion of selected stably resistant cells after transfection.

Cell lines SW620, LS174T, Colo205, SW480, HCT15, LoVo, HT29, Caco 2, WiDr, KM12, SW48, and DLD-1 were obtained from ATCC. Authentication of the cell lines was verified by short tandem repeat (STR) genotyping at the DSMZ (German Collection of Microorganisms and Cell Cultures; Braunschweig, Germany). All cell lines were tested regularly for the absence of mycoplasma. The cell lines were cultured in recommended culture medium, supplemented with 10% FBS (all Life Technologies, Carlsbad, CA, USA). Cells were grown in sterile conditions in a humidified incubator (37 °C, 5% CO_2, 95% humidity). Lyophilized recombinant human DKK1 (rDKK1) protein (R&D Systems, Minneapolis, MN, USA) was dissolved in PBS, supplemented with 1% BSA (Sigma, St. Louis, MO, USA). Cells were treated for 24 h with the indicated rDKK1 protein concentrations. Control cells were treated with the same amounts of 1% BSA solution alone.

2.2. Microarray Analysis of the S100A4-Induced Transcriptome

The competitive hybridization cDNA microarrays were performed at the Center for Cancer Research/NCI (National Cancer Institute, Frederick, MD, USA). Each experiment consisted of two identical microarrays containing reciprocally labeled cDNAs from test samples (HAB92/S100A4) and control samples (HAB92 or HAB92/vector, respectively), giving 4 arrays for analysis of expression differences. The test sample was stained with Cy5 (red fluorescence) and the control sample with Cy3 (green fluorescence). In reciprocal arrays, test samples were stained with Cy3 and controls were stained with Cy5. In brief, isolated total RNA from HAB92, HAB92/vector, and HAB92/S100A4 cells was reverse transcribed and labeled with either Cy5 or Cy3 dye. Test samples were combined with their respective control samples and hybridized onto Human OncoChip arrays (NCI). Fluorescence intensities were determined with a GenePix 4100A microarray scanner. The data were analyzed by GenePix Pro 4.1 software, and the microarray intensities were normalized by setting the ratio of medians to 1. Data were analyzed with available tools on mAdB (https://madb.nci.nih.gov) (accessed on 30 April 2011) and online tools from the 'Database for Annotation, Visualization and Integrated Discovery' (DAVID) [34,35].

2.3. Quantitative Real-Time RT-PCR (qRT-PCR)

Total RNA from cultured cells was extracted with Trizol RNA extraction reagent (Life Technologies). Total RNA from micro-dissected tumor tissues was isolated using the Universal RNA Purification Kit (Roboklon, Berlin, Germany). RNA was reverse transcribed as described previously [18]. cDNA quantification of target genes was performed with the following primers and probes: S100A4_fow: 5′-ctcagcgcttcttcttc-3′, S100A4_rev: 5′-gggtcagcagctccttta-3′, S100A4_FITC: 5′-tgtgatggtgtccaccttccacaagt-3′, S100A4_LCRed640: 5′-tcgggcaaagagggtgacaagt-3′; DKK1_fow: 5′-tagcaccttggatgggtattc-3′, DKK1_rev: 5′-agcctcctcctcacacctcctc-3′, DKK1_FITC: 5′-gtctccggtcatgagactgtgcc-3′, DKK1_LCRed640: 5′-aggattgtgttgtgctagacacctctgg-3′. The hG6PDH Kit (Roche, Basel, Switzerland) was used for cDNA quantification of the housekeeping gene G6PDH. Quantitative real-time RT PCR was performed in a LightCycler480 (Roche). Gene-specific standard curves and a calibrator in each run were used to quantify and normalize the samples. Each run was performed in duplicates and repeated at least twice with independent biological replicates.

2.4. Western Blot (WB) Analysis and Enzyme-Linked Immunosorbent Assay (ELISA)

Western blot analysis was performed as previously described [11]. Briefly, cells were lysed with RIPA buffer (Roche) for total protein extraction. Immunoblotting was performed with antibodies against hS100A4 (rabbit; 1:1000; Agilent, Santa Clara, CA, USA) and hGAPDH (goat; 1:1000; Santa Cruz Biotechnology, Dallas, TX, USA).

Secreted DKK1 was quantified with the DuoSet human DKK-1 ELISA System (R&D Systems). In brief, 4×10^5 cells were plated into 6-well plates, and the cell-free supernatant was harvested after 24 h. The supernatant was diluted with blocking reagent (1:4 and 1:8; PBS with 1% BSA) before entering the previously blocked wells. rDKK1, dissolved in blocking reagent, was used as a standard. Each experiment was performed in duplicate with at least two different dilutions to assure that ELISA reaction occurred in the linear range of sensitivity. The mean values of secreted DKK1 from each supernatant were normalized to the amount of total protein extracted from the respective cells.

2.5. Chromatin Immunoprecipitation Assay (ChIP)

A total of 1×10^6 cells were plated in 15 cm dishes 24 h prior to performing the assay. Cells were incubated with 13.5% formaldehyde for 10 min at room temperature to assure reversible cross-linking of proteins, washed twice with ice-cold PBS, and lysed according to the manufacturer's instructions (Magna ChIP HiSens; Millipore, Burlington, MA, USA). Cell lysates were sonicated for 20 pulses at 100% output and centrifuged at 10,000 rpm at 4 °C for 10 min. The upernatant was transferred to a new tube and aliquoted in 50 µL aliquots for incubation with antibodies. A total of 5 µL of supernatant was stored at −20 °C and used as an input control. Each ChIP was incubated with 10 µg antibody or 10 µg control IgG overnight at 4 °C. Non-bound proteins were washed, followed by elution of the protein-DNA complex from the beads according to the manufacturer's instructions. Cross-linking of protein and DNA was reversed, and PCR amplification of the DKK1-promoter was performed with a limit of 35 cycles, using the following primer set: pDKK1-fow: 5′-cgactaagcaagggagggg-3′; pDKK1-rev: 5′-gcctttataccgcgggcc-3′. PCR product was analyzed via 2% agarose gel electrophoresis.

2.6. Luciferase-Based Reporter Assay

For transient transfection, cells were seeded at a density of 4×10^4 cells in a 24-well plate and directly transfected with 500 ng reporter plasmid using TransIT-2020 (MirusBio, Madison, WI, USA) according to the manufacturer's instructions. After 48 h, cells were transfected with a mix of 100 ng DKK1-promoter plasmids (firefly luciferase) and 20 ng renilla luciferase plasmid (Promega) as an internal control. Cells were lysed 24 h after transfection, and reporter assay was performed using the Dual Luciferase Assay Kit (Promega) according to the manufacturer's instructions. Firefly and Renilla luciferase activities were measured using an infiniteM200Pro (Tecan, Männedorf, Switzerland) plate reader.

2.7. Boyden Chamber Transwell Migration Assaya

Filter membranes of 12 µm pore size (Millipore) were used to analyze the migratory ability of HCT116/vector and HCT116/S100A4 cells. A total of 2.5×10^5 cells were seeded into each transwell chamber, treated with 100 ng/mL rDKK1 or control solution, and incubated for 24 h to migrate through the membrane. After insert removal, cells at the bottom chamber were trypsinized and counted in a Neubauer chamber (LO Laboroptik, Friedrichsdorf, Germany). Each well was counted ten times. The experiments were performed in duplicates and repeated twice.

2.8. mRNA Expression Analysis of Xenograft CRC Mouse Tumor Tissue

Animal experiments were performed in accordance with the United Kingdom Coordinated Committee on Cancer Research (UKCCCR) guidelines and were approved by the responsible local authorities (State Office of Health and Social Affairs, Berlin, Germany), with the registration number A0010/19. mRNA samples of intrasplenically xenografted CRC mouse tumors were obtained after systemic treatment with shRNA expression plasmids. Experimental procedures were previously described [17]. In brief, NOD/SCID mice were intrasplenically transplanted with HCT116 cells and repeatedly treated with S100A4-

shRNA expressing plasmids via tail vein injection. Mice were sacrificed, and spleens and livers were removed. Cryosections of the tumor tissue (spleen) were used to isolate total RNA samples.

2.9. Immunohistochemistry of Xenograft CRC Mouse Tumor Tissue

Cryosections of the tumor tissue (spleen) were fixed with 4% paraformaldehyde, quenched with 0.1 M glycine/PBS, and residual cellular peroxidase activity was blocked with 0.9% H_2O_2/PBS. Cells were permeabilized with 0.5% Triton-X-100/PBS and unspecific binding sites blocked with 1% horse serum/PBS. Target-specific antibodies (S100A4, Dako, 1:400; DKK1, CellSignalling, 1:400) were applied overnight in 0.1% horse serum/PBS and detected with a rabbit-specific DAB kit (Vectastain, Vector Laboratories, Inc., Burlingame, CA, USA) according to the manufacturer's instructions. Nuclei were stained with hematoxylin, and pictures were taken with a BZ-X800 microscope (Keyence, Neu-Isenburg, Germany) at 20× and 40× magnification. Quantification of IHC signal intensities was performed with ImageJ (v1.53).

2.10. Data Mining of Expression Microarray Data

Publicly available expression data of CRC tumor microarrays were obtained from Gene Expression Omnibus (www.ncbi.nlm.nih.gov/geo) (accessed on 10 December 2018). Expression data of target genes were normalized to G6PDH and analyzed for direct or inverse correlation. Expression data of the following sets were combined after normalizing: GDS2201 [36]; GDS4381 [37]; GDS4513 [38]; GDS4515 [39]; and GDS4718 [40].

2.11. Patient Material

Primary tumors were obtained from all patients with informed written consent. The analyses of patient samples, in accordance with the Declaration of Helsinki, were performed with their consent to participate and were approved by the responsible local authorities (State Office of Health and Social Affairs, Berlin, Germany), with the registration number AA3/03/45. Primary tumor tissues were collected immediately after surgical removal and snap-frozen in liquid nitrogen according to internal protocols. In addition to routine pathological examination of the tumor tissue, the histopathology of each sample used for experimental analysis was reviewed by an experienced pathologist to confirm diagnosis, tissue composition, and tumor content. Tumor staging and typing were performed according to UICC and WHO guidelines. The patients were preoperatively untreated, had no history of familial CRC, did not suffer from a second tumor, and underwent R0 resection. One cohort consists of tumor samples from 41 CRC patients at stages I–IV. For the second cohort, CRC tumor tissues were obtained from 60 CRC patients at stages I, II, or III, i.e., without distant metastases at the time point of diagnosis. Detailed information on patients and tumor tissue of both cohorts are provided in previous reports [41,42]. All tumors were R0 resected, were fresh frozen in liquid nitrogen, and the areas of tumor cells were micro-dissected after preparation of serial consecutive cryosections.

2.12. Statistical Analysis

Student's *t*-test was used to compare two groups of data. Comparison of more than two groups was performed by one-way analysis of variance (ANOVA) and Bonferroni post hoc multiple comparisons, or one-way ANOVA on ranks and Tukey post hoc multiple comparison, if the normality test of the data failed. Pearson correlation analysis was used to identify expression correlations. Survival rates were calculated with Kaplan–Meier estimator, with multiple comparisons (pairwise over strata) if indicated. The cut-offs to distinguish low and high expression levels were determined using Receiver–operator-characteristics (ROC) analysis by taking the value with the highest Youden-Index. *p*-values less than 0.05 were defined as statistically significant. All computations were performed using IBM SPSS Statistics 21.

3. Results

3.1. Inverse Expression Correlation of Wnt/β-Catenin Targets S100A4 and DKK1 in CRC Cells

3.1.1. Identification of the S100A4-Induced Transcriptome

Although many protein–protein interaction partners of S100A4 have been identified that sustain the pro-metastatic action of S100A4 [5], much less is known about changes in the transcription of metastasis-associated genes upon elevated S100A4 expression level. To identify the transcriptional mechanism underlying S100A4-driven metastasis formation, we compared the expression profiles of the HCT116-derived isogenic cell lines HAB92, HAB92/vector, and HAB92/S100A4. HAB92 contains only the wild-type allele for β-catenin, resulting in reduced Wnt pathway activity and very low levels of S100A4 [11]. Ectopic overexpression of S100A4 in these cells was achieved by stable transfection of S100A4 cDNA. Competitive hybridization of cDNA from HAB92, HAB92/vector, and HAB92/S100A4 cells onto spotted microarrays identified 195 functionally annotated genes to be differentially expressed >4-fold on average ($n \geq 3$).

The results of four microarrays were combined and subsequently analyzed. A total of 324 transcripts were found differentially expressed in dependency of S100A4 overexpression, with 195 transcripts showing a more than four-fold difference. A total of 32 of the functionally annotated genes in this set were up-regulated, and 140 were down-regulated (Figure 1a). When we clustered the S100A4-associated genes according to their annotations using DAVID/EASE, we found high enrichment scores in topics related to transcription regulation (nuclear localization, DNA-protein complex assembly, chromatin modification, mRNA processing) and cell motility (Figure 1b). Interestingly, we observed a number of Wnt pathway factors and target genes differentially regulated in HAB92/S100A4 cells, indicating a previously unreported regulatory mechanism of S100A4 on Wnt signaling pathway activity (Appendix A).

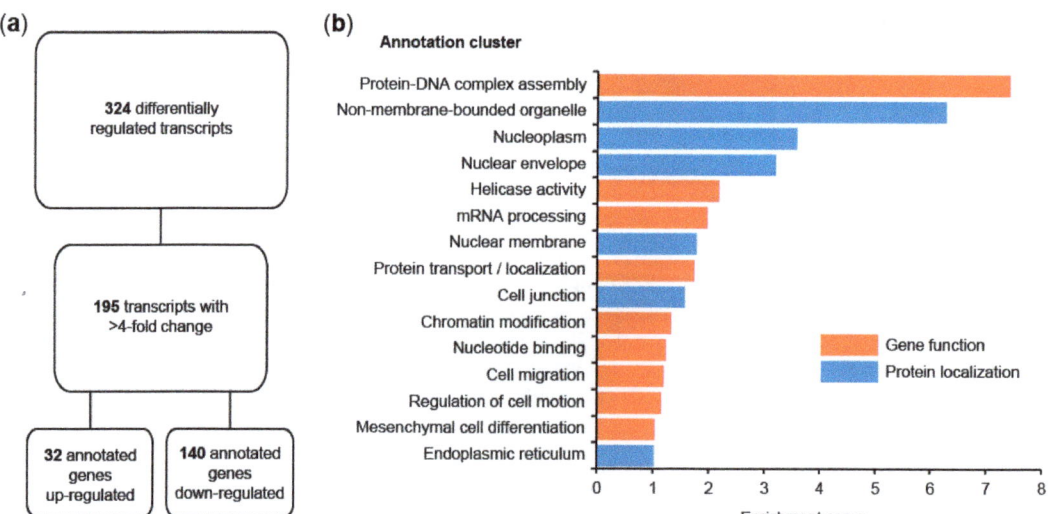

Figure 1. S100A4-dependent transcriptome analysis in HAB92 CRC cells. (**a**) Two color microarray analyses of differentially expressed genes in HAB92/S100A4 cells vs. HAB92 and HAB92/vector cells. (**b**) Annotation cluster analysis of 195 transcripts with a more than four-fold change in expression, classified by gene function and protein localization.

3.1.2. S100A4 Inhibits Expression of the Wnt Pathway Antagonist DKK1

One of the most highly and consistently down-regulated genes in the arrays was DKK1 (Figure 2a). This result was validated by qRT PCR and WB. HAB92/S100A4 cells express 14.4-fold more S100A4 than HAB92 cells, both shown for mRNA and protein levels ($p = 0.003$; Figures 2b and S1a,b), whereas mRNA levels of DKK1 were reduced to 40% in these cells, compared to HAB92 cells ($p < 0.001$; Figure 2c). By quantifying the amount of secreted DKK1 protein via ELISA, we observed a similar decrease to 34% in HAB92/S100A4 cells compared to HAB92 cells ($p < 0.001$; Figure 2d). These data confirm an S100A4-mediated decrease in DKK1. Although both S100A4 and DKK1 are target genes of canonical Wnt signaling, their expression pattern inversely differs in CRC tumors [22]. Therefore, we compared the levels of both genes in HCT116 cells, as well as in its derivatives HAB68 and HAB92. S100A4 expression was found to be 1.2-fold higher in HAB68 cells, harboring only mutant β-catenin, compared to HCT116 cells. In contrast, in HAB92 cells, with only wild-type β-catenin, S100A4 mRNA expression was reduced to 8% ($p < 0.001$; Figures 2e and S1c,d). These data were supported by changes in protein expression, thereby confirming our previous finding [11]. In contrast, we observed an inverse expression pattern of DKK1 in those cells. HAB92 cells expressed nine-fold more DKK1 on the mRNA level compared to HCT116 cells ($p < 0.001$; Figure 2f). We validated the mRNA expression levels of DKK1 with the amount of secreted DKK1 protein in the surrounding medium and found a 5.3-fold increase of extracellular DKK1 from HAB92 cells, compared to HCT116 cells ($p < 0.001$; Figure 2g).

3.1.3. Inverse Expression Correlation of S100A4 and DKK1 in Further CRC Cell Lines

In order to determine if the observation of inverse expression of S100A4 and DKK1 extended to other CRC cell lines, we compared the mRNA levels of both genes in a panel of 12 additional lines. A nearly reciprocal increase of either S100A4 or DKK1 expression was identified when normalized to HCT116 cells (Figure 3a). S100A4 mRNA levels in SW620, LS174T, Colo205, and SW480 cells were similar or higher than in HCT116 cells, and all these cell lines presented with very low levels of DKK1 mRNA. In contrast, HCT15, Lovo, HT29, HAB92, and Caco-2 cells expressed similar or higher levels of DKK1 than HCT116 cells and very low levels of S100A4 mRNA. The mRNA levels of both genes were low in WiDr, KM12, SW48, and DLD1 cells. The expression levels of S100A4 and DKK1 mRNA were significantly inversely correlated (Pearson correlation coefficient, $\rho = -0.566$; $p = 0.041$). The differences in mRNA expression levels were verified at the protein level by either WB for S100A4 (Figures 3b and S1e–h) or ELISA for secreted DKK1 (Figure 3c).

3.1.4. Expression Regulation of DKK1 in CRC Cells Involves the Transcription Factor ATF5

By determining the S100A4-induced transcriptome in CRC cells, we were interested in which transcription factors are involved in the respective expression regulation of differentially expressed transcripts, focusing on the 140 down-regulated genes (Figure 1a). An in silico approach employed the iRegulon module in the Cytoscape analysis platform [43,44]. ATF5 was the only transcription factor predicted for DKK1 expression regulation (NES 3.37; $p = 0.045$), on the basis of ChIPseq data from Lovo cells (GSM1208713) [45]. We validated the binding of ATF5 to the DKK1 promoter via ATF5-specific ChIP assays in the HAB68 and HAB92 cell pair with differential expression of S100A4 and DKK1 (Figure 4a). We observed a higher abundance of DKK1 promoter fragments after precipitating RNA polymerase II in HAB92 cells, confirming the higher DKK1 transcription in these cells. In addition, precipitating ATF5 also resulted in increased band intensity after amplification of the DKK1-specific promoter fragment. To confirm the transcriptional regulation of DKK1 by ATF5 and S100A4 on promoter level, we used the previously described reporter plasmids containing truncated versions of the human DKK1 promoter [22]. We observed significantly increased luciferase reporter activity in HAB92 cells for all promoter fragments (Appendix B) and used the longest and shortest fragment for further analyses. Overexpression of ATF5 in HAB68 cells resulted in significantly increased reporter activity for the longest promoter fragment (2.35 kb; $p = 0.026$; Figure 4b), with a lesser extent for the shortest promoter fragment. In turn, ectopic expression of S100A4 in HAB92 did lead to a significant decrease in DKK1 promoter-driven luciferase activity ($p = 0.014$; Figure 4b).

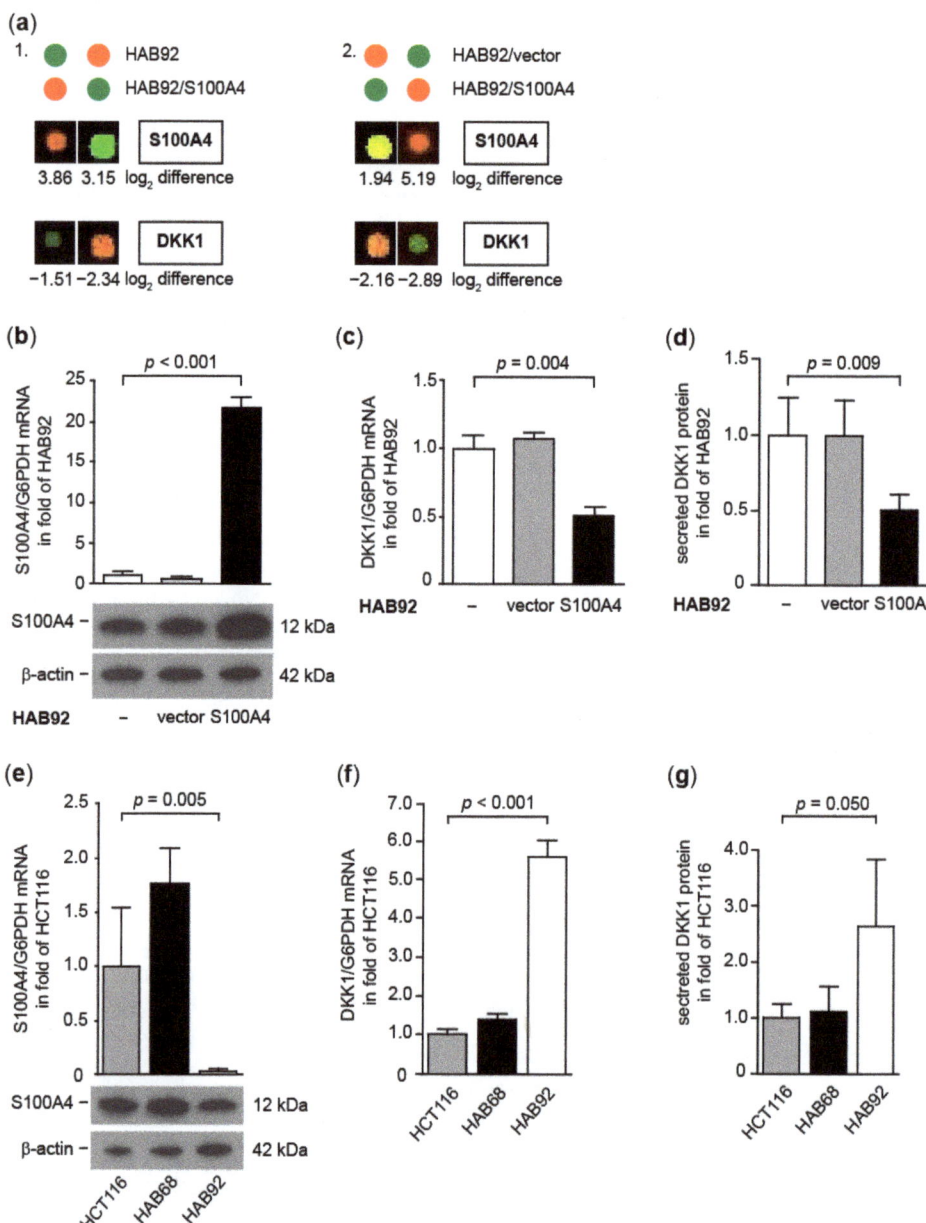

Figure 2. S100A4-induced expression alterations of DKK1 in CRC cell lines HCT116, HAB92, and HAB68. (**a**) Increased S100A4 expression and decreased DKK1 expression in HAB92/S100A4 cells vs. HAB92 cells (part 1) and HAB92/S100A4 cells vs. HAB92/vector cells (part 2). (**b**) Overexpression of S100A4 in HAB92/S100A4 cells on mRNA and protein level. Down-regulation of DKK1 mRNA expression (**c**) and of extracellular DKK1 (**d**) in HAB92/S100A4 cells. (**e**) S100A4 expression in HCT116, HAB68, and HAB92 cells on mRNA and protein levels; lowest S100A4 expression in HAB92 cells. Differential expression of DKK1 in HCT116, HAB68, and HAB92 cells on mRNA (**f**) and extracellular protein (**g**) levels; highest expression in HAB92 cells.

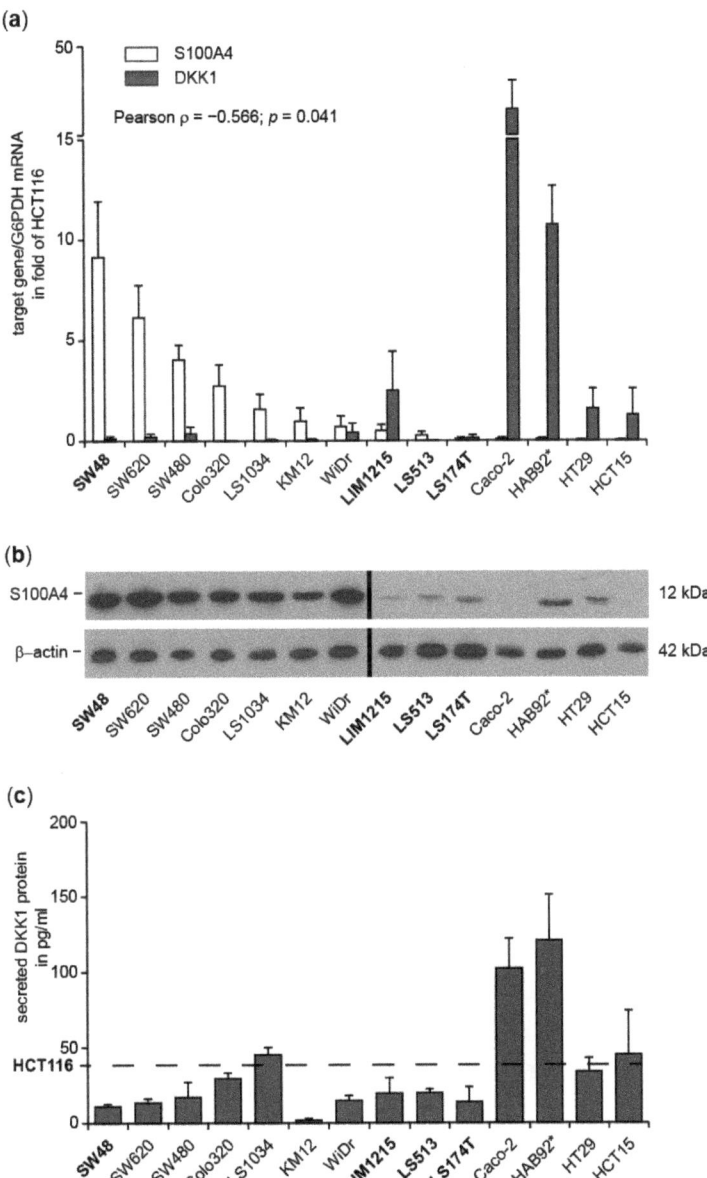

Figure 3. Inverse expression correlation of S100A4 and DKK1 in a panel of 13 CRC cell lines. (a) Relative mRNA expression level of S100A4 and DKK1 determined by gene-specific qRT PCR. (b) Western blot analysis of S100A4 expression. GAPDH served as loading control. (c) ELISA of extracellular amounts of human DKK1 in culture medium in the fold of HCT116. Names in bold indicate mutated β-catenin: HCT116—S45Δ, SW48—S33Y, LIM1215—T41A, LS513—A5-80Δ, LS174T—S45F. * indicates wt for both APC and β-catenin (Figure S1e–h).

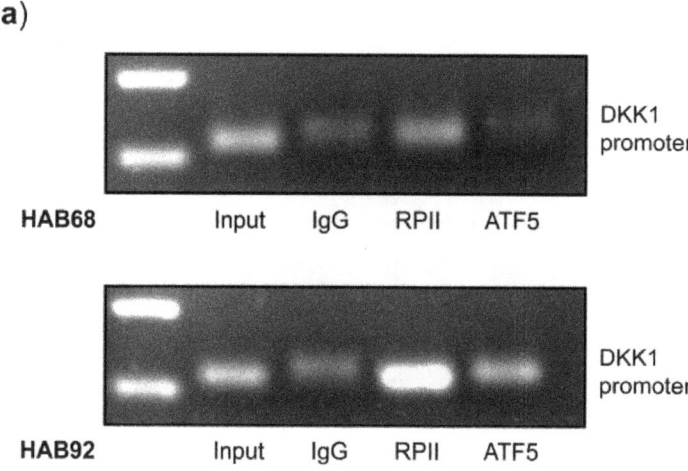

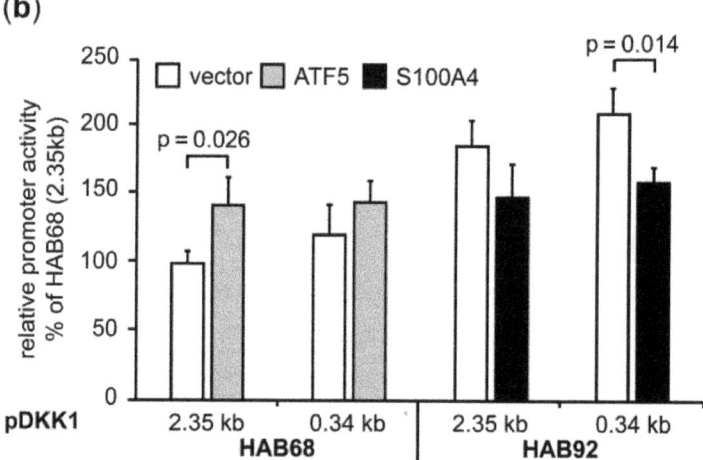

Figure 4. Expression regulation of DKK1 in CRC cells involves the transcription factor ATF5 and S100A4 but on different sites of the promoter. (**a**) ChIP assays of gene-specific pull-downs in HAB68 and HAB92 cells confirm the binding of ATF5 to the DKK1 promoter. Unspecific immunoglobulin served as the negative control and RNA polymerase II as an indicator of general DKK1 transcription. (**b**) Ectopic ATF5 expression in HAB68 cells increased DKK1 promoter-driven luciferase activity, while ectopic expression of S100A resulted in decreased reporter signal. DKK1 promoter fragments: −2238 bp–+112 bp (2.35 kb); −231 bp–+112 bp (0.34 kb).

3.1.5. Transcriptional Cross-Regulation of DKK1 and S100A4 Affects S100A4 Phenotype

Since S100A4 overexpression inhibits the expression of DKK1 in CRC cells, we analyzed the functional consequences of this gene regulation. We transfected HAB92 cells with DKK1-specific shRNA plasmids, generating HAB92/shDKK1 cells. DKK1 mRNA expression in HAB92/shDKK1 cells was reduced to 9% of HAB92/shCtrl cells ($p = 0.009$; Figure 5a). The knock-down of DKK1 mRNA subsequently decreased the amount of secreted DKK1 protein in HAB92/shDKK1 cells to 47%, compared to the control cells ($p = 0.022$; Figure 5b). In turn, we observed a 4.2-fold increase in the S100A4 mRNA level of HAB92/shDKK1 cells, compared to control shRNA-transfected cells (p = 0.015) and an increase in S100A4 protein levels in HAB92/shDKK1 (Figures 5c and S1i,j).

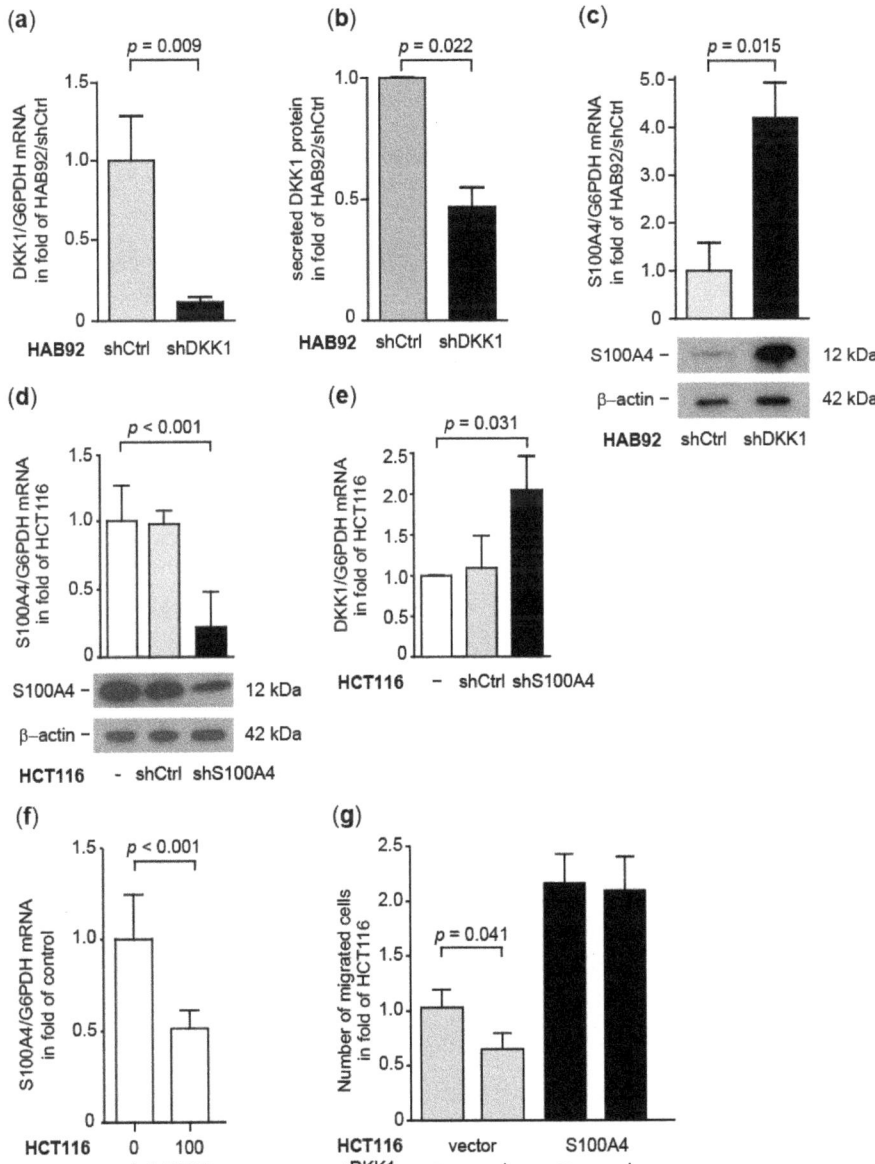

Figure 5. Transcriptional cross-regulation of DKK1 and S100A4 affects cellular motility. Relative DKK1 mRNA expression (**a**) and DKK1 protein secretion (**b**) in HAB92/shDKK1 cells. (**c**) Increase of S100A4 mRNA and protein expression in HAB92/shDKK1 cells. (**d**) Relative S100A4 mRNA and protein expression in HCT116/shS100A4 cells. (**e**) Increase of relative DKK1 mRNA expression in HCT116/shS100A4 cells. (**f**) Decrease of S100A4 mRNA expression level following treatment with rDKK1. (**g**) Decrease of cellular motility by rDKK1 treatment in HCT/vector cells is rescued by ectopic S100A4 expression in HCT116/S100A4 cells.

Next, we hypothesized that a reduction of S100A4 expression would result in increased expression of DKK1. We knocked down S100A4 in HCT116 cells by stably transfecting expression plasmids for either S100A4-specific shRNA (HCT116/shS100A4) or a non-targeting control shRNA (HCT116/shCtrl). HCT116/shS100A4 cells express 56% less S100A4 mRNA, compared to the control cells HCT116 and HCT116/shCtrl, which was confirmed at the protein level ($p < 0.001$; Figure 5d and S1k,l). When we determined the expression of DKK1 in these cells, we observed a 2.0-fold increase in DKK1 mRNA levels in HCT116/shS100A4, compared to the control cells ($p = 0.031$; Figure 5e). Since DKK1 protein is secreted to exert its function as a Wnt pathway antagonist, we treated the HCT116 cells with rDKK1 and analyzed the S100A4 expression in those cells. Treatment with rDKK1 for 24 h reduced the S100A4 mRNA level in a concentration-dependent manner. Cells treated with 25 ng/mL rDKK1 expressed 85% ($p < 0.01$) less S100A4 mRNA, whereas treatment with 100 ng/mL rDKK1 reduced the S100A4 mRNA level to 68% ($p < 0.001$; Figure 5f). Treatment with rDKK1 also reduced cellular motility. Compared to untreated HCT116/vector cells, the migratory ability was diminished to 65% by the application of 100 ng/mL rDKK1 ($p = 0.041$; Figure 5g). Treatment with rDKK1 did not reduce the S100A4-mediated cell migration in cells with ectopic overexpression of S100A4.

3.1.6. Knock-Down of Wnt Target Gene S100A4 Countermands Inhibition of DKK1

To validate the transcriptional cross-regulation of S100A4 and DKK1 in vivo, we analyzed the S100A4-regulated DKK1 expression in tumor tissue of xenograft mice after intrasplenic transplantation of HCT116 cells. These animals were systemically treated with S100A4-specific shRNA expression plasmids (versus non-targeting control shRNA, [18]). We found significantly reduced S100A4 mRNA expression in tumor tissues of mice, treated with S100A4-specific shRNA plasmids (median = 1.78), compared to treatment with control shRNA plasmids (median = 17.52; $p = 0.021$; Figure 6a). Interestingly, we observed an inverse correlation for DKK1 mRNA expression levels when compared to S100A4 mRNA. Tumors of animals treated with S100A4-specific shRNA plasmids expressed increased levels of DKK1 mRNA (median = 5.19) compared to animals treated with control shRNA, showing only low DKK1 expression levels (median = 1.26; $p = 0.057$; Figure 6b). This result was confirmed by IHC, staining S100A4 and DKK1 protein in sequential cryo-sections of the tumor tissues (Figure 6c–e). After quantification of the protein signals, we determined a reduction in S100A4 protein in tumors treated with S100A4-specific shRNA plasmids (median = 36.69), compared to treatment with control-shRNA plasmids (median = 78.01, $p < 0.001$, Figure 6f). In turn, we found a significant increase of DKK1 protein expression in the tumor tissues with reduced S100A4 expression (median = 35.94), compared to control treatment (median = 27.54, $p = 0.024$, Figure 6g).

The reciprocal expression regulation of S100A4 and DKK1 in vivo was further validated by a lower abundance of human DKK1 in mouse plasma when ectopic S100A4 expression was induced in transplanted HAB92 cells (Appendix C).

3.2. Transcriptional Cross-Regulation of S100A4 and DKK1 Has Prognostic Value for CRC Patient Survival

3.2.1. Inverse Expression Correlation of S100A4 and DKK1 in CRC Microarray Datasets

In order to evaluate the inverse expression correlation of S100A4 and DKK1 in patient tumors, we exploited several publicly available mRNA expression data generated by microarray analyses of CRC patient cohorts, using the GEO database from NCBI [36–40]. Expression values of S100A4 and DKK1 were normalized to G6PDH, and the five datasets were combined after normalization ($n = 224$). The inverse correlation of S100A4 and DKK1 mRNA expression in CRC patient tumors was confirmed by Pearson correlation analysis ($\rho = 0.151$; $p = 0.024$; Figure 7).

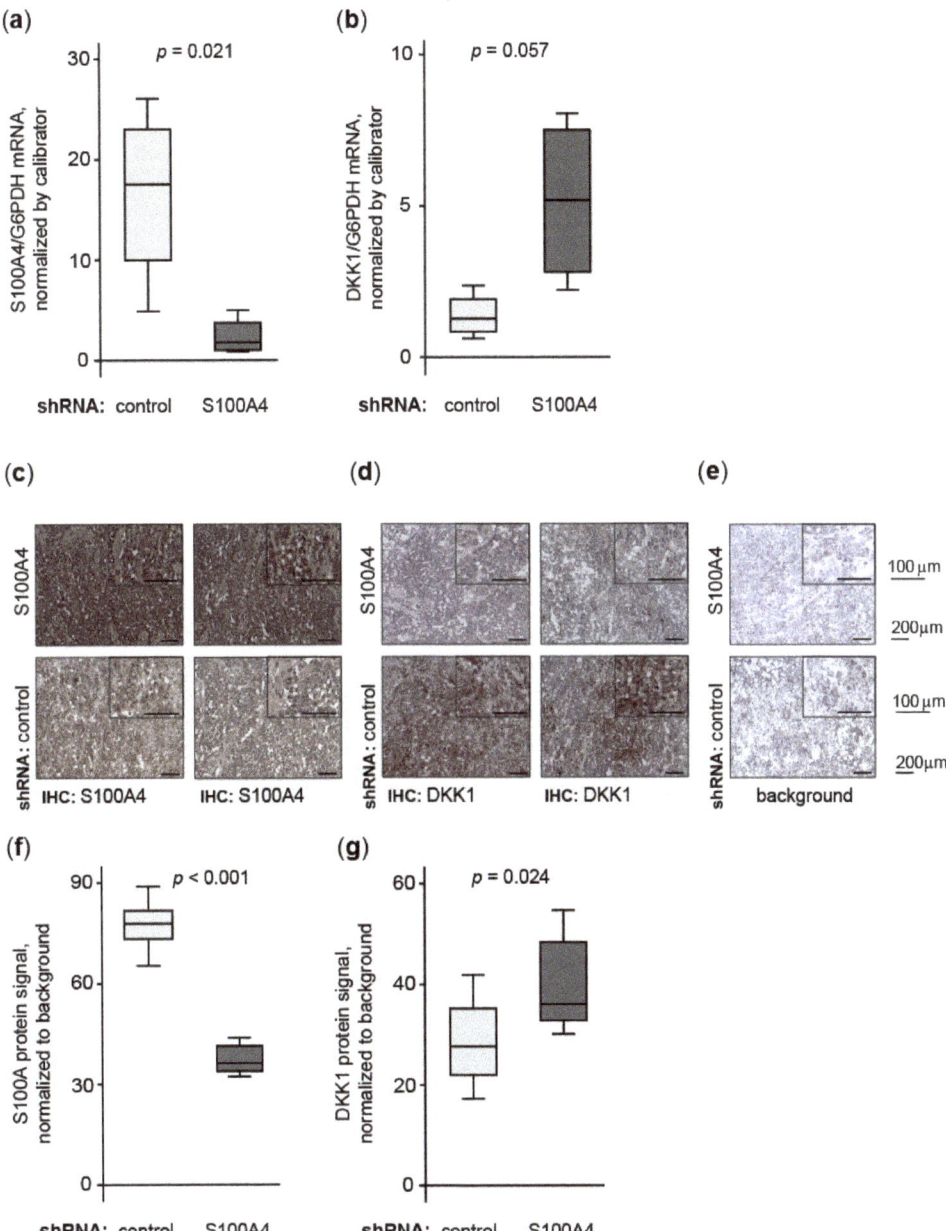

Figure 6. S100A4 reduction restores endogenous DKK1 expression in vivo. Relative mRNA expression of S100A4 (**a**) and DKK1 (**b**) in intrasplenic tumor tissue of xenografted mice receiving the systemic application of S100A4-specific shRNA expression plasmids. Immunostaining of S100A4 (**c**), DKK1 (**d**), and background control (**e**) of two independent samples per group of intrasplenic xenograft tumor tissue. Images were taken at 20× and 40× magnification, and scale bars represent 200 μm and 100 μm, respectively. Quantification of protein-specific immunostaining confirms the cross-regulation of S100A4 (**f**) and DKK1 (**g**) in vivo. Quantified expression of target genes occurred in triplicates of eight independent animal tumors.

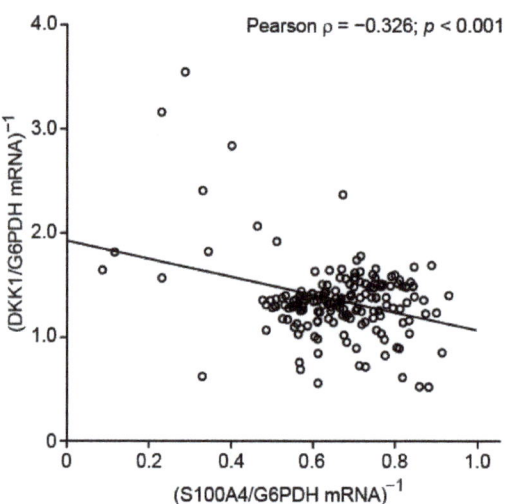

Figure 7. Correlation analysis of S100A and DKK1 mRNA expression of combined GEO datasets of CRC microarray analyses. Expression levels of target genes were normalized to G6PDH.

3.2.2. Prognostic Value of Combining S100A4 and DKK1 Expression in CRC Tumor Samples

Next, we determined the mRNA levels of S100A4 and DKK1 in micro-dissected primary tumor tissues of two independent patient cohorts by gene-specific qRT PCR. One cohort consisted of 41 CRC patients in stages I–IV [42]. Based on gene-expression levels and using ROC-based cut-off values, we calculated the rates for patients' OS by Kaplan–Meier analysis. For S100A4, expression below the cut-off correlated significantly with better outcome in OS ($p = 0.016$; Figure 8a). The five-year OS was 90% (± 4.6%) for low S100A4 expression and 50% (± 2.5%) for S100A4 levels above the cut-off. On the contrary, patients benefited from higher expression levels of the Wnt antagonist DKK1 in longer OS (Figure 8b). The five-year OS was 87% (± 7.0%) for high DKK1 levels and 71% (± 14.3%) for low DKK1 expression.

The second cohort consisted of 60 CRC patients in stages I, II, and III (R0, no metastases at time of diagnosis) [41]. For S100A4, gene expression below the cut-off correlated significantly with better outcomes in both OS (Figure 9a) and MFS (Figure 9b). The five-year OS was 88% (± 5.5%) for low S100A4 expression and 65% (± 9.3%) for S100A4 expression levels above the cut-off. For MFS, the five-year survival rates were 65% (± 7.3%) and 41% (± 11.9%), respectively. On the contrary, patients benefited from higher expression levels of the Wnt antagonist DKK1 in OS (Figure 9c) and MFS (Figure 9d). The five-year OS was 63% (± 11.1%) for low DKK1 expression and 85% (± 5.5%) for high DKK1 levels. Likewise, the five-year MFS of 37% (± 11.1%) for patients with low DKK1 levels increased to 68% (± 7.3%) for DKK1 high expressers.

With the above-reported transcriptional cross-regulation of S100A4 and DKK1 expression in mind, we combined the survival analyses of S100A4 and DKK1 expression. The correlation for patients' OS and their expression levels of the respective genes increased the significance when based on a combinatorial analysis of S100A4 and DKK1. If patients expressed low levels of S100A4 and high levels of DKK1 in the tumor, the five-year survival was 90% (± 7.0%) in the first cohort (Figure 8c) and 91% (± 6.1%) in the second cohort (Figure 9e). Expression of both genes below the respective cut-off resulted in a five-year survival rate of 79% (± 13.4%) in the first cohort and 83% (± 10.8%) in the second cohort. Patients with S100A4 and DKK1 expression above the respective cut-off resulted in a five-year survival rate of 67% (± 27.2%) in the first cohort and 79% (± 9.4%) in the second cohort. Patients with high S100A4 and low DKK1 expression levels showed the poorest five-year

OS in both cohorts. No patient in the first cohort lived longer than five years, and the rate for the second cohort was 29% (±17.1%). When focused on MFS, the combination of S100A4 and DKK1 expression increased the significance with respect to DKK1 expression alone (Figure 9f). Patients expressing low levels of S100A4 and high levels of DKK1 showed a five-year MFS of 74% (±7.9%). Having both genes above the respective cut-off reduced the five-year MFS to 50% (±15.8%). If both genes are below the cut-off, a five-year MFS of 42% (±14.2%) was observed. High S100A4 and low DKK1 expression levels in the primary tumor resulted in a five-year MFS of 29% (±17.1%).

Taken together, the combination of S100A4 and DKK1 expression enables more powerful prognostication of patients' outcomes. Patients with high S100A4 and low DKK1 expression levels in the primary tumor can be classified as high risk for OS. For MFS, patients with low intratumoral S100A4 expression become high-risk patients when the DKK1 expression is also decreased.

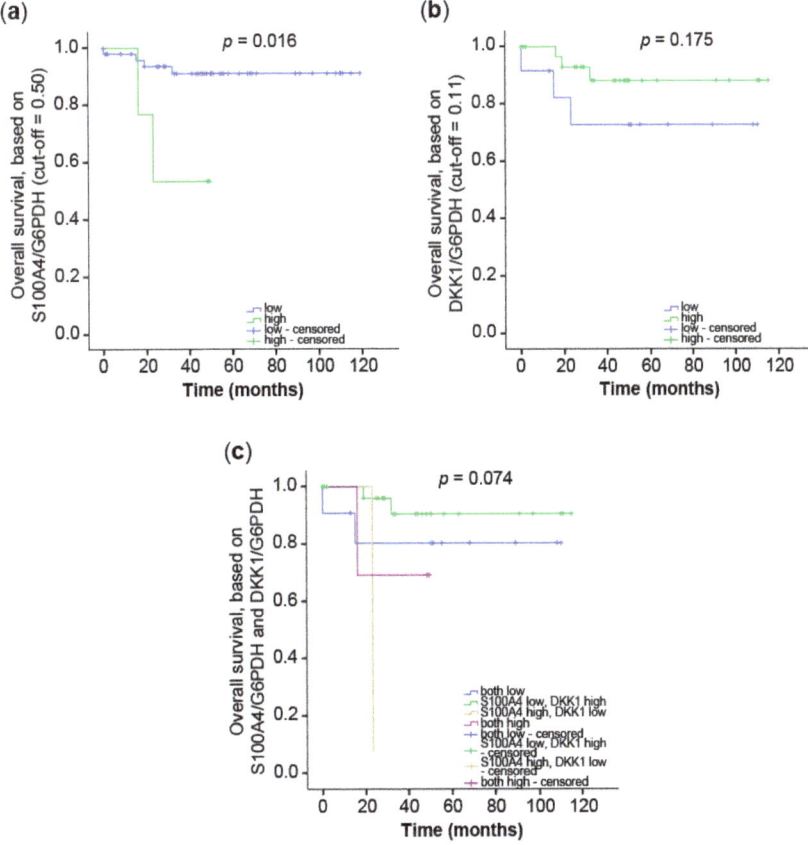

Figure 8. Combination of S100A4 and DKK1 for improved prognosis of OS CRC patients. DKK1, as well as S100A4, mRNA expression levels were determined by qRT PCR in micro-dissected tumor cell populations of primary tumors of stages I–IV ($n = 41$). The cut-off values to distinguish low and high expression levels were determined by ROC analyses. (**a**) OS of CRC patients, based on the S100A4 mRNA expression in the primary tumor. (**b**) OS of CRC patients, based on the DKK1 mRNA expression in the primary tumor. (**c**) OS of CRC patients, based on the combination of S100A4 and DKK1 expression in the tumor. Cut-off values for the respective gene and analysis are indicated by the axis labels.

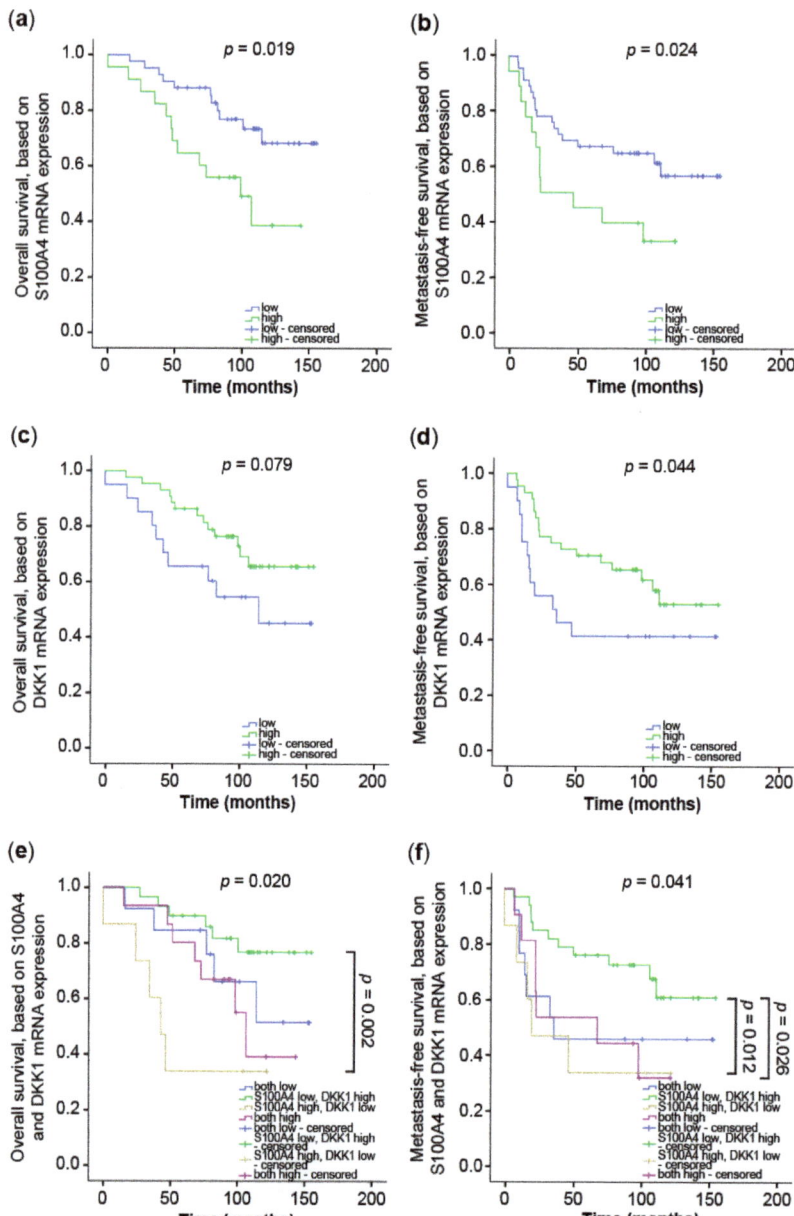

Figure 9. Combination of S100A4 and DKK1 for improved prognosis of OS and MFS of CRC patients. DKK1 and S100A4 mRNA expression levels were determined by qRT PCR in micro-dissected tumor cell populations of primary, not yet metastasized, tumors of stages I, II, and III ($n = 60$). The cut-off values to distinguish low and high expression levels were determined by ROC analyses (highest Youden index: S100A4—2.68; DKK1—0.21). Survival analysis was performed with the Kaplan–Meier estimator, with a chi-square multiple comparison. OS (**a**) and MFS (**b**) of CRC patients, based on the S100A4 mRNA expression in the primary tumor. OS (**c**) and MFS (**d**) of CRC patients, based on the DKK1 mRNA expression in the primary tumor. OS (**e**) and MFS (**f**) of CRC patients, based on the combination of S100A4 and DKK1 expression in the tumor.

4. Discussion

Here we report the transcriptional cross-regulation of the Wnt target genes S100A4 and DKK1 by exploring the first S100A4-regulated transcriptome in CRC. Knock-down of S100A4 under constitutive active Wnt signaling restored the expression of DKK1 in vitro and in vivo. As overexpression of S100A4 reduced DKK1 mRNA and protein levels, S100A4 can be seen as the predominant factor in this feedback loop in Wnt signaling modulation. The inverse correlation of S100A4 and DKK1 was validated in publicly available CRC expression datasets. Combining the intratumoral expression levels of S100A4 and DKK1 increased OS and MFS prognostication and identification of CRC patients at high risk.

S100A4 expression is a marker for malignancy in several cancer types, including CRC [46,47]. Some effort has been made to understand the cellular mechanisms that regulate S100A4 expression. In CRC, the expression of S100A4 is mainly driven by constitutively active Wnt signaling [11]. By comparing transcripts of CRC cell lines that differed exclusively in the expression level of S100A4, we found that the Wnt antagonist DKK1 was inversely expressed. DKK1 itself is also a Wnt target gene, and it is up-regulated by highly active Wnt signaling [22,48]. Secreted DKK1 acts as a Wnt pathway antagonist by interacting with the membranous co-receptor LRP 5/6, which is subsequently sequestered from the Wnt/frizzled signaling complex [49,50]. This decrease in Wnt pathway activity creates a negative feedback loop in normal tissue. With our finding of high S100A4 levels upon active Wnt signaling, suppression of the pathway antagonist DKK1 should reduce the negative feedback loop allowing for sustained Wnt signaling. Indeed, the transcriptional up-regulation of DKK1 by active Wnt signaling has been lost in many cases of CRC [51–53]. The inverse correlation of S100A4 and DKK1 expression in CRC tumors was found significant when we analyzed the combination of several existing microarray datasets [36–40]. When we overexpressed S100A4 in CRC cells with wild-type β-catenin (HAB92), we observed a significant decrease in DKK1 expression along with AMOTL2, also described as a Wnt signaling inhibitor. Interestingly, we found a subset of other Wnt signaling target genes, such as CCND1, PTK2, and MET, down-regulated upon ectopic S100A4 expression in HAB92 cells with restored Wnt signaling pathway. A potential mechanism is the induced expression of APC itself, which can affect cytoplasmic and nuclear β-catenin levels, and thus, activity. In turn, a knock-down of DKK1 in these cells showed re-expression of endogenous S100A4. When we compared the transcriptional cross-regulation of S100A4 and DKK1 in cells harboring mutated β-catenin, the knock-down of S100A4 expression has a stronger effect on DKK1 expression than the treatment of the cells with 100 ng/mL rDKK1 on S100A4 expression. We conclude that S100A4 plays a dominant role in the regulation of DKK1 expression by preventing the normal negative feedback loop induced by DKK1, thus maintaining an activated Wnt pathway and stabilizing (or even increasing) its own expression level.

A recent publication by Park et al. describes remaining susceptibility to Wnt signaling pathway regulation by Wnt stimulation or APC regulation even in the presence of an S45Δ-β-catenin gain-of-function mutation, such as in HCT116 cells [54]. The proposed model of 'just-right' Wnt signaling activation in CRC cells is supported by our finding that S100A4 can modulate Wnt/β-catenin transcriptional activity even in the context of aberrantly active Wnt signaling.

We found ATF5, a member of the ATF/cAMP response element-binding protein family, involved in the regulation of DKK1 expression in CRC cell lines, depending on the activity of the Wnt/β-catenin signaling pathway. ATF5 itself has been related to cell enhanced invasion of fibrosarcoma and breast cancer cells [55], and its therapeutic targeting strongly reduced cancer cell survival, except for pancreatic cancer and CRC [56,57]. ATF5 is able to bind to CRE consensus sequences but prefers binding sites with a core sequence of CYTCTYCCTTW [58]. Interestingly, the promoter of GSK3β, a modulator of Wnt/β-catenin signaling activity, harbors a predicted ATF5 binding site, and it can regulate the levels of ATF5 itself [59,60]. With the here-reported regulation of DKK1 expression, ATF5 becomes further involved in the modulation of Wnt/β-catenin-mediated target gene expression, and thus cancer progression and metastasis also for CRC.

While constitutively active Wnt signaling in the colon gives rise to adenocarcinoma, elevated levels of S100A4 in the primary tumor drives cancer progression up to the formation of distant metastases [12,13]. S100A4 is, therefore, widely used as a prognostic marker to stratify patients' risks to CRC [61,62]. In CRC, high DKK1 expression levels correlate with lower tumor stages, less metastasis, and increased five-year survival of patients [33,63,64].

The diagnosis of metastasized CRC is correlated with the worst prognosis for CRC patients [65]. With the reported transcriptional cross-regulation in expression regulation of S100A4 and DKK1, their combination in expression analyses should improve the prognostication for CRC patients. In our cohorts, patients with high S100A4 expression combined with low DKK1 expression showed the lowest five-year survival rates for both OS and MFS. High DKK1 expression in the tumor tissue or microenvironment seems to compensate for the aggressive phenotype of elevated S100A4 expression in OS. In the case of tumors with low S100A4 expression, patients' outcome in MFS is strongly determined by the expression status of DKK1. The combination of both S100A4 and DKK1 clearly improves the prognostic value in CRC compared to each tumor marker alone.

Therapeutic approaches to restore the expression of DKK1 in tumors, with subsequent reduction of up-regulated Wnt target genes, combined with a reduction of S100A4 expression, could improve the outcome of S100A4-driven CRC. In recent reports, DKK1 expression in CRC cells was restored by treatment with Genistein or targeting the vitamin D receptor, leading to reduced Wnt target gene expression [66,67]. Further, pharmacological inhibitors, such as niclosamide and sulindac, are reported, which decrease S100A4 expression by intervening in the Wnt signaling, resulting in restricted metastasis formation [18,19].

5. Conclusions

Taken together, the identification of S100A4-mediated transcriptome revealed the transcriptional cross-regulation of the metastasis-inducing S100A4 and the Wnt antagonist DKK1, dominated by S100A4, which leads to increased cell motility, cancer progression and metastasis, and decreased survival of CRC patients. By combining both genes in expression analyses of CRC tumors, we were able to identify high-risk patients who might benefit from adapted cancer therapy.

Supplementary Materials: The following are available online at https://www.mdpi.com/article/10.3390/cancers14010037/s1, Figure S1: Western Blots.

Author Contributions: Conceptualization, U.S. and R.H.S.; methodology, U.S., A.M., E.D.H. and M.D.; formal analysis, M.D. and U.S.; investigation, M.D., D.K., F.K. and P.H.; resources, W.K., S.B., W.W., R.H.S. and U.S.; data curation, M.D., M.O. and D.K.; writing—original draft preparation, M.D.; writing—review and editing, M.D., U.S., D.K. and W.W.; visualization, M.D., M.O. and F.K.; supervision, U.S.; funding acquisition, U.S., W.W. and R.H.S. All authors have read and agreed to the published version of the manuscript.

Funding: This work was supported by the Deutsche Forschungsgemeinschaft (DFG, grant number STE 671/8-1), the Alexander von Humboldt Stiftung, and the Deutsches Konsortium für Translationale Krebsforschung (DKTK). This project has been funded in whole or in part with federal funds from the National Cancer Institute, National Institutes of Health, under Contract No. HHSN261200800001E. The content of this publication does not necessarily reflect the views or policies of the Department of Health and Human Services, nor does the mention of trade names, commercial products, or organizations imply endorsement by the U.S. Government. This research was also supported in part by the Developmental Therapeutics Program in the Division of Cancer Treatment and Diagnosis of the National Cancer Institute.

Institutional Review Board Statement: The analyses of patient samples, in accordance with the Declaration of Helsinki, were performed with their consent to participate and were approved by the responsible local authorities (State Office of Health and Social Affairs, Berlin, Germany), with the registration number AA3/03/45. Animal experiments were performed in accordance with the United

Kingdom Co-ordinated Committee on Cancer Research (UKCCCR) guidelines and were approved by the responsible local authorities (State Office of Health and Social Affairs, Berlin, Germany), with the registration number A0010/19.

Informed Consent Statement: Informed consent was obtained from all subjects involved in the study.

Data Availability Statement: Data are available on request via the corresponding author.

Acknowledgments: We are grateful to Todd Waldman (Georgetown University, Washington, DC, USA) for providing the HCT116 cells and its β-catenin knock-out derivatives HAB68 and HAB92. We thank Nicole Fer (Frederick National Laboratory for Cancer Research, MD) for help with the microarray analyses. DKK1 promoter-driven luciferase reporter constructs were kindly provided by Alberto Munoz (Instituto de Investigaciones Biomedicas 'Alberto Sols', Consejo Superior de Investigaciones Cientıficas-Universidad Autonoma de Madrid, Madrid, Spain).

Conflicts of Interest: The authors declare no conflict of interest.

Appendix A

Table A1. List of differentially expressed Wnt signaling pathway-related factors or target genes upon ectopic expression of S100A4 in HAB92 cells with restored Wnt signaling pathway activity.

log2-Fold Change	StDev	Gene Name	Description
5.04	1.21	APC	Promotes rapid degradation of β-catenin and participates in Wnt signaling as a negative regulator.
4.29	0.82	TBL1Y	Plays an essential role in transcription activation mediated by nuclear receptors.
−1.72	0.22	CAMK2D	Calcium/calmodulin-dependent protein kinase involved in the regulation of Ca^{2+} homeostasis.
−1.72	0.36	CD44	Cell-surface receptor that plays a role in cell–cell interactions, cell adhesion, and migration.
−1.73	0.36	HDAC2	Responsible for the deacetylation of lysine residues on the N-terminal part of the core histones (H2A, H2B, H3, and H4).
−1.84	0.57	CCND1	Regulatory component of the cyclin D1-CDK4 (DC) complex that regulates the cell cycle during G_1/S transition.
−1.99	0.43	EPCAM	Plays a role in embryonic stem cells proliferation and differentiation.
−2.13	0.35	PTK2	Non-receptor protein-tyrosine kinase that plays an essential role in regulating cell migration, adhesion, formation, and disassembly of focal adhesions and cell protrusions, cell cycle progression, cell proliferation, and apoptosis.
−2.23	0.57	DKK1	Antagonizes canonical Wnt signaling by inhibiting LRP5/6 interaction with Wnt and by forming a ternary complex with the transmembrane protein KREMEN that promotes internalization of LRP5/6.
−2.26	0.22	MET	Receptor tyrosine kinase that transduces signals from the extracellular matrix into the cytoplasm by binding to hepatocyte growth factor/HGF ligand. Regulates many physiological processes, including proliferation, scattering, morphogenesis, and survival.
−2.50	0.80	AMOTL2	Regulates the translocation of phosphorylated SRC to peripheral cell-matrix adhesion sites. Inhibits the Wnt/β-catenin signaling pathway, probably by recruiting β-catenin to recycling endosomes, and hence preventing its translocation to the nucleus.
−5.22	3.81	TBL1XR1	F-box-like protein involved in the recruitment of the ubiquitin/19S proteasome complex to nuclear receptor-regulated transcription units. Plays an essential role in transcription activation mediated by nuclear receptors.

Appendix B

To investigate in which region of the DKK1 promoter an ectopic expression of S100A4 and ATF5 in HAB92 and HAB68 cells, respectively, will affect DKK1 transcription, we employed previously reported luciferase reporter constructs, driven by DKK1 promoter fragments of different sizes (kind gift of Alberto Munoz; Gonzalez-Sancho et al., Oncogene 2005). A schematic view of the promoter fragments and their predicted binding sites of TCF and CREB-transcription factor family members is depicted in Figure A1a. Relative luciferase reporter activity from each DKK1 promoter fragment is displayed in Figure A1b. Luciferase activity is not significantly altered within each CRC cell line, but we observed significantly higher reporter activity in HAB92 cells compared to HAB68 cells (Figure A1b). As this reflects the observed difference in DKK1 expression between these two cell lines, we focused on the region around the transcription start site (0.34 kb fragment) in comparison to the longest fragment (2.34 kb).

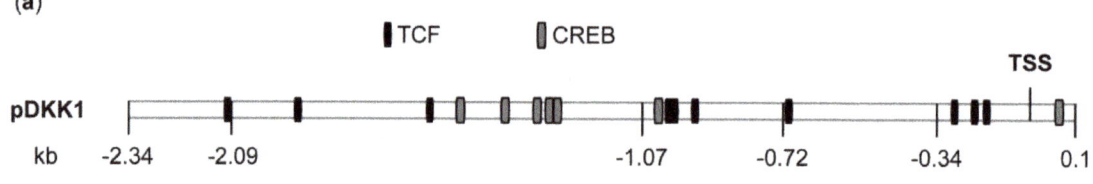

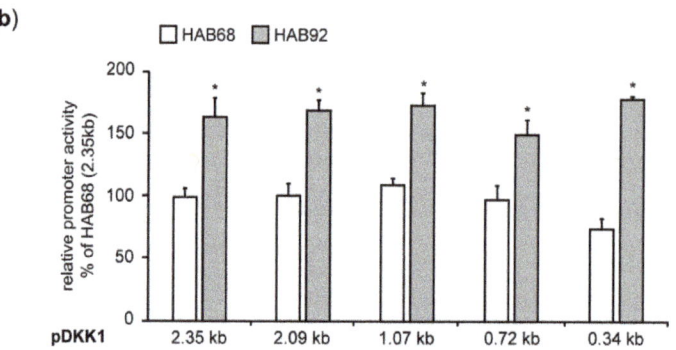

Figure A1. Expression regulation of DKK1 in HAB68 and HAB92 cells occurs near the transcription start site. (**a**) Graphical representation of the human DKK1 promoter. Predicted binding sites of transcription factor complexes containing TCF and CREB-family members are indicated in black and grey, respectively. (**b**) Relative DKK1 promoter-driven luciferase activity in HAB68 cells is significantly lower for all DKK1 promoter constructs compared to HAB92 cells. * statistically significant.

Appendix C

To confirm the expression regulation of DKK1 by ectopic expression of S100A4 in vivo, we generated a doxycycline-induced S100A4 expression vector (tetON-S100A4-AIRES-nLUC; Figure A2a) for lentiviral transduction. This vector and a control vector without the S100A4 coding sequence (tetON-ctrl-AIRES-nLUC) were transduced via lentiviral particles into HAB92 cells, generating HAB92/tetON-S100A4 and HAB92/tetON-ctrl cells, respectively. A total of 1×10^6 cells of each cell line were transplanted into the spleens of NOG mice, and for half of each group, 6 mg/kg of doxycycline was supplied in the drinking water. Plasma samples were taken after 15 days, and equal protein amounts were analyzed for the abundance of human DKK1 via WB. We observed a distinct reduction of hDKK1 in the plasma samples of doxycycline-treated mice harboring HAB92/tetON-S100A4 cells, compared to untreated mice from the same group (Figures A2b and S1m).

Mice with transplanted HAB92/tetON-ctrl cells showed only a minor decrease of hDKK1 in their plasma after doxycycline treatment, which points to a mild unspecific treatment effect. The animal experiment was performed in accordance with the United Kingdom Co-ordinated Committee on Cancer Research (UKCCCR) guidelines and was approved by the responsible local authorities (State Office of Health and Social Affairs, Berlin, Germany), with the registration number G0030/15.

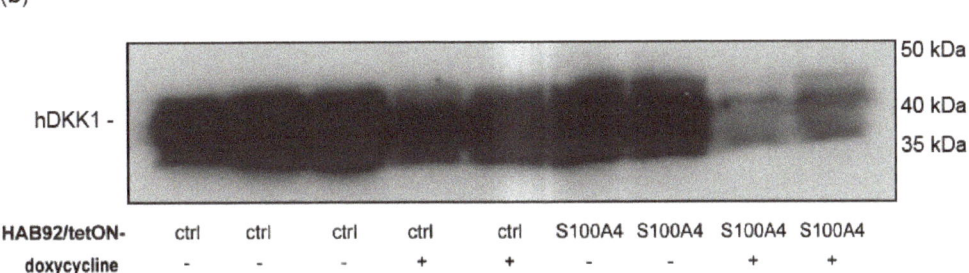

Figure A2. Induced ectopic expression of S100A4 in xenograft tumors results in a reduced abundance of human DKK1 in mouse plasma. (**a**) Schematic representation of the lentiviral vector for doxycycline-induced S100A4 expression. The respective control vector was generated without the coding sequence for S100A4 (not shown). Either vector was lentivirally transduced into HAB92 cells. (**b**) Plasma samples of mice intrasplenically transplanted with HAB92/tetON-S100A4 or HAB92/tetON-ctrl cells were taken after 15 days with or without doxycycline treatment. Immunostaining with human-specific DKK1 antibodies after WB showed reduced hDKK1 abundance in plasma samples of mice with induced S100A4 expression in the xenograft tumors.

References

1. Siegel, R.L.; Miller, K.D.; Jemal, A. Cancer statistics, 2020. CA. *Cancer J. Clin.* **2020**, *70*, 7–30. [CrossRef] [PubMed]
2. Nucci, M.R.; Robinson, C.R.; Longo, P.; Campbell, P.; Hamilton, S.R. Phenotypic and genotypic characteristics of aberrant crypt foci in human colorectal mucosa. *Hum. Pathol.* **1997**, *28*, 1396–1407. [CrossRef]
3. Sancho, E.; Batlle, E.; Clevers, H. Signaling pathways in intestinal development and cancer. *Annu. Rev. Cell Dev. Biol.* **2004**, *20*, 695–723. [CrossRef] [PubMed]
4. Barker, N. The canonical Wnt/beta-catenin signalling pathway. *Methods Mol. Biol.* **2008**, *468*, 5–15. [CrossRef]
5. Sack, U.; Stein, U. Wnt up your mind—Intervention strategies for S100A4-induced metastasis in colon cancer. *Gen. Physiol. Biophys.* **2009**, *28*, F55–F64. [PubMed]
6. Fearon, E.R. Molecular genetics of colorectal cancer. *Annu. Rev. Pathol.* **2011**, *6*, 479–507. [CrossRef] [PubMed]
7. Morin, P.J.; Sparks, A.B.; Korinek, V.; Barker, N.; Clevers, H.; Vogelstein, B.; Kinzler, K.W. Activation of beta-catenin-Tcf signaling in colon cancer by mutations in beta-catenin or APC. *Science* **1997**, *275*, 1787–1790. [CrossRef]
8. Herbst, A.; Jurinovic, V.; Krebs, S.; Thieme, S.E.; Blum, H.; Göke, B.; Kolligs, F.T. Comprehensive analysis of β-catenin target genes in colorectal carcinoma cell lines with deregulated Wnt/β-catenin signaling. *BMC Genom.* **2014**, *15*, 74. [CrossRef] [PubMed]
9. Segditsas, S.; Tomlinson, I. Colorectal cancer and genetic alterations in the Wnt pathway. *Oncogene* **2006**, *25*, 7531–7537. [CrossRef] [PubMed]
10. Rebouissou, S.; Franconi, A.; Calderaro, J.; Letouzé, E.; Imbeaud, S.; Pilati, C.; Nault, J.-C.; Couchy, G.; Laurent, A.; Balabaud, C.; et al. Genotype-phenotype correlation of CTNNB1 mutations reveals different ß-catenin activity associated with liver tumor progression. *Hepatology* **2016**, *64*, 2047–2061. [CrossRef] [PubMed]

11. Stein, U.; Arlt, F.; Walther, W.; Smith, J.; Waldman, T.; Harris, E.D.; Mertins, S.D.; Heizmann, C.W.; Allard, D.; Birchmeier, W.; et al. The metastasis-associated gene S100A4 is a novel target of beta-catenin/T-cell factor signaling in colon cancer. *Gastroenterology* 2006, *131*, 1486–1500. [CrossRef]
12. Mishra, S.K.; Siddique, H.R.; Saleem, M. S100A4 calcium-binding protein is key player in tumor progression and metastasis: Preclinical and clinical evidence. *Cancer Metastasis Rev.* 2012, *31*, 163–172. [CrossRef] [PubMed]
13. Boye, K.; Maelandsmo, G.M. S100A4 and metastasis: A small actor playing many roles. *Am. J. Pathol.* 2010, *176*, 528–535. [CrossRef]
14. Dahlmann, M.; Okhrimenko, A.; Marcinkowski, P.; Osterland, M.; Herrmann, P.; Smith, J.; Heizmann, C.W.; Schlag, P.M.; Stein, U. RAGE mediates S100A4-induced cell motility via MAPK/ERK and hypoxia signaling and is a prognostic biomarker for human colorectal cancer metastasis. *Oncotarget* 2014, *5*, 3220–3233. [CrossRef]
15. Maelandsmo, G.M.; Hovig, E.; Skrede, M.; Engebraaten, O.; Flørenes, V.A.; Myklebost, O.; Grigorian, M.; Lukanidin, E.; Scanlon, K.J.; Fodstad, O. Reversal of the in vivo metastatic phenotype of human tumor cells by an anti-CAPL (mts1) ribozyme. *Cancer Res.* 1996, *56*, 5490–5498.
16. Takenaga, K.; Nakamura, Y.; Sakiyama, S. Expression of antisense RNA to S100A4 gene encoding an S100-related calcium-binding protein suppresses metastatic potential of high-metastatic Lewis lung carcinoma cells. *Oncogene* 1997, *14*, 331–337. [CrossRef]
17. Dahlmann, M.; Sack, U.; Herrmann, P.; Lemm, M.; Fichtner, I.; Schlag, P.M.; Stein, U. Systemic shRNA mediated knock-down of S100A4 in colorectal cancer xenografted mice reduces metastasis formation. *Oncotarget* 2012, *3*, 783–797. [CrossRef]
18. Sack, U.; Walther, W.; Scudiero, D.; Selby, M.; Kobelt, D.; Lemm, M.; Fichtner, I.; Schlag, P.M.; Shoemaker, R.H.; Stein, U. Novel effect of antihelminthic Niclosamide on S100A4-mediated metastatic progression in colon cancer. *J. Natl. Cancer Inst.* 2011, *103*, 1018–1036. [CrossRef] [PubMed]
19. Stein, U.; Arlt, F.; Smith, J.; Sack, U.; Herrmann, P.; Walther, W.; Lemm, M.; Fichtner, I.; Shoemaker, R.H.; Schlag, P.M. Intervening in β-catenin signaling by sulindac inhibits S100A4-dependent colon cancer metastasis. *Neoplasia* 2011, *13*, 131–144. [CrossRef]
20. Sack, U.; Walther, W.; Scudiero, D.; Selby, M.; Aumann, J.; Lemos, C.; Fichtner, I.; Schlag, P.M.; Shoemaker, R.H.; Stein, U. S100A4-induced cell motility and metastasis is restricted by the Wnt/β-catenin pathway inhibitor calcimycin in colon cancer cells. *Mol. Biol. Cell* 2011, *22*, 3344–3354. [CrossRef]
21. Lemos, C.; Sack, U.; Schmid, F.; Juneja, M.; Stein, U. Anti-metastatic treatment in colorectal cancer: Targeting signaling pathways. *Curr. Pharm. Des.* 2013, *19*, 841–863. [CrossRef] [PubMed]
22. González-Sancho, J.M.; Aguilera, O.; García, J.M.; Pendás-Franco, N.; Peña, C.; Cal, S.; García de Herreros, A.; Bonilla, F.; Muñoz, A. The Wnt antagonist DICKKOPF-1 gene is a downstream target of beta-catenin/TCF and is downregulated in human colon cancer. *Oncogene* 2005, *24*, 1098–1103. [CrossRef]
23. Mao, B.; Wu, W.; Li, Y.; Hoppe, D.; Stannek, P.; Glinka, A.; Niehrs, C. LDL-receptor-related protein 6 is a receptor for Dickkopf proteins. *Nature* 2001, *411*, 321–325. [CrossRef] [PubMed]
24. Bafico, A.; Liu, G.; Yaniv, A.; Gazit, A.; Aaronson, S.A. Novel mechanism of Wnt signalling inhibition mediated by Dickkopf-1 interaction with LRP6/Arrow. *Nat. Cell Biol.* 2001, *3*, 683–686. [CrossRef]
25. Tian, E.; Zhan, F.; Walker, R.; Rasmussen, E.; Ma, Y.; Barlogie, B.; Shaughnessy, J.D. The Role of the Wnt-Signaling Antagonist DKK1 in the Development of Osteolytic Lesions in Multiple Myeloma. *N. Engl. J. Med.* 2003, *349*, 2483–2494. [CrossRef] [PubMed]
26. Rachner, T.D.; Göbel, A.; Benad-Mehner, P.; Hofbauer, L.C.; Rauner, M. Dickkopf-1 as a mediator and novel target in malignant bone disease. *Cancer Lett.* 2014, *346*, 172–177. [CrossRef] [PubMed]
27. Thudi, N.K.; Martin, C.K.; Murahari, S.; Shu, S.T.; Lanigan, L.G.; Werbeck, J.L.; Keller, E.T.; McCauley, L.K.; Pinzone, J.J.; Rosol, T.J. Dickkopf-1 (DKK-1) stimulated prostate cancer growth and metastasis and inhibited bone formation in osteoblastic bone metastases. *Prostate* 2011, *71*, 615–625. [CrossRef]
28. Mariz, K.; Ingolf, J.-B.; Daniel, H.; Teresa, N.J.; Erich-Franz, S. The Wnt inhibitor dickkopf-1: A link between breast cancer and bone metastases. *Clin. Exp. Metastasis* 2015, *32*, 857–866. [CrossRef] [PubMed]
29. Zhuang, X.; Zhang, H.; Li, X.; Li, X.; Cong, M.; Peng, F.; Yu, J.; Zhang, X.; Yang, Q.; Hu, G. Differential effects on lung and bone metastasis of breast cancer by Wnt signalling inhibitor DKK1. *Nat. Cell Biol.* 2017, *19*, 1274–1285. [CrossRef] [PubMed]
30. Malladi, S.; Macalinao, D.G.; Jin, X.; He, L.; Basnet, H.; Zou, Y.; de Stanchina, E.; Massagué, J. Metastatic Latency and Immune Evasion through Autocrine Inhibition of WNT. *Cell* 2016, *165*, 45–60. [CrossRef]
31. Liu, Y.; Tang, W.; Xie, L.; Wang, J.; Deng, Y.; Peng, Q.; Zhai, L.; Li, S.; Qin, X. Prognostic significance of dickkopf-1 overexpression in solid tumors: A meta-analysis. *Tumour Biol.* 2014, *35*, 3145–3154. [CrossRef] [PubMed]
32. Gurluler, E.; Tumay, L.V.; Guner, O.S.; Kucukmetin, N.T.; Hizli, B.; Zorluoglu, A. The role of preoperative serum levels for Dickkopf-related protein 1 as a potential marker of tumor invasion in patients with stage II and III colon cancer. *Eur. Rev. Med. Pharmacol. Sci.* 2014, *18*, 1742–1747. [PubMed]
33. Sui, Q.; Zheng, J.; Liu, D.; Peng, J.; Ou, Q.; Tang, J.; Li, Y.; Kong, L.; Jiang, W.; Xiao, B.; et al. Dickkopf-related protein 1, a new biomarker for local immune status and poor prognosis among patients with colorectal liver Oligometastases: A retrospective study. *BMC Cancer* 2019, *19*, 1210. [CrossRef] [PubMed]
34. Hosack, D.A.; Dennis, G.J.; Sherman, B.T.; Lane, H.C.; Lempicki, R.A. Identifying biological themes within lists of genes with EASE. *Genome Biol.* 2003, *4*, R70. [CrossRef] [PubMed]
35. Dennis, G.J.; Sherman, B.T.; Hosack, D.A.; Yang, J.; Gao, W.; Lane, H.C.; Lempicki, R.A. DAVID: Database for Annotation, Visualization, and Integrated Discovery. *Genome Biol.* 2003, *4*, P3. [CrossRef]

36. Laiho, P.; Kokko, A.; Vanharanta, S.; Salovaara, R.; Sammalkorpi, H.; Järvinen, H.; Mecklin, J.-P.; Karttunen, T.J.; Tuppurainen, K.; Davalos, V.; et al. Serrated carcinomas form a subclass of colorectal cancer with distinct molecular basis. *Oncogene* 2007, *26*, 312–320. [CrossRef]
37. Uronis, J.M.; Osada, T.; McCall, S.; Yang, X.Y.; Mantyh, C.; Morse, M.A.; Lyerly, H.K.; Clary, B.M.; Hsu, D.S. Histological and molecular evaluation of patient-derived colorectal cancer explants. *PLoS ONE* 2012, *7*, e38422. [CrossRef] [PubMed]
38. Gröne, J.; Lenze, D.; Jurinovic, V.; Hummel, M.; Seidel, H.; Leder, G.; Beckmann, G.; Sommer, A.; Grützmann, R.; Pilarsky, C.; et al. Molecular profiles and clinical outcome of stage UICC II colon cancer patients. *Int. J. Colorectal Dis.* 2011, *26*, 847–858. [CrossRef] [PubMed]
39. Alhopuro, P.; Sammalkorpi, H.; Niittymäki, I.; Biström, M.; Raitila, A.; Saharinen, J.; Nousiainen, K.; Lehtonen, H.J.; Heliövaara, E.; Puhakka, J.; et al. Candidate driver genes in microsatellite-unstable colorectal cancer. *Int. J. Cancer* 2012, *130*, 1558–1566. [CrossRef]
40. Tsukamoto, S.; Ishikawa, T.; Iida, S.; Ishiguro, M.; Mogushi, K.; Mizushima, H.; Uetake, H.; Tanaka, H.; Sugihara, K. Clinical Significance of Osteoprotegerin Expression in Human Colorectal Cancer. *Clin. Cancer Res.* 2011, *17*, 2444–2450. [CrossRef] [PubMed]
41. Stein, U.; Walther, W.; Arlt, F.; Schwabe, H.; Smith, J.; Fichtner, I.; Birchmeier, W.; Schlag, P.M. MACC1, a newly identified key regulator of HGF-MET signaling, predicts colon cancer metastasis. *Nat. Med.* 2009, *15*, 59–67. [CrossRef]
42. Ilm, K.; Kemmner, W.; Osterland, M.; Burock, S.; Koch, G.; Herrmann, P.; Schlag, P.M.; Stein, U. High MACC1 expression in combination with mutated KRAS G13 indicates poor survival of colorectal cancer patients. *Mol. Cancer* 2015, *14*, 38. [CrossRef] [PubMed]
43. Janky, R.; Verfaillie, A.; Imrichová, H.; Van de Sande, B.; Standaert, L.; Christiaens, V.; Hulselmans, G.; Herten, K.; Naval Sanchez, M.; Potier, D.; et al. iRegulon: From a gene list to a gene regulatory network using large motif and track collections. *PLoS Comput. Biol.* 2014, *10*, e1003731. [CrossRef] [PubMed]
44. Demchak, B.; Hull, T.; Reich, M.; Liefeld, T.; Smoot, M.; Ideker, T.; Mesirov, J.P. Cytoscape: The network visualization tool for GenomeSpace workflows. *F1000Research* 2014, *3*, 151. [CrossRef] [PubMed]
45. Parker, T.; Rudeen, A.; Neufeld, K. Oncogenic Serine 45-Deleted β-Catenin Remains Susceptible to Wnt Stimulation and APC Regulation in Human Colonocytes. *Cancers* 2020, *12*, 2114. [CrossRef]
46. Yan, J.; Enge, M.; Whitington, T.; Dave, K.; Liu, J.; Sur, I.; Schmierer, B.; Jolma, A.; Kivioja, T.; Taipale, M.; et al. Transcription factor binding in human cells occurs in dense clusters formed around cohesin anchor sites. *Cell* 2013, *154*, 801–813. [CrossRef]
47. Taylor, S.; Herrington, S.; Prime, W.; Rudland, P.S.; Barraclough, R. S100A4 (p9Ka) protein in colon carcinoma and liver metastases: Association with carcinoma cells and T-lymphocytes. *Br. J. Cancer* 2002, *86*, 409–416. [CrossRef] [PubMed]
48. Helfman, D.M.; Kim, E.J.; Lukanidin, E.; Grigorian, M. The metastasis associated protein S100A4: Role in tumour progression and metastasis. *Br. J. Cancer* 2005, *92*, 1955–1958. [CrossRef] [PubMed]
49. Niida, A.; Hiroko, T.; Kasai, M.; Furukawa, Y.; Nakamura, Y.; Suzuki, Y.; Sugano, S.; Akiyama, T. DKK1, a negative regulator of Wnt signaling, is a target of the beta-catenin/TCF pathway. *Oncogene* 2004, *23*, 8520–8526. [CrossRef] [PubMed]
50. Glinka, A.; Wu, W.; Delius, H.; Monaghan, A.P.; Blumenstock, C.; Niehrs, C. Dickkopf-1 is a member of a new family of secreted proteins and functions in head induction. *Nature* 1998, *391*, 357–362. [CrossRef] [PubMed]
51. Semënov, M.V.; Tamai, K.; Brott, B.K.; Kühl, M.; Sokol, S.; He, X. Head inducer Dickkopf-1 is a ligand for Wnt coreceptor LRP6. *Curr. Biol.* 2001, *11*, 951–961. [CrossRef]
52. Aguilera, O.; Fraga, M.F.; Ballestar, E.; Paz, M.F.; Herranz, M.; Espada, J.; García, J.M.; Muñoz, A.; Esteller, M.; González-Sancho, J.M. Epigenetic inactivation of the Wnt antagonist DICKKOPF-1 (DKK-1) gene in human colorectal cancer. *Oncogene* 2006, *25*, 4116–4121. [CrossRef] [PubMed]
53. Sato, H.; Suzuki, H.; Toyota, M.; Nojima, M.; Maruyama, R.; Sasaki, S.; Takagi, H.; Sogabe, Y.; Sasaki, Y.; Idogawa, M.; et al. Frequent epigenetic inactivation of DICKKOPF family genes in human gastrointestinal tumors. *Carcinogenesis* 2007, *28*, 2459–2466. [CrossRef] [PubMed]
54. Huang, Z.; Li, S.; Song, W.; Li, X.; Li, Q.; Zhang, Z.; Han, Y.; Zhang, X.; Miao, S.; Du, R.; et al. Lysine-specific demethylase 1 (LSD1/KDM1A) contributes to colorectal tumorigenesis via activation of the Wnt/β-catenin pathway by down-regulating Dickkopf-1 (DKK1) [corrected]. *PLoS ONE* 2013, *8*, e70077. [CrossRef]
55. Nukuda, A.; Endoh, H.; Yasuda, M.; Mizutani, T.; Kawabata, K.; Haga, H. Role of ATF5 in the invasive potential of diverse human cancer cell lines. *Biochem. Biophys. Res. Commun.* 2016, *474*, 509–514. [CrossRef]
56. Karpel-Massler, G.; Horst, B.A.; Shu, C.; Chau, L.; Tsujiuchi, T.; Bruce, J.N.; Canoll, P.; Greene, L.A.; Angelastro, J.M.; Siegelin, M.D. A Synthetic Cell-Penetrating Dominant-Negative ATF5 Peptide Exerts Anticancer Activity against a Broad Spectrum of Treatment-Resistant Cancers. *Clin. Cancer Res.* 2016, *22*, 4698–4711. [CrossRef]
57. Angelastro, J.M. Targeting ATF5 in Cancer. *Trends Cancer* 2017, *3*, 471–474. [CrossRef] [PubMed]
58. Li, G.; Li, W.; Angelastro, J.M.; Greene, L.A.; Liu, D.X. Identification of a novel DNA binding site and a transcriptional target for activating transcription factor 5 in c6 glioma and mcf-7 breast cancer cells. *Mol. Cancer Res.* 2009, *7*, 933–943. [CrossRef] [PubMed]
59. Reddiconto, G.; Toto, C.; Palamà, I.; De Leo, S.; de Luca, E.; De Matteis, S.; Dini, L.; Passerini, C.G.; Di Renzo, N.; Maffia, M.; et al. Targeting of GSK3β promotes imatinib-mediated apoptosis in quiescent CD34+ chronic myeloid leukemia progenitors, preserving normal stem cells. *Blood* 2012, *119*, 2335–2345. [CrossRef] [PubMed]

60. McCubrey, J.A.; Steelman, L.S.; Bertrand, F.E.; Davis, N.M.; Abrams, S.L.; Montalto, G.; D'Assoro, A.B.; Libra, M.; Nicoletti, F.; Maestro, R.; et al. Multifaceted roles of GSK-3 and Wnt/β-catenin in hematopoiesis and leukemogenesis: Opportunities for therapeutic intervention. *Leukemia* **2014**, *28*, 15–33. [CrossRef]
61. Gongoll, S.; Peters, G.; Mengel, M.; Piso, P.; Klempnauer, J.; Kreipe, H.; von Wasielewski, R. Prognostic significance of calcium-binding protein S100A4 in colorectal cancer. *Gastroenterology* **2002**, *123*, 1478–1484. [CrossRef] [PubMed]
62. Liu, Y.; Tang, W.; Wang, J.; Xie, L.; Li, T.; He, Y.; Qin, X.; Li, S. Clinicopathological and prognostic significance of S100A4 overexpression in colorectal cancer: A meta-analysis. *Diagn. Pathol.* **2013**, *8*, 181. [CrossRef] [PubMed]
63. Hao, J.-M.; Chen, J.-Z.; Sui, H.-M.; Si-Ma, X.-Q.; Li, G.-Q.; Liu, C.; Li, J.-L.; Ding, Y.-Q.; Li, J.-M. A five-gene signature as a potential predictor of metastasis and survival in colorectal cancer. *J. Pathol.* **2010**, *220*, 475–489. [CrossRef] [PubMed]
64. Qi, L.; Sun, B.; Liu, Z.; Li, H.; Gao, J.; Leng, X. Dickkopf-1 inhibits epithelial-mesenchymal transition of colon cancer cells and contributes to colon cancer suppression. *Cancer Sci.* **2012**, *103*, 828–835. [CrossRef] [PubMed]
65. Stein, U.; Schlag, P.M. Clinical, biological, and molecular aspects of metastasis in colorectal cancer. *Recent Results Cancer Res.* **2007**, *176*, 61–80. [CrossRef] [PubMed]
66. Wang, H.; Li, Q.; Chen, H. Genistein affects histone modifications on Dickkopf-related protein 1 (DKK1) gene in SW480 human colon cancer cell line. *PLoS ONE* **2012**, *7*, e40955. [CrossRef] [PubMed]
67. Pendás-Franco, N.; Aguilera, O.; Pereira, F.; González-Sancho, J.M.; Muñoz, A. Vitamin D and Wnt/beta-catenin pathway in colon cancer: Role and regulation of *DICKKOPF* genes. *Anticancer Res.* **2008**, *28*, 2613–2623. [PubMed]

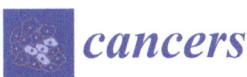

Review

Insights into the Role of Matrix Metalloproteinases in Precancerous Conditions and in Colorectal Cancer

Zahra Pezeshkian [1], Stefania Nobili [2,3], Noshad Peyravian [1], Bahador Shojaee [1], Haniye Nazari [4], Hiva Soleimani [5], Hamid Asadzadeh-Aghdaei [1], Maziar Ashrafian Bonab [6], Ehsan Nazemalhosseini-Mojarad [7,*] and Enrico Mini [8,9,*]

[1] Basic and Molecular Epidemiology of Gastrointestinal Disorders Research Center, Research Institute for Gastroenterology and Liver Diseases, Shahid Beheshti University of Medical Sciences, Tehran 19835-178, Iran; zahrapezeshkian@yahoo.com (Z.P.); peyravian.n@iums.ac.ir (N.P.); bahadorshojaee@ufl.edu (B.S.); hamid.asadzadeh@sbmu.ac.ir (H.A.-A.)
[2] Department of Neurosciences, Imaging and Clinical Sciences, "G. D'Annunzio" University of Chieti-Pescara, 66100 Chieti, Italy; stefania.nobili@unich.it
[3] Center for Advanced Studies and Technology (CAST), University "G. D'Annunzio" Chieti-Pescara, 66100 Chieti, Italy
[4] Department of Microbiology, Faculty of Advanced Science and Technology, Tehran Medical Science, Islamic Azad University, Tehran 19395-1495, Iran; hani7311926@gmail.com
[5] Department of General Biology, Faculty of Fundamental Science, Islamic Azad University of Shahr-E-Qods, Tehran 37515-374, Iran; M_hivi@yahoo.com
[6] School of Medicine, University of Sunderland, City Campus, Chester Road, Sunderland SR1 3SD, UK; maziar.bonab@sunderland.ac.uk
[7] Gastroenterology and Liver Diseases Research Center, Research Institute for Gastroenterology and Liver Diseases, Shahid Beheshti University of Medical Sciences, Tehran 19835-178, Iran
[8] Department of Health Sciences, University of Florence, 50139 Florence, Italy
[9] DENOTHE Excellence Center, University of Florence, 50139 Florence, Italy
* Correspondence: E.nazemalhosseini@sbmu.ac.ir (E.N.-M.); enrico.mini@unifi.it (E.M.)

Simple Summary: Colorectal cancer (CRC) is one of the most common cancer worldwide. CRC is derived from polyps and many factors, such as Matrix Metalloproteinases (MMPs) can gain the progression of colorectal carcinogenesis. Many investigations have indicated the role of MMPs in CRC development while there is not enough knowledge about the function of MMPs in precancerous conditions. This review summarizes the current information about the role of MMPs in polyps and CRC progression.

Abstract: Colorectal cancer (CRC) is the third and second cancer for incidence and mortality worldwide, respectively, and is becoming prevalent in developing countries. Most CRCs derive from polyps, especially adenomatous polyps, which can gradually transform into CRC. The family of Matrix Metalloproteinases (MMPs) plays a critical role in the initiation and progression of CRC. Prominent MMPs, including MMP-1, MMP-2, MMP-7, MMP-8, MMP-9, MMP-12, MMP-13, MMP-14, and MMP-21, have been detected in CRC patients, and the expression of most of them correlates with a poor prognosis. Moreover, many studies have explored the inhibition of MMPs and targeted therapy for CRC, but there is not enough information about the role of MMPs in polyp malignancy. In this review, we discuss the role of MMPs in colorectal cancer and its pathogenesis

Keywords: Matrix Metalloproteinases (MMPs); polyp; colorectal cancer; TIMPs; MMP polymorphisms; MMP targeting

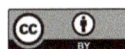

1. Introduction

At approximately 11% of all diagnosed cancer cases, CRC is the third most common cancer and the second most lethal cancer worldwide [1,2]. It is today well known that several factors contribute to the CRC pathogenesis, driving complex genetic and epigenetic processes that, ultimately, transform normal colonic mucosa to cancerous tissue [3]. CRC may initiate from benign polyps with the mucosal origin and can develop into carcinoma. Colorectal polyps, especially adenomas, are proliferative lesions that have been defined as the precursor of CRC. Therefore, the early detection and removal of these polyps can interrupt the progression of the adenoma-carcinoma sequence [4,5].

Many molecular signaling pathways are involved in CRC initiation and progression, such as ERK/MAPK, TGF-β, PI3K/Akt, Src/FAK, and β-catenin pathways. These pathways can promote the hallmarks of cancer such as inflammation, angiogenesis, metastasis, and invasion, also via the activation and overexpression of MMPs [6,7]. Thus, MMPs have been suggested as potential prognostic factors for the malignancy risk of colorectal polyps. MMPs are proteolytic enzymes implicated in the degradation of stromal connective tissues and of the extracellular matrix (ECM), a complex network that plays a key role in sustaining signaling transduction and thus cancer development and progression [8]. As such, MMPs have key roles in tumor initiation, progression, and metastasis and can affect tumor cell behavior by cleaving proapoptotic agents and producing an aggressive phenotype [9]. Because of these roles, MMPs have been detected as biomarkers in CRC progression [10]. A new challenge in CRC treatment is finding an effective pharmacological and therapeutic method for suppression of MMPs and targeted therapy of CRC [11]. This review will deal with the role of MMPs in colorectal carcinogenesis from colorectal polyps to CRC.

2. CRC Pathogenesis and Molecular Classification

Colorectal polyps result from atypical cell proliferation in the colorectal tissue. Based on histological and morphological features, colorectal polyps are divided into neoplastic (adenoma) and non-neoplastic (hyperplastic, hamartomatous, and inflammatory) types [5,12]. Neoplastic polyps, also known as adenomatous polyps, are subclassified by their histological characteristics as tubular, villous, or tubulovillous adenomas. Previous investigations demonstrated that approximately 5–10% of neoplastic polyps are villous adenomas and most of them show dysplasia. Approximately 10–15% of neoplastic polyps show morphological features of both villous and tubular types [13]. Adenomas are not usually transformed to carcinoma, but there is evidence that the adenoma-carcinoma sequence originates from adenomatous polyps [14]. Also, hyperplastic polyps may possess malignancy potential [15]. CRC is caused by the misregulation of some oncogenes such as *KRAS* and *c-MYC* and tumor suppressor genes such as *P53* and APC, which control cellular signal transduction [16–18].

2.1. Molecular Mechanism of CRC

Specific features characterize CRC and its pathogenesis based on genetic, epigenetic, and transcriptomic factors. Three main molecular abnormalities are involved in CRC carcinogenesis:

A. Microsatellite instability (MSI): it consists of mutations in DNA mismatch repair (MMR) genes such as *MSH2, MLH1, PMS2, MLH3, MSH3, PMSI*, and *EXO1*; MSI is rare in polyps but it is always found in serrated polyps and about 15–20% of all CRC cases are derived from MSI [19,20].

B. Chromosomal instability (CIN): this abnormality is identified in 85% of CRC cases and consists of a gain (1q, 7p, 8q, 13q, 2pq) or loss (8q, 15q, 17p, 18p) of chromosomal genes, activation of proto-oncogenes (*KRAS, SRC, c-MYC*), and inactivation of tumor suppressor genes (*P53, APC*) [21].

C. CpG Islands Methylator Phenotype (CIMP): these regions, located in the gene promoter, could disturb the activation of tumor suppressor genes. CIMP phenotype is represented by hypermethylation of CpG dinucleotides and premalignant serrated polyps are correlated with CIMP [22,23].

2.2. Molecular Classification Based on Transcriptomic Analysis

Based on gene expression profiles, CRC has been classified into subgroups with distinct molecular and clinical features [24].

A. Consensus molecular subtype (CMS) classification: CMS classification provides biological insight into metastatic colorectal cancer (mCRC) carcinogenesis and predicts CRC prognosis [25].
  - CMS1 (14%) indicates MSI, CIMP, and *BRAF* mutation and immune activation.
  - CMS2 (37%) shows Wingless-Type MMTR integration site family member (WNT), MYC signaling activation, and epithelial involvement.
  - CMS3 (13%) demonstrates MSI, CIMP, and *KRAS* mutations and metabolic involvement.
  - CMS4 (23%) includes invasion, metastatic situations, and TGF-β signaling co-activation and angiogenesis. Also, epithelial-mesenchymal transition (EMT) is a crucial event in colorectal carcinogenesis and is involved in CMS4 status. EMT can result in advanced-stage CRC, poor patient survival, and worst clinical features [26,27] and CMS4 subgroup shows the most unfavorable prognosis.

B. CRC intrinsic subtypes (CRIS): CRIS is a unique classification exclusively based on the cancer cell-specific transcriptome of CRC since the extrinsic factors of the stroma have not been analyzed. It classifies CRC into five novel transcriptional groups that, thus, further clarify biological understanding of CRC heterogeneity.
  - CRIS-A is enriched for *BRAF*-mutated MSI tumors and *KRAS*-mutated MSS tumors that are without targeted therapeutic options.
  - CRIS-B is related to invasive tumors with poor prognosis and high TGF-ß signaling. CRIS-B is unconnected to the CMS4 mesenchymal subtype, which also indicates aggressive tumors with TGF-ß pathway activation.
  - CRIS-C is dependent on EGFR signals and is sensitive to anti-EGFR monoclonal antibody treatment.
  - CRIS-D shows IGF2 overexpression. This occurrence has been involved in desensitization to the EGFR blockade in patients with *KRAS* wild-type tumors.
  - CRIS-E indicates *KRAS*-mutated, Paneth cell-like CIN tumors refractory to anti-EGFR antibody treatment [28].

3. Structure and Function of MMPs

MMPs are a family of zinc-dependent endopeptidases consisting of a propeptide sequence, a catalytic domain, a hinge region, and a hemopexin (PEX) domain [29]. The propeptide domain is highly conserved and can regulate the sequence that interacts with Zn^{2+}. Also, cystine within this area permits the MMPs to be in the active or inactive status [30]. The catalytic domain possesses a conserved zinc-binding motif which, in the active condition, will disconnect from the propeptide domain. Movement between the catalytic and PEX domain is done via hinge regions [29]. According to their structural domains, MMPs have been categorized into collagenase, gelatinase, stromelysin, matrilysin, and membrane-bound MMPs (MT-MMPs) [31,32].

MMPs play a crucial role in the remodeling of the ECM by digestion of ECM components, stimulation of cell surface proteins. Also, they can control the activity of other proteinases, growth factors, chemokines, and cell receptors, and moderate many biological functions [33]. MMPs can regulate cellular growth, migration, survival, and adhesion in biological and pathological statuses (Table 1, Figure 1). Due to the MMP's key roles, the dysregulation of their expression levels and their activation lead cancerous cells to proliferation, angiogenesis, survival, invasion, malignant transitions, and immune dysregulation [34–36]. Also, the tissue inhibitors of metalloproteinase (TIMPs) control the activation of MMPs and have a critical action in precancerous conditions, CRC progression, and metastasis (Table 2, Figure 2) [11,37].

Table 1. Matrix Metallopeptidases Features in Humans.

MMP Gene	Chromosomal Location	Enzyme	Substrate
MMP-1	11q22.2	Collagenase-1	Col I, II, III, VII, VIII, X, Gelatin
MMP-8	11q22.2	Collagenase-2	Col I, II, III, VII, VIII, X, Gelatin, Aggrecan
MMP-13	11q22.2	Collagenase-3	Col I, II, III, VII, VIII, X, Gelatin
MMP-2	16q12.2	Gelatinase A	Gelatin, Col I, II, III, IV, VII
MMP-9	20q13.12	Gelatinase B	Gelatin, Col IV, V
MMP-3	11q22.3	Stromelysin-1	Col II, III, IV, IX, X, proteoglycans, fibronectin, laminin, and elastin.
MMP-10	11q22.2	Stromelysin-2	Col II, III, IV, IX, X, proteoglycans, fibronectin, laminin, and elastin
MMP-7	11q22.2	Marilysin-1	Fibronectin, Laminin, Col I, Gelatin
MMP-14	14q11.2	MT-MMP	Gelatin, Fibronectin, Laminin
MMP-12	11q22.2	Metalloelastase	Gelatin, Fibronectin, Col IV
MMP-21	10q26.2	XMMP	Aggrecan

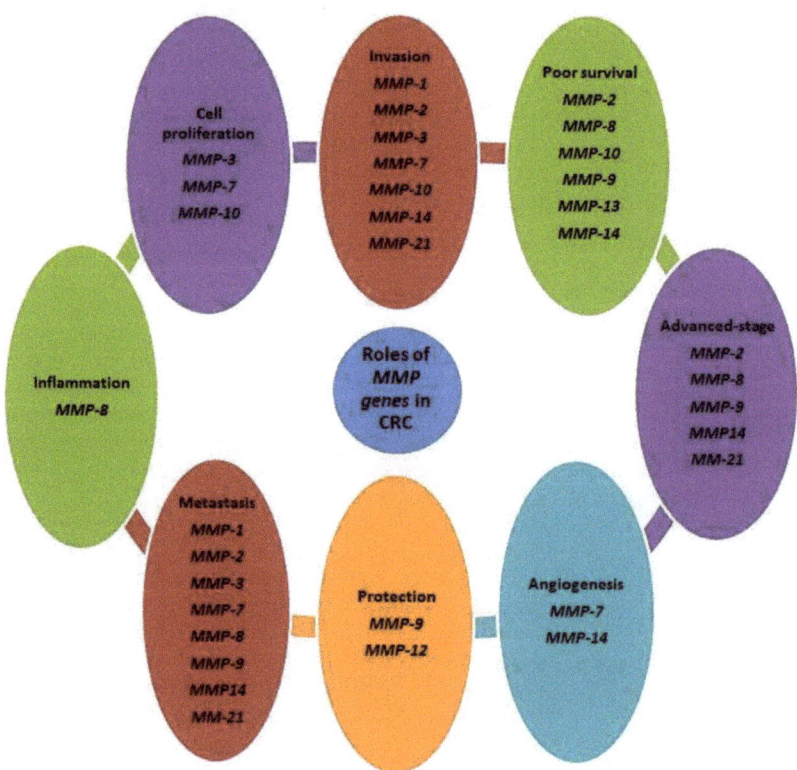

Figure 1. Summary of the prominent *MMP* genes in CRC. MMPs play different functions in CRC.

Table 2. Summary of Investigations about the Roles of MMP Genes and Proteins in Colorectal Polyps and Cancer.

References	Gene/Protein Expression	Samples	Methods	Results
Huang X., et al., 2021 [38]	MMP-7, MMP-9, MMP-11, TIMP-1, TIMP-2, CEA	Human polyps and tumor	Enzyme-linked immunosorbent assay	A combined detection model, including MMP-7, TIMP-1, and CEA improved both the specificity and sensitivity for detecting CRC.
Zhou X., et al., 2021 [39]	MMP-7, MMP-9, MMP-11, TIMP-1, TIMP-2, CEA	Human CRC	ELISA and electro-chemiluminescence immunoassay	The miR 135a was downregulated and MMP 13 was increased in samples. Combined detection of the two had a good diagnostic effect on the occurrence of CRC.
Rasool M., et al., 2021 [40]	TGF, VEGF, TNF, ILs, MMP-2, 9, 11, and 19	Human polyps and tumor	ELISA	Significant upregulation of MMP-2, MMP-9, MMP-11, and MMP-19 was reported in polyp and colon cancer samples compared with their MMP profile in normal samples.
Barabás L., et al., 2020 [41]	MMP-2, MMP-7, MMP-9, TIMP-1 and TIMP-2	Human adenomas, and CRC	ELISA	The serum antigen concentrations of MMP-7, MMP-9, TIMP-1, and TIMP-2 were significantly increased in patients with CRC and adenomas compared with the controls. They were also activated in premalignant adenomas.
Hsieh S.L., et al., 2019 [42]	Study of the mechanism of carnosine, TIMP-1, and MMP-9	Human HCT-116 CRC cell line	MTT assay and qPCR	The carnosine inhibits the migration and intravasation of human CRC cells. The regulatory mechanism may occur by suppressing NF-κB activity and modulating MMPs and EMT-related gene expression in HCT-116 cells treated with carnosine. *MMP-9* mRNA and protein levels were decreased. *TIMP-1* mRNA and protein levels were increased.
Kıyak R., et al., 2018 [43]	MMP-7, COX-2, TIMP-1, and CEA protein	Human polyps	ELISA and chemiluminescent enzyme immunometric assay (CEIA)	The plasma TIMP-1 levels were significantly elevated in cancer compared with the polyp group. The plasma MMP-7 levels were decreased in polyps compared with the control group. The plasma CEA and TIMP-1 are valuable biomarker candidates for differentiating CRC from colorectal polyps.
Eiró N., et al., 2017 [44]	*MMP-1, 2, 7, 9, 11, 13* and *14*	Human adenomas and hyperplastic polyps	Real-time PCR and Western-blot, and	The hyperplastic polyps had the lowest levels of *MMP-1* and *MMP-7*. Tubular polyps had high levels of both *MMP-7* and *MMP-14*, and tubulo-villous adenomas had high levels of *MMP-1, 7*, and *14* compared with the normal group.

Table 2. Cont.

References	Gene/Protein Expression	Samples	Methods	Results
Pezeshkian Z., et al., 2017 [45]	MMP-7 and VEGF-A	Human adenomas	Real-time PCR in 50 biopsy samples of adenomas including villous, tubular, and tubulo-villous types, and 20 paired tissue samples	The MMP-7 mRNA expression was significantly higher in villous adenoma with high-grade dysplasia compared with the control group. MMP-7 and VEGF-A are prognostic biomarkers for colorectal adenoma polyp progression to malignancy.
Wernicke A.K., et al., 2016 [46]	Association between grade of dysplasia and MMP-13 expression	Human adenomas and hyperplastic polyps	Immunohistochemistry and immune-reactive score (IRS)	The MMP-13 has been identified as an excellent marker of high-grade intraepithelial neoplasia and CRC. The strength of the association between pathologic stage and immune-reactive MMP-13 scoring emphasizes its potential for diagnosis in precancerous colorectal lesions.
Gimeno-García A., et al., 2016 [47]	MMP-9	Patients' blood, adenomas, hyperplastic polyps, and CRC tissue	Luminex XMAP technology, gelatin zymography, western blot, and SNP analysis in 150 blood and tissue	There was a significant correlation between plasma and tissue levels of MMP-9. Plasma MMP-9 levels in patients with neoplastic lesions were significantly higher than in healthy controls. Also, MMP-9 in CRC was higher than in non-advanced adenomas.
Annaha'zi A., et al., 2016 [48]	MMP-9	Patients' stool samples, adenomas, hyperplastic polyps, and CRC tissue	ELISA	Stool MMP-9 was significantly increased in CRC compared with all the other groups. Stool MMP-9 may be a new noninvasive marker in CRC.
Klupp et al., 2016 [49]	MMP-7, MMP-10, and MMP-12	Serum specimens of patients with colon adenocarcinoma	Luminex based multiplex assay	Expression levels of MMP-7, MMP-10, and MMP-12 in serum of colon cancer patients are different compared with serum specimens of the healthy control group. The upregulation of MMP-7, MMP-10, and MMP-12 in colon cancer patients' serum was associated with a poor prognosis.
Otero-Estévez O., et al., 2015 [50]	MMP-9	Human adenomas and CRC	non-invasive stool immunochemical test (FIT) and ELISA	The MMP-9 levels were higher in advanced adenomas and CRC compared with those reported in samples of healthy individual. Elevated MMP-9 concentration was associated with several lesions, size, and adenoma histology.

Table 2. Cont.

References	Gene/Protein Expression	Samples	Methods	Results
Bengi G., et al., 2015 [51]	MMP-7, TIMP-1, and COX-2	Human adenomas and CRC	Real-time PCR	The expression of TIMP-1, COX-2, and MMP-7 was significantly higher in polyps compared with normal tissue. Overexpression of MMP-7, COX-2, and TIMP-1 determine an important role of these genes in the progression of colon cancer.
Odabasi M., et al., 2014 [52]	MMP-9 and NGAL	Human adenomas and CRC	Immunohistochemistry	The MMP-9 and NGAL overexpression in neoplastic polyps might be used as markers to separate them from non-neoplastic polyps. These genes as immune-histochemical markers determine dysplasia in the early steps of the colorectal adenoma-carcinoma sequence.
Qasim B.J., et al., 2013 [53]	MMP-7	Human adenomas	Immunohistochemistry	MMP-7 was expressed in advanced colorectal adenomatous polyps with large size, severe dysplasia, and villous.
Sheth R.A., et al., 2012 [54]	MMP-2, and MMP-9	Xenograft model of CRC in nude mice	The MMP enzyme activity was measured by an enzyme-activatable optical molecular probe and quantitative fluorescence colonoscopy in nude mice which received celecoxib versus vehicle	There was an apparent linear relationship between measured MMP activity and tumor growth rate.
Murname M.J., et al., 2009 [55]	MMP-2 and MMP-9	Mouse models of CRC and human HT-29 CRC cell line	Gene-expression microarray and ELISA	The plotted receiver operating characteristic (ROC) curves estimated the sensitivity and specificity profiles of MMP-2 and MMP-9 for the identification of CRC.
Jeffery N., et al., 2009 [56]	MMP-1, 2, 3, 7, 9, 13, MT1-MMP, MT2-MMP and TIMP-1, TIMP-2, and IMP-3	Human adenomas and CRC	Immunohistochemistry	MMP-1, MMP-2, MMP-3, TIMP-1, and TIMP-2 showed a significant increase in carcinomatous epithelium compared with adenoma epithelium. The increased expression of MMPs and TIMPs occurred at an early stage of colorectal neoplasia.
Lièvre A., et al., 2006 [57]	The functional gene promoter polymorphisms of MMP1, MMP3, and MMP7	Human adenomas	Real-time PCR allelic discrimination assay	These data showed a relation between MMP-1 -1607 ins/del G and MMP-3 -1612 ins/del A combined polymorphisms and risk of small adenomas.

Table 2. *Cont.*

References	Gene/Protein Expression	Samples	Methods	Results
Tutton M.G., et al., 2003 [58]	MMP-2 and MMP-9	Patients' plasma samples, adenomas, and CRC	Immunohistochemistry, real-time PCR, and ELISA	The expression of MMP-2 and MMP-9 was significantly increased in CRC tissues compared with matched normal tissues. Plasma MMP-2 and MMP-9 levels were significantly elevated at all stages in CRC patients. Plasma levels of these enzymes may be a noninvasive indicator of invasion or metastasis in CRC.

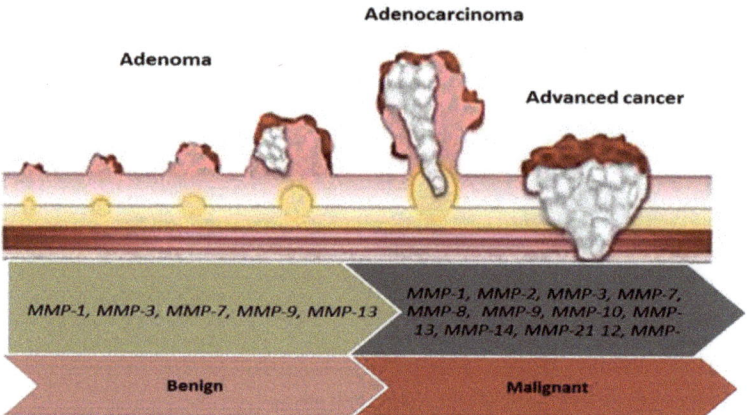

Figure 2. The diagram indicates the role of *MMPs* genes in adenoma development, colorectal adenoma-carcinoma sequence, and tumor progression. *MMP-1*, *MMP-3*, *MMP-7*, *MMP-9*, and *MMP-13* are involved in adenoma development. *MMP-1*, *MMP-2*, *MMP-3*, *MMP-7*, *MMP-8*, *MMP-9*, *MMP-12*, *MMP-13*, *MMP-14*, and *MMP-21* participate in adenoma-carcinoma sequence and tumor progression.

4. The Function of MMPs in Colorectal Polyps and Cancer

4.1. MMP-1, MMP-13, and MMP-8 (Collagenases)

The specific targets for MMP-1 and MMP-13 are in the intestine. MMP-1 can digest type I, II, III, VII, VIII, X collagen, and gelatin. Upregulation of *MMP-1* gene was detected in CRC patients compared to normal tissue [6,59]. Eiro et al., found overexpression of *MMP-1* gene in serrated, villous, and tubulovillous adenomas (i.e., polyps with high potential for transformation to CRC) [44]. Previous investigations demonstrated the correlation between *MMP-1* gene expression and CRC progression: high expression levels of *MMP-1* were associated with invasion, advanced stage metastasis, LNM, and shorter overall survival [60,61]. Wang, et al. investigated the role of MMP-1 in the development of CRC. They found that the downregulation of MMP-1 expression inhibited the progression of CRC in vitro and in vivo by suppressing the PI3K/Akt/c-myc signaling pathway and the EMT [6].

MMP-13, another member of the collagenase category, could degenerate type III collagen. According to the strength of the association between pathologic stage and immunoreactivity scoring (IRS) of MMP-13, in high-grade adenomas and CRC, MMP-13 was observed with a moderate and strong staining intensity, respectively [46]. This result indicated that MMP-13 could help to predict metastatic behavior and prognosis of early-stage cancerous and precancerous colorectal adenoma [46,62]. The study of the association between grade dysplasia and MMP-13 expression in 137 biopsies from patients with cancerous and non-cancerous colorectal adenomas showed that the high expression level of MMP-13 IRS could be helpful to predict metastatic state, prognosis, and recrudescence at an early stage of cancerous and precancerous colorectal adenoma. Moreover, the upregulation of MMP-13 IRS from low to high-grade adenoma was considered an early predictive cancer biomarker [46]. Meanwhile, several studies confirmed that upregulation of MMP-13 was related to advanced CRC and liver metastasis [62–64]. Also, the expression of MMP-13 on the primary tumor cell surface is increased in inflammatory bowel disease. The expression of MMP-13 is closely related to the progression, early relapse, and high mortality of CRC [63,65].

Another member of collagenase enzymes is MMP-8 which is frequently expressed by neutrophils. MMP-8 cleaves many substrates, such as type I, II, and III collagen. This MMP is mainly considered to play a protective role against cancer. However, more recent findings also suggest an oncogenic function of *MMP-8* gene [66,67].

Sirnio et al., found that enhanced-serum MMP-8 level in CRC patients was significantly related to advanced-stage CRC, distant metastasis, lack of MMR, and poor survival. Thus,, they evidenced that MMP-8 is correlated with inflammation and CRC progression [68].

4.2. MMP-2 and MMP-9 (Gelatinase)

MMP-2 and MMP-9, known as gelatinases, can digest type IV collagen and gelatin [69]. Murname et al. showed that MMP-2 protein activity in adenomas with high-grade dysplasia (HGD) was different from adenomas with low-grade dysplasia (LGD). They suggested that the active *MMP-2* gene could predict CRC malignancy risk in patients with adenomatous polyps [70]. Some studies also indicated high expression levels of MMP-9 protein in adenomas with HGD compared to adenomas with LGD and normal tissue. As such, researchers speculated that upregulation of MMP-9 is a primary event in the CRC adenoma-carcinoma sequence [41,71]. High expression levels of MMP-2 protein in CRC tumors compared to normal mucosa have also been reported [41,72]. In addition, a statistically significant relationship between upregulation of *MMP-2* gene with advanced-stage CRC or CRC progression has been observed [41,73–75]. On this basis, *MMP-2* has been suggested as a potential biomarker to detect CRC progression and predict patient survival. Furthermore, overexpression of the *MMP-2* gene was associated with metastasis of lymph nodes and a decrease of cell adhesion in tumors [73].

Finally, also the upregulation of *MMP-9* gene was associated with the advanced stage of CRC and suggested as a biomarker predictive of poor overall survival [41,76]. Chen et al. indicated that the overexpression of *MMP-9* gene promoted CRC metastasis through the MKK-3/p38/NF-κB pro-oncogenic pathway. Furthermore, they suggested *MMP-9* gene as a potential molecular target for targeted therapy to treat metastatic CRC patients [76].

On the contrary, some investigations reported that *MMP-9* gene has a protective role in CRC by stimulating Notch activation resulting in the activation of p21WAF1/Cip1 leading to the suppression of β-catenin [77,78]. In a recent study, although in colitis-associated colon cancer, Walter et al. confirmed this observation by revealing that MMP-9 protein expression was associated with reduced ROS levels, decreased DNA damage, and stimulated mismatch repair pathway [79].

In an interesting study, Wei et al., by analyzing microbiota in tumors obtained by patients with different prognoses, found that the expression of some inflammatory genes, including *MMP-9*, was associated with the abundance of specific bacteria. High levels of *MMP-9* expression were significantly correlated with the high abundance of *B. fragilis* and *F. nucleatum* whereas a high level of *F. prausnitzii* was associated with downregulation of *MMP-9* [80].

4.3. MMP-3, MMP-10 (Stromelysin)

Another member of MMPs family is MMP-3, or stromelysin-1, which degrades collagen (types II, III, IV, IX, and X), proteoglycans, fibronectin, laminin, and elastin in ECM.

Sipos et al., found a positive association between MMP-3 protein expression and the adenoma–dysplasia–carcinoma sequence. In particular, they reported that high-grade dysplastic sessile adenomatous-stage and early-stage CRC conditions can be differentiated based on the stroma expression of MMP3 [81]. Meaningful positive associations between the protein expression level of MMP-3, invasion, lymph node metastasis, histological type of CRC, and poorly differentiated tumor were reported by Islekel et al. [82]. MMP-3 can activate other MMPs, such as MMP-1, MMP-7, and MMP-9, to promote the progression of tumor initiation [83,84].

MMP-10 also belongs to the stromelysin family. It can digest collagen types II, III, IV, IX, X, proteoglycans, fibronectin, laminin, and elastin. Also, MMP-10 enhances cell growth and invasion in CRC, and its upregulation was found to be associated with poor survival [49,85].

4.4. MMP-7 (Matrilysin)

MMP-7, or matrilysin, digests fibronectin, laminin, type I collagen, and gelatin. It can provide the right condition for vascularization via cleavage of ECM [86]. A major ratio of MMP-7 expression in tumor cells has been reported. Qasim et al., found MMP-7 protein overexpression in villous adenomatous polyps compared to other types of polyps and demonstrated that MMP-7 protein overexpression is an initial event in CRC carcinogenesis that could lead adenomas to CRC [53]. In our laboratory, we observed high expression levels of *MMP-7* and *VEGF-A* mRNA in adenomatous polyps compared to normal tissue. We found that the expression levels of *MMP-7* and *VEGF-A* genes were higher in villous adenoma than in other types of adenomas. Thus, we concluded that the *MMP-7* gene overexpression has a critical role in colorectal adenoma angiogenesis and could be a primary event in the adenoma-carcinoma sequence [45].

MMP-7 gene can enhance tumor growth and metastasis [87]. Also, MMP-7 activates other MMPs, such as proMMP9 and proMMP2 [88] In addition. MMP-7 exerts a wide spectrum of activities not only as an enzyme but also as a signaling molecule. In fact, it has been shown that MMP-7 trans-activates EGFR by releasing the heparin-binding epidermal growth factor (HB-EGF) in CRC cells, with consequent cell proliferation and apoptosis regulation [89,90].

4.5. MMP-12 (Metalloelastase)

MMP-12, or metalloelastase, can digest different substrates. Several studies considered *MMP-12* gene as an anti-metastatic agent [91,92]. Also, it could inhibit angiogenesis by downregulation of *VEGF* and enhancement of the endogenous angiogenesis inhibitor angiostatin. Overall, the role of *MMP-12* in tumor suppression and increase in overall survival has been widely recognized [93–95].

Importantly, Klupp et al., found higher levels of MMP-12 protein expression in sera of CRC patients compared with those of healthy individuals. Also, they suggested an association between MMP-12 protein expression levels and CRC advanced disease and vascular invasion. Furthermore, a significant correlation between the upregulation of MMP-12 expression and poor survival was shown [49].

4.6. MMP-21 (XMMP)

MMP-21 (XMMP) can degenerate aggrecan (cartilage-specific proteoglycan core protein) in the internal region of ECM [96]. Overexpression of MMP-21 protein in CRC compared with normal tissue was shown in many studies [97,98]. Furthermore, significant associations between MMP-21 protein expression and CRC tumor invasion, lymph node metastasis, and distant metastasis were found [97,99]. Wu et al., showed that MMP-21 not only affected CRC progression but also was an independent prognostic biomarker in patients with stage II and stage III CRC cancer. Taken together, these facts led them to conclude that MMP-21 could be used for targeted therapy in CRC [97]. Huang et al., demonstrated that the upregulation of MMP-21 protein was related to shorter overall survival in patients with CRC [98].

4.7. MMP-14 (MT1-MMP)

MMP-14, called MT1-MMP, acts on matrix substrates, such as collagens I, II, III, and gelatin. The *MMP-14* gene plays a crucial role in many biological and pathological conditions and activation of proMMP2 [92,100]. The role of *MMP-14* in angiogenesis and cancer invasion has been identified by previous investigations [101–103]. Cui et al., observed statistically significant associations between the overexpression of *MMP-14* gene in CRC compared to normal mucosa. Their analysis indicated that high expression levels of *MMP-14* were associated with advanced-stage CRC, lymph node metastasis, and poor overall survival. They concluded that the *MMP-14* gene is an oncogene and may represent a potential prognostic biomarker in CRC [104].

Yang et al., showed in an in vivo CRC model that the STAT3 phosphorylation activity and the overexpression of MMP14 protein were enhanced by the overexpression of Hes1 gene. Also, they suggested that Hes1 promoted the invasion of colorectal cancerous cells via the STAT3-MMP14 pathway [103]. It was reported that the overexpression of MMP-14 protein was associated with Prox1 gene. When Prox1 gene was deleted, MMP14 protein was increased, and the mice showed slow-growing, matrix-rich, chemotherapy-resistance, and cancerous cells with malignant stromal features, including activation of fibroblasts, blood vessels dysfunction, and lack of cytotoxic T cells [105].

5. The Effects of Polymorphisms of *MMP* Genes on Colorectal Carcinogenesis

Single-nucleotide polymorphisms (SNPs) are a common genetic variation involving a single base pair in DNA. SNPs are mostly located in the gene promoter region and may have an impact on gene and protein expression levels. The effects of MMP polymorphisms have been observed in many cancers such as CRC and hepatocellular carcinoma [106,107].

In a Japanese population, the *MMP-1* 1G/2G polymorphism was detected and associated with the development of CRC [108]. In the Iranian population, Kouhkan et al., demonstrated that *MMP-1* 2G/2G genotype polymorphism was correlated with invasion risk of CRC, especially in smoker men [109]. In the Netherlands, *MMP-2*-1306C>T SNP was detected in CRC patients, and the T/T genotype was found to be associated with poor overall survival whereas C/C and C/T genotypes showed better outcomes. No difference in overall survival was instead observed among patients with different genotypes of the *MMP-9*-1562C>T SNP [110]. Also, in a cohort study of Taiwanese CRC patients, Ting et al. indicated that patients carrying the A/A genotype of the *MMP-2*-1575G>A SNP had a higher risk to develop distant metastasis compared with patients carrying the T/T genotype [111]. In a Polish population with CRC, individuals with the G/G variant genotype of *MMP-7*-181A>G SNP had a higher risk of lymph node involvement and advanced tumor infiltration than patients carrying the A/A genotype [112]. A Chinese study showed that the *MMP-9* R279Q SNP relative to the R/R genotype was correlated with a higher risk of CRC compared with the QQ genotype. Also, the allele frequency of the *MMP-1* 16071G/2G and *MMP-7* 181 A/G polymorphisms were not associated with CRC [113]. In a Korean population, the homozygous *MMP-9*-1562C/C genotype was significantly more frequent in CRC cases than in the control group [114]. In Sweden, researchers found that the A/A genotype of *MMP-12*-82A>G increased the risk of disseminated malignancy in CRC patients while the A/A genotype of *MMP-13*-82A>G was not correlated to invasion [115].

Lièvre et al., investigated *MMP-3*, *MMP-7*, and *MMP-1* genes promoter polymorphisms in 295 patients with large adenomas and 302 patients with small adenomas. The analysis revealed a significant association between *MMP-3*-1612 ins/del A, *MMP-1*-1607 ins/del G polymorphism, and small adenomas; also, adenomas were associated with the combined genotype 2G/2G-6A/6A. However, no significant association between *MMP-7* polymorphism and the development of adenomas was found. The authors suggested that only the study *MMP-3* and *MMP-1* gene promoter polymorphisms had potential roles in the development of adenomas from normal colon epithelial cells or in the earliest steps of CRC [57].

Tai et al., showed that *MMP-8* rs11225395 related to the risk of CRC and worst outcomes in a subpopulation of the Han Chinese population. On this basis, they suggested *MMP-8* rs11225395 polymorphism as a potential biomarker predictive of CRC susceptibility [116].

6. Targeting MMPs in CRC Treatment

6.1. Pharmacological Inhibition

Several pharmacological inhibitors of MMPs (MMPIs) have been studied and tested in phase I-III clinical trials, but to date, none of these drugs has been approved for the treatment of cancer, including CRC. Overall, the late stages of the clinical experimentation failed because of the substantial toxicity and weak selectivity of MMPIs [117]. Mainly, candidate MMPIs are represented by small molecules, peptides, and antibodies [118]. Currently, only one broad-spectrum MMPI has been approved by FDA but it has not indication in cancer (i.e., the small molecule periostat) [117,119]. Other MMPIs, such as the small molecule prinomastat, selective for MMP-1, MMP-2, and MMP-9 [120–123] and the GA-5745/andecaliximab, a selective anti-body against MMP-9, have reached the phase III [124,125]. However, none of these trials includes CRC.

6.2. Inhibition of MMPs by TIMPs

Since MMPs are naturally inhibited by TIMPs, these proteins have also been widely investigated mainly to exploit their ability to discover potential strategies for MMP inhibition [126]. The TIMP family consists of four members of proteins (TIMP1-4) that form a 1:1 complex with MMPs. Dysregulation of this complex due to the increased expression of MMPs or a decreased control by TIMPs has been observed in several diseases, including cancer. TIMPs control the activity of MMPs via binding to them (Figure 3) [126–128].

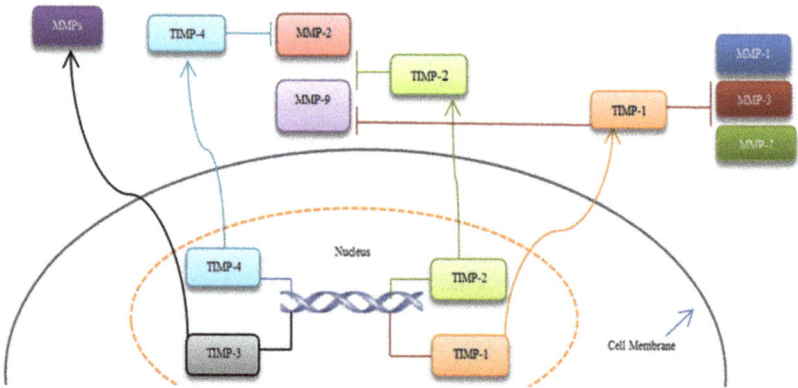

Figure 3. MMPs inhibition by TIMPs. TIMP-1 inhibits MMP-1, 3, 7, 9. TIMP-2 can suppress MMP-2 and 9, and TIMP-4 blocks MMP-2. These inhibitions result in the primary tumor transitioning to advanced CRC. Moreover, TIMP-3 has a protective effect on CRC cases and could bind to several MMPs [126–128].

TIMP-1 inhibits MMP-1, 3, 7, 9 and affects angiogenesis [37,129]. Previous investigations considered a dual activity for the *TIMP-1* gene: in particular, *TIMP-1* was associated with tumor growth at the early stages of colon cancer, and decreased activity of *TIMP-1* could lead to tumor invasion [130,131].

TIMP-2 can suppress MMP-2, MMP-9, and microvascularization [129,132]. Also, downregulation of TIMP-2 is related to invasive CRC [133]. Wang et al., reported that downregulation of *TIMP-2* in CRC tumor tissues was meaningfully correlated with the depth of invasion, lymph node metastasis, tumor stage, and poor survival [134].

TIMP-3 is known as a tumor suppressor gene and inhibits several MMPs. TIMP-3 downregulation is associated with advanced CRC [135]. Lin et al., represented that, adenovirus-mediated *TIMP-3* transduction in CT26 colon cancer cell line suppressed cell growth and stimulated apoptosis. Also, *TIMP-3* transduction inhibited migration and invasion. In vivo data indicated that *TIMP-3* prevented in vivo tumor growth and liver metastasis [136].

TIMP-4 protein suppresses MMP-2, and one study showed that overexpression of TIMP-4 increased the survival rate of rectal cancer [128].

Currently, no drug mimicking the TIMP activity has been obtained as well as no gene therapeutic approach able to modulate the activity of TIMPs is available.

6.3. MMPs Regulation by microRNA

MicroRNAs, a class of small, endogenous RNAs of 21–25 nucleotides in length, control gene and protein regulation via binding and digesting target mRNA (Table 3). Suppression of MMPs by microRNAs is a suggested way for CRC treatment. Some evidence has been provided. In particular, microRNA-34 (miR-34a) plays a role as a tumor suppressor, and its overexpression could suppress *MMP-1*, *MMP-9*, and tumor cell proliferation, migration, and invasion via acetylation of *P53* in CRC [137–139]. The upregulation of miR-139 reduces proliferation, migration, and invasion by suppression of the IGF-IR/MEK/ERK signaling and *MMP-2* gene in CRC patients [140]. Upregulation of miR-29a increases CRC metastasis via suppression of KLF4 (Kruppel-like factor 4), transcription factor, and upregulation of *MMP-2* gene [141]. Also, miR-29b suppresses CRC metastasis, reduces angiogenesis and EMT by targeting the *MMP-2* gene [142]. Overexpression of miR-143 can suppress the *MMP-7* gene directly and prevent colorectal tumor cell proliferation and invasion [143].

Table 3. MMPs are Regulated by microRNAs in CRC.

MicroRNA	MMP	Result
miR-34a	MMP-1, MMP-9	miR-34a overexpression prevents tumor cell proliferation, migration, and invasion [138,139].
miR-139	MMP-2	Downregulation of miR-139 reduces proliferation, migration, and invasion [140].
miR-29a	MMP-2	Upregulation of miR-29a increases metastasis [141].
miR-29b	MMP-2	Upregulation of miR-29b increases metastasis [142].
miR-143	MMP-7	Upregulation of miR-143 enhances tumor cell proliferation and invasion [143].

6.4. MMPs Regulation by Long Non-Coding RNAs

Long non-coding RNAs (lncRNAs) can regulate gene expression and have key roles in cell proliferation, migration, invasion, apoptosis, metastasis, and EMT in CRC. In this regard, lncRNA-targeted therapy is today considered a potential promising strategy for CRC treatment [144]. In fact, based on mechanistic studies investigating the complex lncRNA-mediated sponge interactions in CRC, potential therapeutic targets for the treatment of this cancer may be identified. Among the available findings, Tian et al., demonstrated that the suppression of *TUG1* by shRNA prevented *MMP-14* expression, proliferation, invasion, and EMT in colon cancer [145]. Sun et al., found a significant association between XIST inhibition and suppression of *c-Myc*, *cyclinD1*, and *MMP-7* expression through inactivation of Wnt/β-catenin signaling pathway [146]. A recent investigation showed a meaningful correlation between the overexpression of LINC00963 and the upregulation of *MMP-2* and *MMP-9*, proliferation, migration, and invasion of CRC cells [147]. Duan et al., revealed that the inhibition of the CCEPR lncRNA reduced the expression levels of *MMP-2* and *MMP-9*, and prevented EMT in CRC cells [148]. Pan et al., realized that the expression level of MMP-2 protein was notably decreased when PCA3 was knocked out. In addition, suppression of PCA3 inhibited colon cancer cell invasion and migration [149].

7. Conclusions

In summary, MMPs genes and proteins, through complex mechanisms involving the induction of many molecular signaling pathways and the EMT process, play a relevant role in the transition from pre-cancerous lesions and polyps to advanced CRC. However, further investigation is needed to understand how MMPs exactly work. This would improve the selectivity of MMPIs that could be exploited in a dual-mode: to treat CRC alone or in combination with targeted agents and/or chemotherapy and to prevent CRC development.

Author Contributions: Conceptualization, investigation, writing—original draft, designed tables and figures Z.P.; editing, validation, and revise, S.N.; writing, design table, and investigation, N.P.; revise, B.S.; investigation, H.N. and H.S.; validation, H.A.-A. and E.M.; supervision, validation, and revise E.N.-M. and M.A.B. All authors have read and agreed to the published version of the manuscript.

Funding: This research was supported by Fondo Beneficenza Intesa Sanpaolo S.p.A. (Milan, Italy) and Associazione Giacomo Onlus (Castiglioncello, Italy) to E.M.

Acknowledgments: The authors would like to thank all the staff of the Department of Cancer at the Research Institute for Gastroenterology and Liver Diseases, Shahid Beheshti University of Medical Sciences, Tehran, Iran.

Conflicts of Interest: The authors declare no conflict of interest.

References

1. Sung, H.; Ferlay, J.; Siegel, R.L.; Laversanne, M.; Soerjomataram, I.; Jemal, A.; Bray, F. Global Cancer Statistics 2020: GLOBOCAN Estimates of Incidence and Mortality Worldwide for 36 Cancers in 185 Countries. *CA Cancer J. Clin.* **2021**, *71*, 209–249. [CrossRef] [PubMed]
2. Vogelstein, B.; Fearon, E.R.; Hamilton, S.R.; Kern, S.E.; Preisinger, A.C.; Leppert, M.; Nakamura, Y.; White, R.; Smits, A.M.; Bos, J.L. Genetic alterations during colorectal-tumor development. *N. Engl. J. Med.* **1988**, *319*, 525–532. [CrossRef] [PubMed]
3. Kasi, A.; Handa, S.; Bhatti, S.; Umar, S.; Bansal, A.; Sun, W. Molecular Pathogenesis and Classification of Colorectal Carcinoma. *Curr. Colorectal Cancer Rep.* **2020**, *16*, 97–106. [CrossRef] [PubMed]
4. Huck, M.B.; Bohl, J.L. Colonic Polyps: Diagnosis and Surveillance. *Clin. Colon Rectal Surg.* **2016**, *29*, 296–305. [CrossRef]
5. Smit, W.L.; Spaan, C.N.; de Boer, R.J.; Ramesh, P.; Garcia, T.M.; Meijer, B.J.; Vermeulen, J.L.M.; Lezzerini, M.; MacInnes, A.W.; Koster, J.; et al. Driver mutations of the adenoma-carcinoma sequence govern the intestinal epithelial global translational capacity. *Proc. Natl. Acad. Sci. USA* **2020**, *117*, 25560. [CrossRef]
6. Wang, K.; Zheng, J.; Yu, J.; Wu, Y.; Guo, J.; Xu, Z.; Sun, X. Knockdown of MMP-1 inhibits the progression of colorectal cancer by suppressing the PI3K/Akt/c–myc signaling pathway and EMT. *Oncol. Rep.* **2020**, *43*, 1103–1112. [CrossRef]
7. Yuan, X.; Sun, X.; Shi, X.; Wang, H.; Wu, G.; Jiang, C.; Yu, D.; Zhang, W.; Xue, B.; Ding, Y. USP39 promotes colorectal cancer growth and metastasis through the Wnt/β-catenin pathway. *Oncol. Rep.* **2017**, *37*, 2398–2404. [CrossRef]
8. Quintero-Fabián, S.; Arreola, R.; Becerril-Villanueva, E.; Torres-Romero, J.C.; Arana-Argáez, V.; Lara-Riegos, J.; Ramírez-Camacho, M.A.; Alvarez-Sánchez, M.E. Role of Matrix Metalloproteinases in Angiogenesis and Cancer. *Front. Oncol.* **2019**, *9*, 1370. [CrossRef]
9. Yadav, L.; Puri, N.; Rastogi, V.; Satpute, P.; Ahmad, R.; Kaur, G. Role of Matrix Metalloproteinases in Angiogenesis and Cancer. *Asian Pac. J. Cancer Prev.* **2014**, *15*, 1085–1091. [CrossRef]
10. Ligi, D.; Mannello, F. Do matrix metalloproteinases represent reliable circulating biomarkers in colorectal cancer? *Br. J. Cancer* **2016**, *115*, 633–634. [CrossRef]
11. Yeh, Y.-C.; Sheu, B.-S. Matrix metalloproteinases and their inhibitors in the gastrointestinal cancers: Current knowledge and clinical potential. *Met. Med.* **2014**, *1*, 3–13. [CrossRef]
12. Wu, Z.; Liu, Z.; Ge, W.; Shou, J.; You, L.; Pan, H.; Han, W. Analysis of potential genes and pathways associated with the colorectal normal mucosa-adenoma-carcinoma sequence. *Cancer Med.* **2018**, *7*, 2555–2566. [CrossRef]
13. Bertelson, N.L.; Kalkbrenner, K.A.; Merchea, A.; Dozois, E.J.; Landmann, R.G.; De Petris, G.; Young-Fadok, T.M.; Etzioni, D.A. Colectomy for Endoscopically Unresectable Polyps: How Often Is It Cancer? *Dis. Colon Rectum* **2012**, *55*, 1111–1116. [CrossRef]
14. Shussman, N.; Wexner, S.D. Colorectal polyps and polyposis syndromes. *Gastroenterol. Rep.* **2014**, *2*, 1–15. [CrossRef]
15. Liljegren, A.; Lindblom, A.; Rotstein, S.; Nilsson, B.; Rubio, C.; Jaramillo, E. Prevalence and incidence of hyperplastic polyps and adenomas in familial colorectal cancer: Correlation between the two types of colon polyps. *Gut* **2003**, *52*, 1140–1147. [CrossRef]
16. Malki, A.; ElRuz, R.A.; Gupta, I.; Allouch, A.; Vranic, S.; Al Moustafa, A.E. Molecular Mechanisms of Colon Cancer Progression and Metastasis: Recent Insights and Advancements. *Int. J. Mol. Sci.* **2020**, *22*, 130. [CrossRef]
17. Kato, S.; Lippman, S.M.; Flaherty, K.T.; Kurzrock, R. The Conundrum of Genetic "Drivers" in Benign Conditions. *J. Natl. Cancer Inst.* **2016**, *108*, djw036. [CrossRef]
18. Mustjoki, S.; Young, N.S. Somatic Mutations in "Benign" Disease. *N. Engl. J. Med.* **2021**, *384*, 2039–2052. [CrossRef]
19. Nojadeh, J.N.; Behrouz Sharif, S.; Sakhinia, E. Microsatellite instability in colorectal cancer. *EXCLI J.* **2018**, *17*, 159–168. [CrossRef]

20. Arabsorkhi, Z.; Sadeghi, H.; Gharib, E.; Rejali, L.; Asadzadeh-Aghdaei, H.; Nazemalhosseini-Mojarad, E. Can *hypoxia-inducible factor-1α* overexpression discriminate human colorectal cancers with different microsatellite instability? *Genes Genet. Syst.* 2021, 96, 1–6. [CrossRef]
21. Pino, M.S.; Chung, D.C. The chromosomal instability pathway in colon cancer. *Gastroenterology* 2010, 138, 2059–2072. [CrossRef]
22. Colussi, D.; Brandi, G.; Bazzoli, F.; Ricciardiello, L. Molecular pathways involved in colorectal cancer: Implications for disease behavior and prevention. *Int. J. Mol. Sci.* 2013, 14, 16365–16385. [CrossRef]
23. Grady, W.M.; Markowitz, S.D. The molecular pathogenesis of colorectal cancer and its potential application to colorectal cancer screening. *Dig. Dis. Sci.* 2015, 60, 762–772. [CrossRef]
24. Sadanandam, A.; Lyssiotis, C.A.; Homicsko, K.; Collisson, E.A.; Gibb, W.J.; Wullschleger, S.; Ostos, L.C.; Lannon, W.A.; Grotzinger, C.; Del Rio, M.; et al. A colorectal cancer classification system that associates cellular phenotype and responses to therapy. *Nat. Med.* 2013, 19, 619–625. [CrossRef]
25. Guinney, J.; Dienstmann, R.; Wang, X.; de Reyniès, A.; Schlicker, A.; Soneson, C.; Marisa, L.; Roepman, P.; Nyamundanda, G.; Angelino, P.; et al. The consensus molecular subtypes of colorectal cancer. *Nat. Med.* 2015, 21, 1350–1356. [CrossRef]
26. Thanki, K.; Nicholls, M.E.; Gajjar, A.; Senagore, A.J.; Qiu, S.; Szabo, C.; Hellmich, M.R.; Chao, C. Consensus Molecular Subtypes of Colorectal Cancer and their Clinical Implications. *Int. Biol. Biomed. J.* 2017, 3, 105–111.
27. McCorry, A.M.; Loughrey, M.B.; Longley, D.B.; Lawler, M.; Dunne, P.D. Epithelial-to-mesenchymal transition signature assessment in colorectal cancer quantifies tumour stromal content rather than true transition. *J. Pathol.* 2018, 246, 422–426. [CrossRef]
28. Isella, C.; Brundu, F.; Bellomo, S.E.; Galimi, F.; Zanella, E.; Porporato, R.; Petti, C.; Fiori, A.; Orzan, F.; Senetta, R.; et al. Selective analysis of cancer-cell intrinsic transcriptional traits defines novel clinically relevant subtypes of colorectal cancer. *Nat. Commun.* 2017, 8, 15107. [CrossRef]
29. Cui, N.; Hu, M.; Khalil, R.A. Biochemical and biological attributes of matrix metalloproteinases. *Prog. Mol. Biol. Transl. Sci.* 2017, 147, 1–73. [CrossRef]
30. Morgunova, E.; Tuuttila, A.; Bergmann, U.; Isupov, M.; Lindqvist, Y.; Schneider, G.; Tryggvason, K. Structure of human pro-matrix metalloproteinase-2: Activation mechanism revealed. *Science* 1999, 284, 1667–1670. [CrossRef]
31. Laronha, H.; Caldeira, J. Structure and function of human matrix metalloproteinases. *Cells* 2020, 9, 1076. [CrossRef] [PubMed]
32. Sternlicht, M.D.; Werb, Z. How matrix metalloproteinases regulate cell behavior. *Annu. Rev. Cell. Dev. Biol.* 2001, 17, 463–516. [CrossRef] [PubMed]
33. Baker, A.H.; Edwards, D.R.; Murphy, G. Metalloproteinase inhibitors: Biological actions and therapeutic opportunities. *J. Cell Sci.* 2002, 115, 3719–3727. [CrossRef] [PubMed]
34. Hua, H.; Li, M.; Luo, T.; Yin, Y.; Jiang, Y. Matrix metalloproteinases in tumorigenesis: An evolving paradigm. *Cell Mol. Life Sci.* 2011, 68, 3853–3868. [CrossRef]
35. Alaseem, A.; Alhazzani, K.; Dondapati, P.; Alobid, S.; Bishayee, A.; Rathinavelu, A. Matrix Metalloproteinases: A challenging paradigm of cancer management. *Semin. Cancer Biol.* 2019, 56, 100–115. [CrossRef]
36. Gonzalez-Avila, G.; Sommer, B.; Mendoza-Posada, D.A.; Ramos, C.; Garcia-Hernandez, A.A.; Falfan-Valencia, R. Matrix metalloproteinases participation in the metastatic process and their diagnostic and therapeutic applications in cancer. *Crit. Rev. Oncol. Hematol.* 2019, 137, 57–83. [CrossRef]
37. Herszényi, L.; Hritz, I.; Lakatos, G.; Varga, M.Z.; Tulassay, Z. The behavior of matrix metalloproteinases and their inhibitors in colorectal cancer. *Int. J. Mol. Sci.* 2012, 13, 13240–13263. [CrossRef]
38. Huang, X.; Lan, Y.; Li, E.; Li, J.; Deng, Q.; Deng, X. Diagnostic values of MMP-7, MMP-9, MMP-11, TIMP-1, TIMP-2, CEA, and CA19-9 in patients with colorectal cancer. *J. Int. Med. Res.* 2021, 49, 1–11. [CrossRef]
39. Zhou, X.; Yang, D.; Ding, X.; Xu, P. Clinical value of microRNA-135a and MMP-13 in colon cancer. *Oncol. Lett.* 2021, 22, 583. [CrossRef]
40. Rasool, M.; Malik, A.; Waquar, S.; Ain, Q.T.; Rasool, R.; Asif, M.; Anfinan, N.; Haque, A.; Alam, H.; Ahmed, S.; et al. Assessment of clinical variables as predictive markers in the development and progression of colorectal cancer. *Bioengineered* 2021, 12, 2288–2298. [CrossRef]
41. Barabás, L.; Hritz, I.; István, G.; Tulassay, Z.; Herszényi, L. The Behavior of MMP-2, MMP-7, MMP-9, and Their Inhibitors TIMP-1 and TIMP-2 in Adenoma-Colorectal Cancer Sequence. *Dig. Dis.* 2021, 39, 217–224. [CrossRef]
42. Hsieh, S.L.; Hsieh, S.; Lai, P.Y.; Wang, J.J.; Li, C.C.; Wu, C.C. Carnosine Suppresses Human Colorectal Cell Migration and Intravasation by Regulating EMT and MMP Expression. *Am. J. Chin. Med.* 2019, 47, 477–494. [CrossRef]
43. Kıyak, R.; Keles, D.; Bengi, G.; Yalcin, M.; Topalak, Ö.; Oktay, G. The Importance of Fecal and Plasma CEA, COX-2, MMP-7, and TIMP-1 in the Diagnosis of Colorectal Cancer. *J. Basic Clin. Health Sci.* 2018, 2, 7–14. [CrossRef]
44. Eiró, N.; Gonzalez, L.; Cid, S.; Andicoechea, A.; Vizoso, F. Matrix metalloproteases expression in different histological types of colorectal polyps. *Rev. Esp. Enferm. Dig.* 2017, 109, 414–420. [CrossRef]
45. Pezeshkian, Z.; Forouzesh, F.; Peyravian, N.; Yaghoob-Taleghani, M.; Asadzadeh-Aghdaei, H.; Zali, M.; Nazemalhosseini-Mojarad, E. Clinicopathological correlations of *VEGF-A* and *MMP-7* genes expression in different types of colorectal adenoma polyps. *WCRJ* 2017, 4, e978.
46. Wernicke, A.-K.; Churin, Y.; Sheridan, D.; Windhorst, A.; Tschuschner, A.; Gattenlöhner, S.; Roderfeld, M.; Roeb, E. Matrix metalloproteinase-13 refines pathological staging of precancerous colorectal lesions. *Oncotarget* 2016, 7, 73552–73557. [CrossRef]

47. Gimeno-García, A.Z.; Triñanes, J.; Quintero, E.; Salido, E.; Nicolás-Pérez, D.; Adrián-de-Ganzo, Z.; Alarcón-Fernández, O.; Abrante, B.; Romero, R.; Carrillo, M.; et al. Plasma matrix metalloproteinase 9 as an early surrogate biomarker of advanced colorectal neoplasia. *Gastroenterol. Hepatol.* **2016**, *39*, 433–441. [CrossRef]
48. Annaházi, A.; Ábrahám, S.; Farkas, K.; Rosztóczy, A.; Inczefi, O.; Földesi, I.; Szűcs, M.; Rutka, M.; Theodorou, V.; Eutamene, H.; et al. A pilot study on faecal MMP-9: A new noninvasive diagnostic marker of colorectal cancer. *Br. J. Cancer* **2016**, *114*, 787–792. [CrossRef]
49. Klupp, F.; Neumann, L.; Kahlert, C.; Diers, J.; Halama, N.; Franz, C.; Schmidt, T.; Koch, M.; Weitz, J.; Schneider, M.; et al. Serum MMP7, MMP10 and MMP12 level as negative prognostic markers in colon cancer patients. *BMC Cancer* **2016**, *16*, 494. [CrossRef]
50. Otero-Estévez, O.; De Chiara, L.; Rodríguez-Girondo, M.; Rodríguez-Berrocal, F.J.; Cubiella, J.; Castro, I.; Hernández, V.; Martínez-Zorzano, V.S. Serum matrix metalloproteinase-9 in colorectal cancer family-risk population screening. *Sci. Rep.* **2015**, *5*, 13030. [CrossRef]
51. Bengi, G.; Keles, D.; Topalak, Ö.; Yalçin, M.; Kiyak, R.; Oktay, G. Expressions of TIMP-1, COX-2 and MMP-7 in Colon Polyp and Colon Cancer. *Euroasian J. Hepatogastroenterol.* **2015**, *5*, 74–79. [CrossRef]
52. Odabasi, M.; Yesil, A.; Ozkara, S.; Paker, N.; Ozkan, S.; Eris, C.; Yildiz, M.K.; Abuoglu, H.H.; Gunay, E.; Tekeşin, K. Role of human neutrophil gelatinase associated lipocalin (NGAL) and Matrix Metalloproteinase-9 (MMP-9) overexpression in neoplastic colon polyps. *Int. J. Clin. Exp. Med.* **2014**, *7*, 2804–2811.
53. Qasim, B.J.; Ali, H.H.; Hussein, A.G. Immunohistochemical expression of matrix metalloproteinase-7 in human colorectal adenomas using specified automated cellular image analysis system: A clinicopathological study. *Saudi J. Gastroenterol.* **2013**, *19*, 23–27. [CrossRef]
54. Sheth, R.A.; Kunin, A.; Stangenberg, L.; Sinnamon, M.; Hung, K.E.; Kucherlapati, R.; Mahmood, U. In vivo optical molecular imaging of matrix metalloproteinase activity following celecoxib therapy for colorectal cancer. *Mol. Imaging* **2012**, *11*, 417–425. [CrossRef] [PubMed]
55. Murnane, M.J.; Cai, J.; Shuja, S.; McAneny, D.; Klepeis, V.; Willett, J.B. Active MMP-2 effectively identifies the presence of colorectal cancer. *Int. J. Cancer* **2009**, *125*, 2893–2902. [CrossRef] [PubMed]
56. Jeffery, N.; McLean, M.H.; El-Omar, E.M.; Murray, G.I. The matrix metalloproteinase/tissue inhibitor of matrix metalloproteinase profile in colorectal polyp cancers. *Histopathology* **2009**, *54*, 820–828. [CrossRef] [PubMed]
57. Lièvre, A.; Milet, J.; Carayol, J.; Le Corre, D.; Milan, C.; Pariente, A.; Nalet, B.; Lafon, J.; Faivre, J.; Bonithon-Kopp, C.; et al. Genetic polymorphisms of MMP1, MMP3 and MMP7 gene promoter and risk of colorectal adenoma. *BMC Cancer* **2006**, *6*, 270. [CrossRef] [PubMed]
58. Tutton, M.G.; George, M.L.; Eccles, S.A.; Burton, S.; Swift, R.I.; Abulafi, A.M. Use of plasma MMP-2 and MMP-9 levels as a surrogate for tumour expression in colorectal cancer patients. *Int. J. Cancer* **2003**, *107*, 541–550. [CrossRef]
59. Jonsson, A.; Falk, P.; Angenete, E.; Hjalmarsson, C.; Ivarsson, M.-L. Plasma MMP-1 Expression as a Prognostic Factor in Colon Cancer. *J. Surg. Res.* **2021**, *266*, 254–260. [CrossRef]
60. Liang, Y.; Lv, Z.; Huang, G.; Qin, J.; Li, H.; Nong, F.; Wen, B. Prognostic significance of abnormal matrix collagen remodeling in colorectal cancer based on histologic and bioinformatics analysis. *Oncol. Rep.* **2020**, *44*, 1671–1685. [CrossRef]
61. Sunami, E.; Tsuno, N.; Osada, T.; Saito, S.; Kitayama, J.; Tomozawa, S.; Tsuruo, T.; Shibata, Y.; Muto, T.; Nagawa, H. MMP-1 is a prognostic marker for hematogenous metastasis of colorectal cancer. *Oncologist* **2000**, *5*, 108–114. [CrossRef]
62. Yamada, T.; Oshima, T.; Yoshihara, K.; Tamura, S.; Kanazawa, A.; Inagaki, D.; Yamamoto, N.; Sato, T.; Fujii, S.; Numata, K.; et al. Overexpression of MMP-13 gene in colorectal cancer with liver metastasis. *Anticancer Res.* **2010**, *30*, 2693–2699.
63. Leeman, M.F.; McKay, J.A.; Murray, G.I. Matrix metalloproteinase 13 activity is associated with poor prognosis in colorectal cancer. *J. Clin. Pathol.* **2002**, *55*, 758–762. [CrossRef]
64. Merchant, N.; Chalikonda, G.; Nagaraju, G.P. Role of Matrix Metalloproteinases in Colorectal Cancer. In *Theranostics Approaches to Gastric and Colon Cancer*; Springer: Singapore, 2020; pp. 49–59. [CrossRef]
65. Yan, Q.; Yuan, Y.; Yankui, L.; Jingjie, F.; Linfang, J.; Yong, P.; Dong, H.; Xiaowei, Q. The Expression and Significance of CXCR5 and MMP-13 in Colorectal Cancer. *Cell Biochem. Biophys.* **2015**, *73*, 253–259. [CrossRef]
66. Korpi, J.T.; Kervinen, V.; Mäklin, H.; Väänänen, A.; Lahtinen, M.; Läärä, E.; Ristimäki, A.; Thomas, G.; Ylipalosaari, M.; Aström, P.; et al. Collagenase-2 (matrix metalloproteinase-8) plays a protective role in tongue cancer. *Br. J. Cancer* **2008**, *98*, 766–775. [CrossRef]
67. Balbín, M.; Fueyo, A.; Tester, A.M.; Pendás, A.M.; Pitiot, A.S.; Astudillo, A.; Overall, C.M.; Shapiro, S.D.; López-Otín, C. Loss of collagenase-2 confers increased skin tumor susceptibility to male mice. *Nat. Genet.* **2003**, *35*, 252–257. [CrossRef]
68. Sirniö, P.; Tuomisto, A.; Tervahartiala, T.; Sorsa, T.; Klintrup, K.; Karhu, T.; Herzig, K.-H.; Mäkelä, J.; Karttunen, T.J.; Salo, T.; et al. High-serum MMP-8 levels are associated with decreased survival and systemic inflammation in colorectal cancer. *Br. J. Cancer* **2018**, *119*, 213–219. [CrossRef]
69. Beutel, B.; Song, J.; Konken, C.P.; Korpos, E.; Schinor, B.; Gerwien, H.; Vidyadharan, R.; Burmeister, M.; Li, L.; Haufe, G.; et al. New in Vivo Compatible Matrix Metalloproteinase (MMP)-2 and MMP-9 Inhibitors. *Bioconjugate Chem.* **2018**, *29*, 3715–3725. [CrossRef]
70. Murnane, M.J.; Cai, J.; Shuja, S.; McAneny, D.; Willett, J.B. Active matrix metalloproteinase-2 activity discriminates colonic mucosa, adenomas with and without high-grade dysplasia, and cancers. *Hum. Pathol.* **2011**, *42*, 688–701. [CrossRef]

71. Gimeno-García, A.Z.; Santana-Rodríguez, A.; Jiménez, A.; Parra-Blanco, A.; Nicolás-Pérez, D.; Paz-Cabrera, C.; Díaz-González, F.; Medina, C.; Díaz-Flores, L.; Quintero, E. Up-regulation of gelatinases in the colorectal adenoma-carcinoma sequence. *Eur. J. Cancer* **2006**, *42*, 3246–3252. [CrossRef]
72. Salem, N.; Kamal, I.; Al-Maghrabi, J.; Abuzenadah, A.; Peer-Zada, A.A.; Qari, Y.; Al-Ahwal, M.; Al-Qahtani, M.; Buhmeida, A. High expression of matrix metalloproteinases: MMP-2 and MMP-9 predicts poor survival outcome in colorectal carcinoma. *Future Oncol.* **2016**, *12*, 323–331. [CrossRef] [PubMed]
73. Langenskiöld, M.; Holmdahl, L.; Falk, P.; Ivarsson, M.-L. Increased plasma MMP-2 protein expression in lymph node-positive patients with colorectal cancer. *Int. J. Colorectal Dis.* **2005**, *20*, 245–252. [CrossRef] [PubMed]
74. Kryczka, J.; Stasiak, M.; Dziki, L.; Mik, M.; Dziki, A.; Cierniewski, C.S. Matrix metalloproteinase-2 cleavage of the β1 integrin ectodomain facilitates colon cancer cell motility. *J. Biol. Chem.* **2012**, *287*, 36556–36566. [CrossRef] [PubMed]
75. Takeuchi, T.; Hisanaga, M.; Nagao, M.; Ikeda, N.; Fujii, H.; Koyama, F.; Mukogawa, T.; Matsumoto, H.; Kondo, S.; Takahashi, C.; et al. The membrane-anchored matrix metalloproteinase (MMP) regulator RECK in combination with MMP-9 serves as an informative prognostic indicator for colorectal cancer. *Clin. Cancer Res.* **2004**, *10*, 5572–5579. [CrossRef] [PubMed]
76. Chen, H.; Ye, Y.; Yang, Y.; Zhong, M.; Gu, L.; Han, Z.; Qiu, J.; Liu, Z.; Qiu, X.; Zhuang, G. TIPE-mediated up-regulation of MMP-9 promotes colorectal cancer invasion and metastasis through MKK-3/p38/NF-κB pro-oncogenic signaling pathway. *Signal Transduct. Target. Ther.* **2020**, *5*, 163. [CrossRef] [PubMed]
77. Garg, P.; Jeppsson, S.; Dalmasso, G.; Ghaleb, A.M.; McConnell, B.B.; Yang, V.W.; Gewirtz, A.T.; Merlin, D.; Sitaraman, S.V. Notch1 regulates the effects of matrix metalloproteinase-9 on colitis-associated cancer in mice. *Gastroenterology* **2011**, *141*, 1381–1392. [CrossRef]
78. Garg, P.; Sarma, D.; Jeppsson, S.; Patel, N.R.; Gewirtz, A.T.; Merlin, D.; Sitaraman, S.V. Matrix metalloproteinase-9 functions as a tumor suppressor in colitis-associated cancer. *Cancer Res.* **2010**, *70*, 792–801. [CrossRef]
79. Walter, L.; Canup, B.; Pujada, A.; Bui, T.A.; Arbasi, B.; Laroui, H.; Merlin, D.; Garg, P. Matrix metalloproteinase 9 (MMP9) limits reactive oxygen species (ROS) accumulation and DNA damage in colitis-associated cancer. *Cell Death Dis.* **2020**, *11*, 767. [CrossRef] [PubMed]
80. Wei, Z.; Cao, S.; Liu, S.; Yao, Z.; Sun, T.; Li, Y.; Li, J.; Zhang, D.; Zhou, Y. Could gut microbiota serve as prognostic biomarker associated with colorectal cancer patients' survival? A pilot study on relevant mechanism. *Oncotarget* **2016**, *7*, 46158–46172. [CrossRef]
81. Sipos, F.; Germann, T.M.; Wichmann, B.; Galamb, O.; Spisák, S.; Krenács, T.; Tulassay, Z.; Molnár, B.; Műzes, G. MMP3 and CXCL1 are potent stromal protein markers of dysplasia-carcinoma transition in sporadic colorectal cancer. *Eur. J. Cancer Prev.* **2014**, *23*, 336–343. [CrossRef]
82. Işlekel, H.; Oktay, G.; Terzi, C.; Canda, A.E.; Füzün, M.; Küpelioğlu, A. Matrix metalloproteinase-9,-3 and tissue inhibitor of matrix metalloproteinase-1 in colorectal cancer: Relationship to clinicopathological variables. *Cell Biochem. Funct.* **2007**, *25*, 433–441. [CrossRef] [PubMed]
83. Jin, X.; Yagi, M.; Akiyama, N.; Hirosaki, T.; Higashi, S.; Lin, C.Y.; Dickson, R.B.; Kitamura, H.; Miyazaki, K. Matriptase activates stromelysin (MMP-3) and promotes tumor growth and angiogenesis. *Cancer Sci.* **2006**, *97*, 1327–1334. [CrossRef] [PubMed]
84. Inuzuka, K.; Ogata, Y.; Nagase, H.; Shirouzu, K. Significance of coexpression of urokinase-type plasminogen activator, and matrix metalloproteinase 3 (stromelysin) and 9 (gelatinase B) in colorectal carcinoma. *J. Surg. Res.* **2000**, *93*, 211–218. [CrossRef] [PubMed]
85. Batra, J.; Robinson, J.; Soares, A.S.; Fields, A.P.; Radisky, D.C.; Radisky, E.S. Matrix metalloproteinase-10 (MMP-10) interaction with tissue inhibitors of metalloproteinases TIMP-1 and TIMP-2: Binding studies and crystal structure. *J. Biol. Chem.* **2012**, *287*, 15935–15946. [CrossRef]
86. Surlin, V.; Ioana, M.; Pleşea, I.E. Genetic patterns of metalloproteinases and their tissular inhibitors—Clinicopathologic and prognostic significance in colorectal cancer. *Rom. J. Morphol. Embryol.* **2011**, *52*, 231–236.
87. Asadzadeh Aghdaei, H.; Pezeshkian, Z.; Abdollahpour-Alitappeh, M.; Nazemalhosseini Mojarad, E.; Zali, M.R. The Role of Angiogenesis in Colorectal Polyps and Cancer, a Review. *Med. Lab. J.* **2018**, *12*, 1–6. [CrossRef]
88. Ii, M.; Yamamoto, H.; Adachi, Y.; Maruyama, Y.; Shinomura, Y. Role of matrix metalloproteinase-7 (matrilysin) in human cancer invasion, apoptosis, growth, and angiogenesis. *Exp. Biol. Med.* **2006**, *231*, 20–27. [CrossRef]
89. Cheng, K.; Xie, G.; Raufman, J.P. Matrix metalloproteinase-7-catalyzed release of HB-EGF mediates deoxycholyltaurine-induced proliferation of a human colon cancer cell line. *Biochem. Pharmacol.* **2007**, *73*, 1001–1012. [CrossRef]
90. Xie, G.; Cheng, K.; Shant, J.; Raufman, J.P. Acetylcholine-induced activation of M3 muscarinic receptors stimulates robust matrix metalloproteinase gene expression in human colon cancer cells. *Am. J. Physiol. Gastrointest. Liver Physiol.* **2009**, *296*, G755–G763. [CrossRef]
91. Decock, J.; Thirkettle, S.; Wagstaff, L.; Edwards, D.R. Matrix metalloproteinases: Protective roles in cancer. *J. Cell Mol. Med.* **2011**, *15*, 1254–1265. [CrossRef]
92. Asano, T.; Tada, M.; Cheng, S.; Takemoto, N.; Kuramae, T.; Abe, M.; Takahashi, O.; Miyamoto, M.; Hamada, J.; Moriuchi, T.; et al. Prognostic values of matrix metalloproteinase family expression in human colorectal carcinoma. *J. Surg. Res.* **2008**, *146*, 32–42. [CrossRef]
93. Yang, W.; Arii, S.; Gorrin-Rivas, M.J.; Mori, A.; Onodera, H.; Imamura, M. Human macrophage metalloelastase gene expression in colorectal carcinoma and its clinicopathologic significance. *Cancer* **2001**, *91*, 1277–1283. [CrossRef]

94. Shi, H.; Xu, J.M.; Hu, N.Z.; Wang, X.L.; Mei, Q.; Song, Y.L. Transfection of mouse macrophage metalloelastase gene into murine CT-26 colon cancer cells suppresses orthotopic tumor growth, angiogenesis and vascular endothelial growth factor expression. *Cancer Lett.* **2006**, *233*, 139–150. [CrossRef]
95. Xu, Z.; Shi, H.; Li, Q.; Mei, Q.; Bao, J.; Shen, Y.; Xu, J. Mouse macrophage metalloelastase generates angiostatin from plasminogen and suppresses tumor angiogenesis in murine colon cancer. *Oncol. Rep.* **2008**, *20*, 81–88. [CrossRef]
96. Beurden, P.; Von den Hoff, J. Zymographic techniques for the analysis of matrix metalloproteinases and their inhibitors. *BioTechniques* **2005**, *38*, 73–83. [CrossRef]
97. Wu, T.; Li, Y.; Liu, X.; Lu, J.; He, X.; Wang, Q.; Li, J.; Du, X. Identification of high-risk stage II and stage III colorectal cancer by analysis of MMP-21 expression. *J. Surg. Oncol.* **2011**, *104*, 787–791. [CrossRef]
98. Huang, Y.; Li, W.; Chu, D.; Zheng, J.; Ji, G.; Li, M.; Zhang, H.; Wang, W.; Du, J.; Li, J. Overexpression of matrix metalloproteinase-21 is associated with poor overall survival of patients with colorectal cancer. *J. Gastrointest. Surg.* **2011**, *15*, 1188–1194. [CrossRef]
99. Zhang, J.; Pan, Q.; Yan, W.; Wang, Y.; He, X.; Zhao, Z. Overexpression of MMP21 and MMP28 is associated with gastric cancer progression and poor prognosis. *Oncol. Lett.* **2018**, *15*, 7776–7782. [CrossRef]
100. Pahwa, S.; Stawikowski, M.J.; Fields, G.B. Monitoring and Inhibiting MT1-MMP during Cancer Initiation and Progression. *Cancers* **2014**, *6*, 416–435. [CrossRef]
101. Devy, L.; Huang, L.; Naa, L.; Yanamandra, N.; Pieters, H.; Frans, N.; Chang, E.; Tao, Q.; Vanhove, M.; Lejeune, A.; et al. Selective Inhibition of Matrix Metalloproteinase-14 Blocks Tumor Growth, Invasion, and Angiogenesis. *Cancer Res.* **2009**, *69*, 1517–1526. [CrossRef]
102. Duan, F.; Peng, Z.; Yin, J.; Yang, Z.; Shang, J. Expression of MMP-14 and prognosis in digestive system carcinoma: A meta-analysis and databases validation. *J. Cancer* **2020**, *11*, 1141–1150. [CrossRef]
103. Yang, B.; Gao, J.; Rao, Z.; Shen, Q. Clinicopathological and prognostic significance of α5β1-integrin and MMP-14 expressions in colorectal cancer. *Neoplasma* **2013**, *60*, 254–261. [CrossRef] [PubMed]
104. Cui, G.; Cai, F.; Ding, Z.; Gao, L. MMP14 predicts a poor prognosis in patients with colorectal cancer. *Hum. Pathol.* **2019**, *83*, 36–42. [CrossRef] [PubMed]
105. Claesson-Welsh, L. How the matrix metalloproteinase MMP14 contributes to the progression of colorectal cancer. *J. Clin. Investig.* **2020**, *130*, 1093–1095. [CrossRef] [PubMed]
106. Decock, J.; Paridaens, R.; Ye, S. Genetic polymorphisms of matrix metalloproteinases in lung, breast and colorectal cancer. *Clin. Genet.* **2008**, *73*, 197–211. [CrossRef] [PubMed]
107. Langers, A.M.; Verspaget, H.W.; Hommes, D.W.; Sier, C.F. Single-nucleotide polymorphisms of matrix metalloproteinases and their inhibitors in gastrointestinal cancer. *World J. Gastrointest. Oncol.* **2011**, *3*, 79–98. [CrossRef] [PubMed]
108. Hinoda, Y.; Okayama, N.; Takano, N.; Fujimura, K.; Suehiro, Y.; Hamanaka, Y.; Hazama, S.; Kitamura, Y.; Kamatani, N.; Oka, M. Association of functional polymorphisms of matrix metalloproteinase (MMP)-1 and MMP-3 genes with colorectal cancer. *Int. J. Cancer* **2002**, *102*, 526–529. [CrossRef]
109. Kouhkan, F.; Motovali-Bashi, M.; Hojati, Z. The influence of interstitial collagenas-1 genotype polymorphism on colorectal cancer risk in Iranian population. *Cancer Investig.* **2008**, *26*, 836–842. [CrossRef]
110. Langers, A.M.J.; Sier, C.F.M.; Hawinkels, L.J.A.C.; Kubben, F.J.G.M.; van Duijn, W.; van der Reijden, J.J.; Lamers, C.B.H.W.; Hommes, D.W.; Verspaget, H.W. MMP-2 geno-phenotype is prognostic for colorectal cancer survival, whereas MMP-9 is not. *Br. J. Cancer* **2008**, *98*, 1820–1823. [CrossRef]
111. Ting, W.-C.; Chen, L.-M.; Pao, J.-B.; Yang, Y.-P.; You, B.-J.; Chang, T.-Y.; Lan, Y.-H.; Lee, H.-Z.; Bao, B.-Y. Genetic Polymorphisms of Matrix Metalloproteinases and Clinical Outcomes in Colorectal Cancer Patients. *Int. J. Med. Sci.* **2013**, *10*, 1022–1027. [CrossRef]
112. Dziki, L.; Przybyłowska, K.; Majsterek, I.; Trzciński, R.; Mik, M.; Sygut, A. A/G Polymorphism of the MMP-7 Gene Promoter Region in Colorectal Cancer. *Pol. Przegl. Chir.* **2011**, *83*, 622–626. [CrossRef]
113. Fang, W.-L.; Liang, W.; He, H.; Zhu, Y.; Li, S.-L.; Gao, L.-B.; Zhang, L. Association of Matrix Metalloproteinases 1, 7, and 9 Gene Polymorphisms with Genetic Susceptibility to Colorectal Carcinoma in a Han Chinese Population. *DNA Cell Biol.* **2010**, *29*, 657–661. [CrossRef]
114. Park, K.S.; Kim, S.J.; Kim, K.H.; Kim, J.C. Clinical characteristics of TIMP2, MMP2, and MMP9 gene polymorphisms in colorectal cancer. *J. Gastroenterol. Hepatol.* **2011**, *26*, 391–397. [CrossRef]
115. Van Nguyen, S.; Skarstedt, M.; LÖFgren, S.; Zar, N.; Andersson, R.E.; Lindh, M.; Matussek, A.; Dimberg, J.A.N. Gene Polymorphism of Matrix Metalloproteinase-12 and -13 and Association with Colorectal Cancer in Swedish Patients. *Anticancer Res.* **2013**, *33*, 3247–3250.
116. Tai, J.; Sun, D.; Wang, X.; Kang, Z. Matrix metalloproteinase-8 rs11225395 polymorphism correlates with colorectal cancer risk and survival in a Chinese Han population: A case-control study. *Aging* **2020**, *12*, 19618–19627. [CrossRef]
117. Vandenbroucke, R.E.; Libert, C. Is there new hope for therapeutic matrix metalloproteinase inhibition? *Nat. Rev. Drug Discov.* **2014**, *13*, 904–927. [CrossRef]
118. Raeeszadeh-Sarmazdeh, M.; Do, L.D.; Hritz, B.G. Metalloproteinases and Their Inhibitors: Potential for the Development of New Therapeutics. *Cells* **2020**, *9*, 1313. [CrossRef]
119. Caton, J.G. Evaluation of Periostat for patient management. *Compend. Contin. Educ. Dent.* **1999**, *20*, 451, 458–460.

120. Bissett, D.; O'Byrne, K.J.; von Pawel, J.; Gatzemeier, U.; Price, A.; Nicolson, M.; Mercier, R.; Mazabel, E.; Penning, C.; Zhang, M.H.; et al. Phase III study of matrix metalloproteinase inhibitor prinomastat in non-small-cell lung cancer. *J. Clin. Oncol.* **2005**, *23*, 842–849. [CrossRef]
121. Scatena, R. Prinomastat, a hydroxamate-based matrix metalloproteinase inhibitor. A novel pharmacological approach for tissue remodelling-related diseases. *Expert Opin. Investig. Drugs* **2000**, *9*, 2159–2165. [CrossRef]
122. Hande, K.R.; Collier, M.; Paradiso, L.; Stuart-Smith, J.; Dixon, M.; Clendeninn, N.; Yeun, G.; Alberti, D.; Binger, K.; Wilding, G. Phase I and pharmacokinetic study of prinomastat, a matrix metalloprotease inhibitor. *Clin. Cancer Res.* **2004**, *10*, 909–915. [CrossRef] [PubMed]
123. Yang, J.-S.; Lin, C.-W.; Su, S.-C.; Yang, S.-F. Pharmacodynamic considerations in the use of matrix metalloproteinase inhibitors in cancer treatment. *Expert Opin. Drug Metab. Toxicol.* **2015**, *12*, 191–200. [CrossRef] [PubMed]
124. Shah, M.A.; Starodub, A.; Sharma, S.; Berlin, J.; Patel, M.; Wainberg, Z.A.; Chaves, J.; Gordon, M.; Windsor, K.; Brachmann, C.B.; et al. Andecaliximab/GS-5745 Alone and Combined with mFOLFOX6 in Advanced Gastric and Gastroesophageal Junction Adenocarcinoma: Results from a Phase I Study. *Clin. Cancer Res.* **2018**, *24*, 3829–3837. [CrossRef] [PubMed]
125. Sandborn, W.J.; Bhandari, B.R.; Randall, C.; Younes, Z.H.; Romanczyk, T.; Xin, Y.; Wendt, E.; Chai, H.; McKevitt, M.; Zhao, S.; et al. Andecaliximab [Anti-matrix Metalloproteinase-9] Induction Therapy for Ulcerative Colitis: A Randomised, Double-Blind, Placebo-Controlled, Phase 2/3 Study in Patients With Moderate to Severe Disease. *J. Crohn's Colitis* **2018**, *12*, 1021–1029. [CrossRef]
126. Murphy, G. Tissue inhibitors of metalloproteinases. *Genome Biol.* **2011**, *12*, 233. [CrossRef]
127. Li, K.; Tay, F.R.; Yiu, C.K.Y. The past, present and future perspectives of matrix metalloproteinase inhibitors. *Pharmacol. Ther.* **2020**, *207*, 107465. [CrossRef]
128. Melendez-Zajgla, J.; Del Pozo, L.; Ceballos, G.; Maldonado, V. Tissue Inhibitor of Metalloproteinases-4. The road less traveled. *Mol. Cancer* **2008**, *7*, 85. [CrossRef]
129. Hayden, D.M.; Forsyth, C.; Keshavarzian, A. The role of matrix metalloproteinases in intestinal epithelial wound healing during normal and inflammatory states. *J. Surg. Res.* **2011**, *168*, 315–324. [CrossRef]
130. Song, G.; Xu, S.; Zhang, H.; Wang, Y.; Xiao, C.; Jiang, T.; Wu, L.; Zhang, T.; Sun, X.; Zhong, L.; et al. TIMP1 is a prognostic marker for the progression and metastasis of colon cancer through FAK-PI3K/AKT and MAPK pathway. *J. Exp. Clin. Cancer Res.* **2016**, *35*, 148. [CrossRef]
131. Noël, A.; Jost, M.; Maquoi, E. Matrix metalloproteinases at cancer tumor-host interface. *Semin. Cell Dev. Biol.* **2008**, *19*, 52–60. [CrossRef]
132. Lu, X.; Duan, L.; Xie, H.; Lu, X.; Lu, D.; Lu, D.; Jiang, N.; Chen, Y. Evaluation of MMP-9 and MMP-2 and their suppressor TIMP-1 and TIMP-2 in adenocarcinoma of esophagogastric junction. *OncoTargets Ther.* **2016**, *9*, 4343–4349. [CrossRef]
133. Groblewska, M.; Mroczko, B.; Gryko, M.; Pryczynicz, A.; Guzińska-Ustymowicz, K.; Kędra, B.; Kemona, A.; Szmitkowski, M. Serum levels and tissue expression of matrix metalloproteinase 2 (MMP-2) and tissue inhibitor of metalloproteinases 2 (TIMP-2) in colorectal cancer patients. *Tumor Biol.* **2014**, *35*, 3793–3802. [CrossRef]
134. Wang, W.; Li, D.; Xiang, L.; Lv, M.; Tao, L.; Ni, T.; Deng, J.; Gu, X.; Masatara, S.; Liu, Y.; et al. TIMP-2 inhibits metastasis and predicts prognosis of colorectal cancer via regulating MMP-9. *Cell Adhes. Migr.* **2019**, *13*, 273–284. [CrossRef]
135. Huang, H.-L.; Liu, Y.-M.; Sung, T.-Y.; Huang, T.-C.; Cheng, Y.-W.; Liou, J.-P.; Pan, S.-L. TIMP3 expression associates with prognosis in colorectal cancer and its novel arylsulfonamide inducer, MPT0B390, inhibits tumor growth, metastasis and angiogenesis. *Theranostics* **2019**, *9*, 6676–6689. [CrossRef]
136. Lin, H.; Zhang, Y.; Wang, H.; Xu, D.; Meng, X.; Shao, Y.; Lin, C.; Ye, Y.; Qian, H.; Wang, S. Tissue inhibitor of metalloproteinases-3 transfer suppresses malignant behaviors of colorectal cancer cells. *Cancer Gene Ther.* **2012**, *19*, 845–851. [CrossRef]
137. Soheilifar, M.H.; Grusch, M.; Keshmiri Neghab, H.; Amini, R.; Maadi, H.; Saidijam, M.; Wang, Z. Angioregulatory microRNAs in Colorectal Cancer. *Cancers* **2019**, *12*, 71. [CrossRef]
138. Wu, J.; Wu, G.; Lv, L.; Ren, Y.; Zhang, X.; Xue, Y.; Li, G.; Lu, X.; Sun, Z.; Tang, K. MicroRNA-34a inhibits migration and invasion of colon cancer cells via targeting to Fra-1. *Carcinogenesis* **2012**, *33*, 519–528. [CrossRef]
139. Abba, M.; Patil, N.; Allgayer, H. MicroRNAs in the Regulation of MMPs and Metastasis. *Cancers* **2014**, *6*, 625–645. [CrossRef]
140. Shen, K.; Liang, Q.; Xu, K.; Cui, D.; Jiang, L.; Yin, P.; Lu, Y.; Li, Q.; Liu, J. MiR-139 inhibits invasion and metastasis of colorectal cancer by targeting the type I insulin-like growth factor receptor. *Biochem. Pharmacol.* **2012**, *84*, 320–330. [CrossRef]
141. Tang, W.; Zhu, Y.; Gao, J.; Fu, J.; Liu, C.; Liu, Y.; Song, C.; Zhu, S.; Leng, Y.; Wang, G.; et al. MicroRNA-29a promotes colorectal cancer metastasis by regulating matrix metalloproteinase 2 and E-cadherin via KLF4. *Br. J. Cancer* **2014**, *110*, 450–458. [CrossRef]
142. Leng, Y.; Chen, Z.; Ding, H.; Zhao, X.; Qin, L.; Pan, Y. Overexpression of microRNA-29b inhibits epithelial-mesenchymal transition and angiogenesis of colorectal cancer through the ETV4/ERK/EGFR axis. *Cancer Cell Int.* **2021**, *21*, 17. [CrossRef] [PubMed]
143. Yu, B.; Liu, X.; Chang, H. MicroRNA-143 inhibits colorectal cancer cell proliferation by targeting MMP7. *Minerva Med.* **2017**, *108*, 13–19. [CrossRef] [PubMed]
144. Schwarzmueller, L.; Bril, O.; Vermeulen, L.; Léveillé, N. Emerging Role and Therapeutic Potential of lncRNAs in Colorectal Cancer. *Cancers* **2020**, *12*, 3843. [CrossRef] [PubMed]
145. Tian, L.; Zhao, Z.F.; Xie, L.; Zhu, J.P. Taurine up-regulated 1 accelerates tumorigenesis of colon cancer by regulating miR-26a-5p/MMP14/p38 MAPK/Hsp27 axis in vitro and in vivo. *Life Sci.* **2019**, *239*, 117035. [CrossRef]
146. Sun, N.; Zhang, G.; Liu, Y. Long non-coding RNA XIST sponges miR-34a to promotes colon cancer progression via Wnt/β-catenin signaling pathway. *Gene* **2018**, *665*, 141–148. [CrossRef]

147. Lv, H.; Zhou, D.; Liu, G. LncRNA LINC00963 promotes colorectal cancer cell proliferation and metastasis by regulating miR–1281 and TRIM65. *Mol. Med. Rep.* **2021**, *24*, 781. [CrossRef]
148. Duan, Y.; Fang, Z.; Shi, Z.; Zhang, L. Knockdown of lncRNA CCEPR suppresses colorectal cancer progression. *Exp. Ther. Med.* **2019**, *18*, 3534–3542. [CrossRef]
149. Pan, Y.; Zhu, L.; Pu, J.; Wang, W.; Qian, W. lncRNA PCA3 plays a key role in colon cancer occurrence and development. *Arch. Med. Sci.* **2020**. [CrossRef]

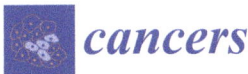

Article

Tackling Tumour Cell Heterogeneity at the Super-Resolution Level in Human Colorectal Cancer Tissue

Fabian Lang [1,†], María F. Contreras-Gerenas [2,3,†], Márton Gelléri [3], Jan Neumann [3], Ole Kröger [4], Filip Sadlo [4], Krzysztof Berniak [5], Alexander Marx [6], Christoph Cremer [3,4,7,‡], Hans-Achim Wagenknecht [1,‡] and Heike Allgayer [2,*,‡]

1. Institute of Organic Chemistry, Karlsruhe Institute of Technology (KIT), Fritz-Haber-Weg 6, Campus Süd, 76131 Karlsruhe, Germany; fabian.lang2@kit.edu (F.L.); hans-achim.wagenknecht@kit.edu (H.-A.W.)
2. Department of Experimental Surgery—Cancer Metastasis, Mannheim Medical Faculty, Ruprecht-Karls University of Heidelberg, Ludolf-Krehl-Straße 13-17, 68167 Mannheim, Germany; mfcontrerasg@gmail.com
3. Institute of Molecular Biology (IMB), Ackermannweg 4, 55128 Mainz, Germany; m.gelleri@imb-mainz.de (M.G.); jan.neumann@mail.de (J.N.); c.cremer@imb-mainz.de (C.C.)
4. Interdisciplinary Centre for Scientific Computing (IWR), University Heidelberg, Mathematikon B, Im Neuenheimer Feld 205, 69120 Heidelberg, Germany; o.kroeger@opensourc.es (O.K.); sadlo@uni-heidelberg.de (F.S.)
5. Department of Cell Biophysics, Faculty of Biochemistry, Biophysics and Biotechnology, Jagiellonian University, Gronostajowa 7 Street, 30-387 Krakow, Poland; kberniak@gmail.com
6. Institute of Pathology, Mannheim Medical Faculty, Ruprecht-Karls University of Heidelberg, Theodor-Kutzer-Ufer 1, 68167 Mannheim, Germany; Alexander.Marx@umm.de
7. Institute of Pharmacy & Molecular Biotechnology, Ruprecht-Karls University of Heidelberg, Im Neuenheimer Feld 364, 69120 Heidelberg, Germany
* Correspondence: heike.allgayer@medma.uni-heidelberg.de; Tel.: +49-(0)621-383-71630 / -1406 / -71635; Fax: +49-(0)621-383-71631
† These authors contributed equally to this work.
‡ These authors contributed equally to this work.

Citation: Lang, F.; Contreras-Gerenas, M.F.; Gelléri, M.; Neumann, J.; Kröger, O.; Sadlo, F.; Berniak, K.; Marx, A.; Cremer, C.; Wagenknecht, H.-A.; et al. Tackling Tumour Cell Heterogeneity at the Super-Resolution Level in Human Colorectal Cancer Tissue. *Cancers* 2021, 13, 3692. https://doi.org/10.3390/cancers13153692

Academic Editor: Yoshinobu Hirose

Received: 7 July 2021
Accepted: 20 July 2021
Published: 22 July 2021

Publisher's Note: MDPI stays neutral with regard to jurisdictional claims in published maps and institutional affiliations.

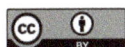

Copyright: © 2021 by the authors. Licensee MDPI, Basel, Switzerland. This article is an open access article distributed under the terms and conditions of the Creative Commons Attribution (CC BY) license (https://creativecommons.org/licenses/by/4.0/).

Simple Summary: Tumour cell heterogeneity is the most fundamental problem in cancer diagnosis and therapy. Micro-diagnostic technologies able to differentiate the heterogeneous molecular, especially metastatic, potential of single cells or cell clones already within early primary tumours of carcinoma patients would be of utmost importance. Single molecule localisation microscopy (SMLM) has recently allowed the imaging of subcellular features at the nanoscale. However, the technology has mostly been limited to cultured cell lines only. We introduce a first-in-field approach for quantitative SMLM-analysis of chromatin nanostructure in individual cells in resected, routine-pathology colorectal carcinoma patient tissue sections, illustrating, as a first example, changes in nuclear chromatin nanostructure and microRNA intracellular distribution within carcinoma cells as opposed to normal cells, chromatin accessibility and microRNAs having been shown to be critical in gene regulation and metastasis. We believe this technology to have an enormous potential for future differential diagnosis between individual cells in the tissue context.

Abstract: Tumour cell heterogeneity, and its early individual diagnosis, is one of the most fundamental problems in cancer diagnosis and therapy. Single molecule localisation microscopy (SMLM) resolves subcellular features but has been limited to cultured cell lines only. Since nuclear chromatin architecture and microRNAs are critical in metastasis, we introduce a first-in-field approach for quantitative SMLM-analysis of chromatin nanostructure in individual cells in resected, routine-pathology colorectal carcinoma (CRC) patient tissue sections. Chromatin density profiles proved to differ for cells in normal and carcinoma colorectal tissues. In tumour sections, nuclear size and chromatin compaction percentages were significantly different in carcinoma versus normal epithelial and other cells of colorectal tissue. SMLM analysis in nuclei from normal colorectal tissue revealed abrupt changes in chromatin density profiles at the nanoscale, features not detected by conventional widefield microscopy. SMLM for microRNAs relevant for metastasis was achieved in colorectal cancer tissue at the nuclear level. Super-resolution microscopy with quantitative image evaluation algorithms provide powerful tools to analyse chromatin nanostructure and microRNAs of individual cells from normal and tumour tissue at the nanoscale. Our new perspectives improve the differential diagnosis of normal and (metastatically relevant) tumour cells at the single-cell level within the heterogeneity of primary tumours of patients.

Keywords: chromatin density; nanoscale; tumour cell heterogeneity; microRNAs; metastasis; super-resolution microscopy

1. Introduction

One of the most challenging problems in oncology, diagnosis and (personalised) tumour therapy still is the huge heterogeneity of carcinoma cells within tumours of patients with malignant diseases. It is estimated that each patient primary tumour comprises millions of different tumour cells/tumour cell clones that differ in their molecular and functional characteristics. Within this huge heterogeneity of cells in tumours, some cancer cells show rather low, some others high potential to promote cancer progression, to give rise to metastasis, which is still the cause of about 90% of cancer-related deaths [1], or to respond, or become resistant, to classical or novel personalised therapeutic strategies [2–4]. This has been shown recently, for example, in our own whole genome sequencing work in which it became apparent that primary tumours and their corresponding metastases originate from a common ancestor clone each, but that metastases still develop further changes already at the genome level as compared to their corresponding primaries, an issue which might impact tremendously therapy response or resistance [5]. Thus, recent years of research, especially in the fields of cancer stem cells, metastasis-initiating cells, single cell analysis [5–8], and others have illustrated how important it will be for individualised diagnosis and therapy to be able to differentiate cells with different molecular, metastatic, and therapeutic potential already at the stage of the primary tumour. Especially, to improve patient prognosis fundamentally and prospectively, it will be highly important to establish micro-diagnostic tools able to detect, ideally, single tumour cell clones that harbour a high risk to lead to later disease recurrence and metastasis, or particular patterns of therapy resistance within the primary tumour, before these cells give rise to macroscopic relapse. This would enable a new generation of targeted therapy design which is capable of preventing crucial tumour cell clones from spreading, growing, and metastasizing.

Nuclear architecture is crucial for determining the levels of gene activation. However, the extent and means by which chromatin structure alters gene expression are not fully understood yet. Early detection of replication "factories" allowed for a simplified nuclear model comprising heterochromatin (dense, inactive chromatin) and euchromatin (loose, transcription factor-enriched chromatin) [9]. Recently, a more detailed model has been proposed which predicts that the nuclear genome is partitioned into two co-aligned regions, an active nuclear compartment with low DNA density and an inactive nuclear compartment with high DNA density. There is also an interchromatin compartment in this model, which consists of channel-like regions mostly with a very low DNA density [10]. Areas of low density have been proposed to harbour loci of active gene transcription [10,11]. Moreover, studies have already suggested that reprogramming the chromatin status and increasing chromatin accessibility by different molecular means in cancer cells is associated with promoting cancer metastasis [12,13]. Moreover, the use of drugs that help recover normal nuclear architecture features has been linked with the recovery of normal cell phenotype [14].

Thus, diagnostic tools that involve high-resolution options within the chromatin nanostructure might be highly interesting to identify cells critical for progression, metastasis, or therapy response, if these tools could be applied directly to histopathological whole sections already of patient primary tumours and further tissues. This would be critical also since structural differences have been observed between cells (or cell lines) in monolayer cultures and the same cells in tissues [15]. However, up to now, attempts in this context to achieve subcellular imaging of the DNA distribution in tumour cells at the nanoscale with SMLM have been rare. In our own preliminary studies, we started to study chromatin distribution by confocal and SMLM [16], whereby the percentage of compact chromatin calculated from confocal microscopy images proved to differ for cells with different functionality. SMLM data in nuclei from normal colorectal tissue revealed abrupt changes in chromatin density profiles at the nanoscale, features not detected by conventional widefield microscopy. These observations highlight the importance of advancing super-resolution techniques like SMLM as individual diagnosis tools of single cell heterogeneity [17], as well as the enormous potential that this can have for answering biological/medical questions such as diagnosing individual cells within an individual patient with different metastatic or therapy response potential.

In the diagnosis of metastatically capable cells, microRNAs (miRs) could play a highly interesting role as well since many of these have been shown, by us and others, to be critical players in the metastatic process [18–22]. MiRs have an average length of 22 nucleotides and belong to the class of small non-coding RNAs. They bind with their seed sequence to the 3' untranslated region (UTR) of their target and then degrade, or block translation of, the target mRNA [23]. More recently, additional nuclear functions of miRs have been elucidated, which include post-transcriptional and transcriptional gene silencing, and the transcriptional activation of genes [24], this potentially links miR-intracellular diagnostics to chromatin diagnostics. Specific aberrant miRNA expression profiles have been identified in different cancer types including colorectal cancer, especially as pro-or antagonists of metastasis at several instances. Towards this end, miR are not only direct regulators of mRNAs for oncogenes, tumour suppressor genes, or metastatically relevant genes, but also are able to, for example, prime metastatic niches systemically via being spread within exosomes by primary cancer cells [25–28]. Therefore, miRNA imaging could play an important role in cancer diagnostics but is a challenge for imaging methods due to the short length and homologues. Several miRNA imaging methods have been developed mainly based on in situ hybridisation (ISH) [29], nucleic acid amplification [30], northern blotting [31], or microarray [32]. These methods have been improved with regard to sensitivity, specificity, and imaging over the past years [33]. Nevertheless, detection of miRNAs with microscopic methods was restricted due to the conventional limit of resolution in optical microscopy. With the help of SMLM, we recently overcame this limitation and showed the detection of single miRNA molecules at the superresolution level in single cells of cultured colorectal cancer cell lines [34]. However, successfully establishing this technology for single cell, single molecule subcellular diagnosis in specific resected tissues of patients still remains undone.

Herein, we present the first successful combination of Fluorescence in situ Hybridisation (FISH) with SMLM based chromatin nanotexture and microRNA analysis in routine-pathology, paraffin-embedded colorectal cancer tissue sections, to characterise cellular heterogeneity in the primary tumour tissue of colorectal cancer patients. We believe that this technology could be interesting for the future to identify tumour cell clones of, for example, higher individual metastatic potential or therapy resistance, given their chromatin texture and intracellular distribution and number of metastatically relevant microRNA molecules.

2. Material and Methods

2.1. Ethics Approval and Colorectal Tissue Samples

Formalin-fixed, paraffin embedded (FFPE) tissue blocks were generously provided by Prof. Alexander Marx (Pathologisches Institut, UMM/Mannheim Medical Faculty of Heidelberg University, Germany). Anonymous colorectal carcinoma and paired corresponding normal (colorectal) tissue blocks were available from the archival material of the same patients. Approval by the institutional ethics board (Ethics board II at UMM, approval no. 2017-806R-MA) was granted to AM, waiving the need for informed consent for this retrospective and fully anonymised analysis of archival pathological samples.

FFPE blocks were cut using a Leica RM2255 fully automated rotary microtome. The first few sections were discharged and 10 µm thick sections were collected on top of previously cleaned coverslips (No. 1.5H, Paul Marienfeld, Lauda-Könishofen, Germany) from a 37 °C water bath. Coverslips were transferred to a 65 °C oven and left there for a minimum of 30 min. Dried slices were kept at 4 °C for not more than a month before further processing (FISH, confocal microscopy or SMLM).

2.2. Fluorescence In Situ Hybridisation (FISH) on Colorectal Tissue Sections

Tissue sections on coverslips were accommodated in a custom-made Teflon coverslip holder and placed for 5-min steps in the following solutions: Roticlear, 1:1 Roticlear: 100% EtOH, ethanol series (100%, 95%, 70%, 50%, 25%), briefly in DI water and PBS. For the antigen retrieval step, 2 mL of a 1 µg/mL of proteinase K (NEB, Ipswich, MA, USA) in 50 mM Tris buffer was added per tissue section in a 6-well plate (15 min, RT, gentle stirring). Two washes followed, one with 0.1% Tween-20/PBS and the second one with PBS. Samples were permeabilised in a 0.5% Triton-X 100/PBS solution (1 h, RT, gentle stirring), followed by two PBS washes and immediate dehydration in ethanol solution steps of increasing concentration (25%, 50%, 70%, 95%, 100%), followed by air drying (5 min each). A boundary was put around the tissue samples using Picondent Twinsil (Picodent, Wipperfürth, Germany). Subsequent volumes were added to an extent that the entire sample was covered (maximum 100 µL). Hybridisation solution (50% *v/v* formamide, 0.75 M NaCl, 75 mM Na-Citrate, 50 mg/mL heparin, 0.5% *v/v* Tween-20) was added to each sample (15 min, 37 °C). Prior to hybridisation, miR probes were denatured at 80 °C for 5 min. The probes were diluted in hybridisation buffer to 200 nM and added to the samples. Hybridisation was performed overnight at 37 °C. Stringent washes were performed twice in 0.2× SSC (10 min each, RT, gentle stirring), for 5 min each at RT under gentle stirring.

2.3. DNA Probe Synthesis and Characterisation

DNA sequences complementary to the four metastatically relevant miRNAs miR-135b, miR-210, miR-21 and miR-31 studied in this work, as well as a positive control (sequence against U6 snRNA) and negative control (scrambled sequence) were synthesised. The most central thymidine was exchanged for a 2'-O-propargyl-uridine (cU) (building block is commercially available from GlenResearch) to enable the post-synthetic modification with fluorophores via copper-catalysed azide-alkyne cycloaddition (CuAAC). The solid-phase phosphoramidite synthesis was performed with an H6 DNA/RNA synthesizer (K&A Laborgeräte, Schaafheim, Germany), using standard protocols. For the incorporation of the cU-phosphoramidite, the reaction time of the coupling step was increased to 4 min. After successful synthesis and cleavage from the solid phase with 24% ammonia solution overnight at 60 °C, the synthesised DNA probes were modified in two separate sets with Cy5-azide and AF488-azide [35]. Cy5 is a well-established fluorophore in confocal microscopy and was chosen for the proof of concept. AF488 has a better blinking behaviour than Cy5 which makes it suitable for superresolution microscopy. After modification, the oligonucleotides were purified via reversed-phase HPLC with a Thermo Fisher UltiMate 3000 (Thermo Fisher Scientific Inc., Waltham, MA, USA) (0–40% acetonitrile in 50 mM ammonium acetate buffer). Spectroscopic measurements were performed with solutions of 2.5 µM FISH-probe, 2.5 µM corresponding RNA, 50 mM Na-P_i buffer, and 250 mM NaCl in water at pH 7. Absorption spectra were measured with a *Varian Cary 100* UV/Vis-spectrometer, and fluorescence spectra were measured with a *HORIBA FluoroMax 4* spectrofluorometer. The used excitation wavelengths were λ_{exc} = 647 nm for Cy5 probes and λ_{exc} = 488 nm for AF488 probes.

2.4. Confocal Microscopy on Colorectal Tissue Sections

Imaging of the tissue sections was carried out on a Leica TCS SP5 STED microscope (used in confocal mode) using either a 40×/1.1 or a 63×/1.2 water immersion objective.

Sytox Orange was excited by using a 561 laser. A HyD detector (nm range) was employed to capture the signals.

2.5. Chromatin Compaction Quantitative Analysis—Confocal Data

A total of 50 nuclei images of each of the colorectal cell types (normal tissue: epithelial cells of the mucosa; stromal cells of the submucosa, and smooth muscle cells of the L. muscularis layer; carcinoma: epithelial-derived tumour cells) were selected from representative confocal images. For the analysis, the area of each nucleus was estimated using an ImageJ's macro. Local intensity maxima were acquired in this area. The number of detected maxima in the nucleus was defined as the number of chromatin domains [36]. To determine the local neighbourhood area for each peak, changes in signal intensity distribution on the image of the stained nucleus were taken into account. All image processing was performed by using an ImageJ algorithm [37]. To obtain the dark area of each nucleus (low chromatin density area), the total area of all recognised domains was subtracted from the size of the whole nucleus.

2.6. miRNA Signal Quantification and Statistical Analysis

Confocal images of samples on which FISH was performed were analysed using Columbus Software (PerkinElmer, Waltham, MA, USA), to identify the miRNA positive (miR+) cells within the tissue. 20× magnification fields of view from the confocal images were analysed. A visual description of the pipeline can be found in Figure S5. Briefly, nuclei were identified from an input image based on the nuclear dye signal intensities. A contour was drawn estimating the cytoplasm region for each identified nucleus. Finally, a list of cells was obtained and filtered exclusively for cells that had a strong probe signal in the cytosolic area (defined as miR+). A strong probe signal was defined as an intensity in the miR channel above or higher than 5. This cut-off value was chosen given that all the measured intensities in the miR channel on negative control samples that were not incubated with miR-probe, but scrambled sequence instead, were below this value as background signals. Quantified values from this analysis are presented as the percentage of miR+ cells in a given tissue area (field of view).

Statistical analysis was performed with R statistical software (version 4.0.0, The R Foundation for Statistical Computing, Vienna, Austria). An unpaired one-sided Wilcoxon test ($p \leq 0.05$ was considered significant) was used to compare the abovementioned quantified values between cancer tissue and its matched normal counterpart.

2.7. SMLM on Colorectal Tissue Specimen

2D single molecule localisation microscopy (SMLM) was performed on an SR GSD setup (Leica Microsystems CMS GmbH, Wetzlar, Germany), based on an inverse widefield microscope DMI AF6000 equipped with an oil immersion objective (160×/1.43). Fluorescent emission was captured and imaged on an EMCCD camera with a pixel size of 100 nm (iXon3 Ultra 897, Andor Technology Ltd., Belfast, UK). Prior to imaging, the tissue sections on coverslips (see colorectal tissue samples) were deparaffinised and rehydrated (see Fluorescence in situ hybridisation on colorectal tissue sections). Samples were permeabilised in 0.5% Triton/PBS for 1 h, covered with 50 nM Sytox Orange in PBS for 1 h, and embedded on freshly prepared GOX/CAT blinking buffer (0.5 mg/mL glucose oxidase (GOX), 40 µg/mL catalase (CAT) and 10% *w/v* glucose, all in PBS) [16]. The coverslip was sealed with a two-part epoxy sealant (Picondent Twinsil, Wipperfürth, Germany) to a glass slide. All the above mentioned steps were executed at room temperature, and three PBS washes were carried out in between steps. Samples were taken to the microscope right after being embedded in the blinking buffer. For Sytox Orange imaging, a 561 nm laser (2.1 mW) and 30,000 frames with 30 ms camera exposure were used. Single molecule reconstructions were generated with ThunderSTORM (Fiji plugin).

2.8. Quantitative Analysis (SMLM)

Chromatin Density Profiles (Binning Analysis)

To compare the chromatin density distributions between colorectal carcinoma and the corresponding normal tissue nuclei, an in-house R script was used to bin single molecule localisation signals in a 50×50 nm^2 grind. The histograms were visualised in the form of violin plots, showing the frequency of bins with a given number of localisation signals. The R script was fed with the localisation tables obtained from ThunderSTORM (Fiji plugin, Prague, Czech Republic). Briefly, a 2D histogram with a given bin size (50×50 nm^2) was generated using the geom_bin2d function. Then, the value of the number of localisations on each bin was transferred into a table.

2.9. Radial Chromatin Density (Ring Analysis)

A region of interest (ROI) was manually drawn, enclosing the nuclear area on each of the reconstructed images generated by ThunderSTORM. An in-house MATLAB (MATLAB version 9.3.0 (2017b), The Mathworks, Natick, MA, USA) code was used to subdivide the cell nucleus into six concentric rings with equal area, and to draw concentric areas following the nuclear contour as a guide [38]. The number of localisation signals in each of these rings served as a basis to calculate the average localisation density per ring.

3. Results

Distinctive regions within whole 10 μm tissue sections of human colorectal carcinomas and matched corresponding normal tissues were analysed in a first-in-field attempt with SMLM super-resolution microscopy at the nanoscale, following confocal resolution imaging. In the following, we present results and images for chromatin density within nuclei of carcinoma, normal epithelial, and further cell types in CRC tissue sections, followed by single molecule microRNA subcellular analysis for selective miRs, which have been shown to play significant roles in different aspects of metastasis [18,20,34]. Altogether, we hypothesise that this technology could be a highly supportive tool to decipher molecular (tumour) cell heterogeneity at the single cell level within any individual tissue context.

3.1. Chromatin Density of Nuclei from Colorectal Carcinoma and Its Corresponding Normal Tissues

3.1.1. Chromatin Density—Confocal Resolution

Nuclei from individual tissue regions depicted in Figure S1 were analysed independently to demonstrate that nuclei from cells with distinctive functions (benign and malignant epithelial cells, stromal cells including smooth muscle cells from different tissue layers) would lead to distinctive chromatin density profiles. Figure S1 shows the three distinctive regions taken for the analysis: mucosa, submucosa, and the muscularis layer. Nuclei analysed within the colorectal carcinoma specimen corresponded to the tumour areas, regions enclosed in blue (Figure S1A).

To obtain a first overview of the different chromatin density distributions and features between cell types, the human colorectal tissue nuclei were stained with Sytox Orange and imaged with a confocal microscope (for details, see Section 2 Materials and Methods). Different nuclear architecture features were observed between (epithelial-derived) carcinoma and normal epithelial cells, as well as between carcinoma, normal epithelial, stromal cells within the submucosa, and smooth muscle cells within the muscularis layer. For each of these cell types, images of 50 nuclei were selected from the confocal images for quantitative analysis. Segmentation analysis was performed using an ImageJ algorithm (see Section 2 Materials and Methods). The area of each nucleus was classified into either a region of high intensity (compact chromatin) or a region of low intensity (loose chromatin). Figure 1 shows representative confocal images and the results after performing the segmentation analysis. Figure 2 shows the nuclear size distributions and percentages of chromatin compaction for the different cell types from a human colorectal carcinoma and the corresponding normal tissue specimen.

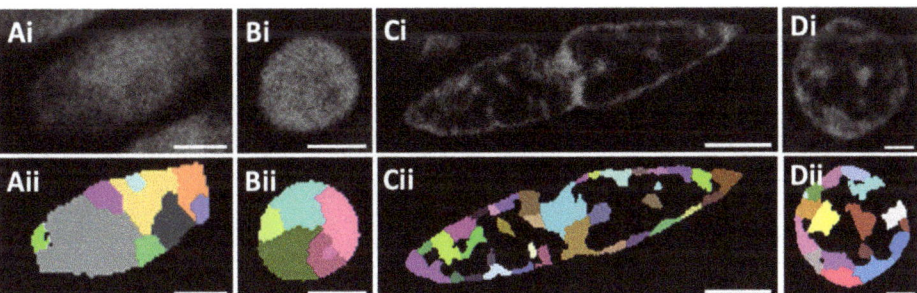

Figure 1. Representative confocal images of human colorectal tissue nuclei stained with Sytox Orange dye. (**Ai–Ci**) Images from a normal colorectal tissue sample comprising a nucleus from the mucosa (normal epithelial cell) (**Ai**), the submucosa (**Bi**) and the muscularis (**Ci**) layer. An image from a colorectal carcinoma tissue sample shows a carcinoma cell nucleus from the tumour region (**Di**). Resulting images for each cell type after the segmentation analysis was performed (**Aii–Dii**). Scale bars: 3 µm.

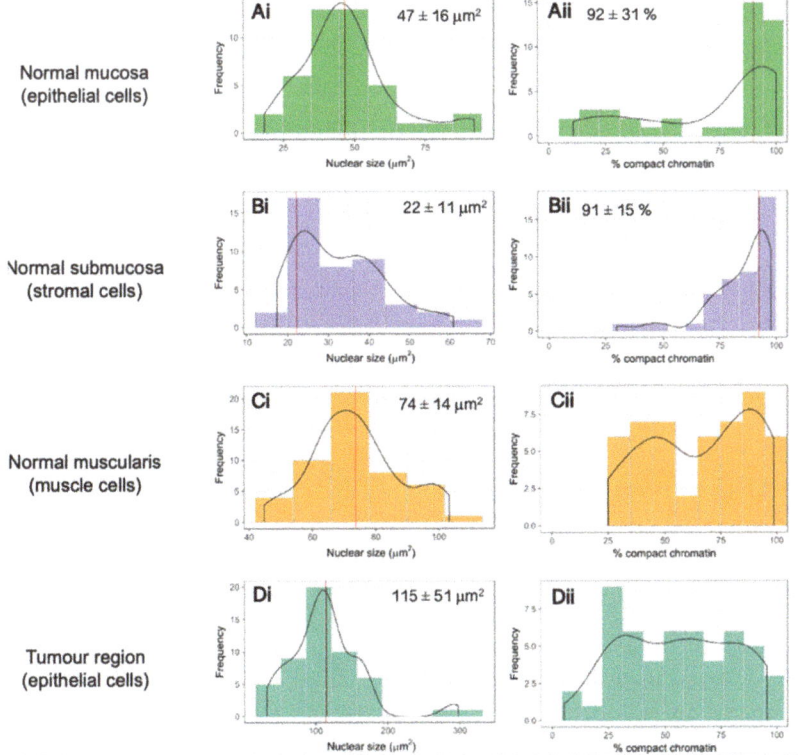

Figure 2. (**Ai–Ci**) Nuclear size distribution of normal colorectal tissue cell types: epithelial cells of the normal mucosa (**Ai**), stromal cells (Tunica submucosa) (**Bi**) and muscle cells (Tunica muscularis) (**Ci**). Nuclear size distribution of epithelial nuclei from a tumour area within a representative example of a colorectal carcinoma tissue specimen (**Di**). (**Aii–Dii**) Percentage of compact chromatin in the same normal and carcinoma colorectal cell types. Solid red vertical lines correspond to the mode from the data. Reported values are the mode ± SD. For normal distributions, the mode coincides with the mean of the distribution. Distributions in (**Cii,Dii**) might correspond to a multimodal distribution ($n = 50$).

To characterise and quantify the differences in chromatin density regions between cells with different functionality (epithelial, submucosa, and muscle) and malignancy (non-malignant epithelial versus carcinoma cells), a quantitative analysis was conducted considering a minimum number of 50 cell nuclei from each of the abovementioned cell types. The two main properties that were analysed were the nuclear size and the percentage of bright nuclear area (coloured domains of Figure 1), which quantifies the chromatin compaction.

Figure 2 shows the sizes of the nuclear cross sections in µm² (Figure 2(Ai–Di)) as well as the quantification of the percentage of compact chromatin per nucleus (Figure 2(Aii–Dii)) in a normal and carcinoma colorectal tissue sample with a thickness of 10 µm. Values shown in the nuclear size distribution graphs correspond to mode values. In the case of a normal distribution, the mode value corresponds to the mean.

Figure 2(Aii–Dii) shows the distribution of compact chromatin percentages in the same types of cells. The vast majority of nuclei from mucosa-derived normal epithelial and submucosal cells had a high percentage (above 90%) of their chromatin compacted (Figure 2(Aii,Bii)). This is in agreement with a publication that showed that specialised somatic cells have denser and more compact chromatin in comparison to, for example, stem cells [39]. In contrast, smooth muscle cell nuclei distribution showed a higher variability and was multimodal (two peaks), so no central value out of a population of 50 nuclei could be reported (Figure 2(Cii)).

The same type of analysis was performed for cells from the corresponding colorectal carcinoma tissue. Here, our attention was focused on cells belonging to a tumour area (Figure S1). These tumour areas were delineated by an experienced pathologist depending on the morphological changes presented by tumour cells, a common current practice in routine pathological diagnosis. Figure 2(Di) shows the size of the nuclear cross sections in µm² from cells in a tumour area within a carcinoma tissue specimen. Nuclei from these cells showed a considerably larger average nuclear size of 115 ± 51 µm² in comparison to their normal mucosa epithelial cell counterparts, 47 ± 16 µm². Not only their size but also their variability within the distribution was higher for the nuclei of carcinoma cells.

We also observed considerable differences in the distribution showing the percentages of chromatin compaction (Figure 2(Aii, Dii)). Nuclei from carcinoma cells in the primary tumour CRC tissue (Figure 2(Dii)) showed a broad distribution, covering cells with values as low as 5% and as high as 96%. In contrast, nuclei from normal mucosa epithelial cells (Figure 2(Aii)) showed a narrow distribution around a mode of 92%.

3.1.2. Chromatin Density at the Nanoscale

Colorectal tissue samples were stained with Sytox Orange, imaged, and the super-resolution data processed as described for SMLM in Materials and Methods. Figure 3 shows representative images of the super-resolution reconstruction images (right) alongside the widefield images of nuclei from either carcinoma cells of the tumour region within a colorectal carcinoma tissue (D), or from normal epithelial, submucosa-derived stromal cells, and muscle cells of the muscle layer of corresponding normal colorectal tissue, respectively (A–C).

The total number of blinking signals for each one of the reconstructed images shown in Figure 3 is 0.98×10^6 (A), 0.55×10^6 (B), 1.34×10^6 (C), and 0.16×10^6 (D), respectively. Tissue background and signals coming from neighbouring tissue nuclei were present but did not interfere with the measurements, since the background signal within the nuclear region was negligible. Tumour regions within cancer tissue samples still had a higher cell density compared to the corresponding normal colorectal tissue, and therefore, the background signals were higher and the number of blinking events lower. Therefore, to isolate the signals coming exclusively from the nuclei of interest, regions of interest (ROIs) were manually drawn on the widefield images, transferred to the reconstructed images, and only localisation events within these ROIs were considered for downstream analysis.

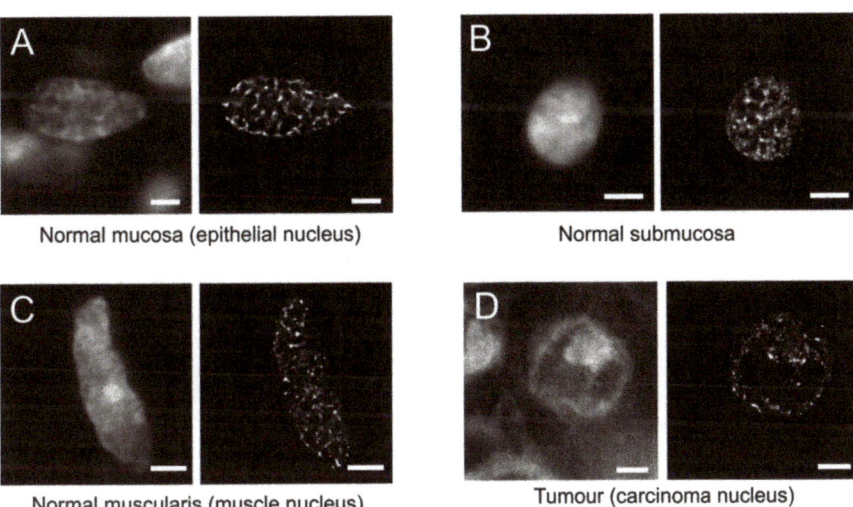

Figure 3. Representative SMLM images of normal colorectal cell nuclei (normal epithelial cell of normal mucosa, submucosa-derived stromal cell, smooth muscle cell within muscular layer) within normal colorectal tissue specimen (**A–C**), and of a carcinoma cell nucleus (**D**). Widefield images (**left**) and SMLM reconstructions (**right**) of nuclei imaged from human colorectal tissue sections. Scale bars: 3 µm.

Figure 4 shows the chromatin density profiles of the muscle nucleus showed in Figure 3C. Two profile lines, a vertical (red) and a horizontal (blue), were drawn in both the widefield image (dashed lines) and the super-resolution reconstruction image (solid lines). Figure 4B shows the intensity profiles (distance vs. intensity) for each one of the profile lines. Intensity values correspond to the widefield image for the dashed lines, and to the super-resolution reconstruction for the solid lines.

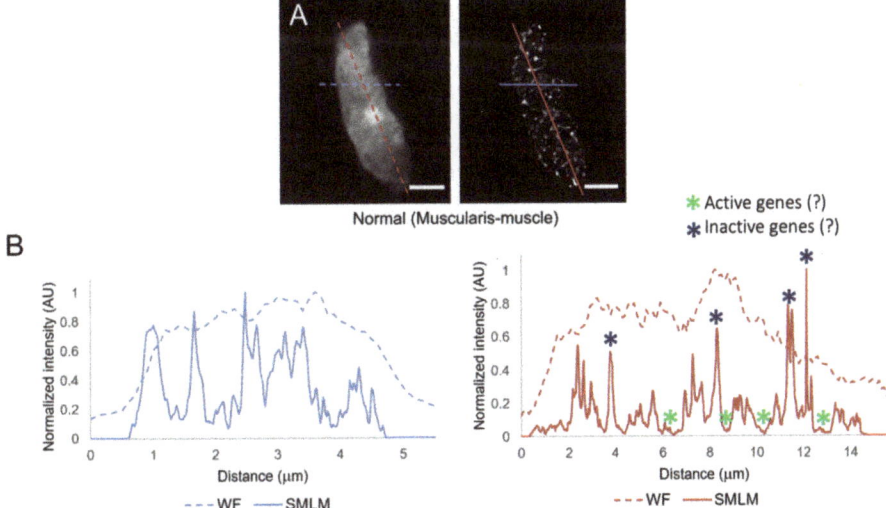

Figure 4. Chromatin density profiles of a normal colorectal muscle nucleus. (**A**) Widefield image and its super-resolved (SMLM) reconstruction. (**B**) Comparison of intensity profiles taken from the widefield image (dotted lines) and the SMLM reconstruction (solid lines). Location of active/inactive genes is hypothesised. Scale bars: 3 µm.

Strong differences in chromatin density changes can be observed when comparing the widefield profiles with the super-resolved ones. There is a similar trend followed by the two profiles for each one of the graphs in Figure 4B. However, the intensity profiles from the widefield images are not able to detect very low density chromatin regions or regions where the chromatin is highly condensed (very strong intensity signals). The location of active genes (in low density and hence more accessible chromatin regions) and inactive genes (in high density chromatin regions) is hypothesised [36,40,41].

The Heterogeneity of Chromatin Density in Human Colorectal (Cancer) Tissue

Given that strong differences in the super-resolved reconstruction (SMLM) images were observed when comparing colorectal carcinoma nuclei with the corresponding ones of epithelial cells in normal colorectal tissue, different ways of quantifying and visually presenting the super-resolution data are shown. Figure 5 shows the chromatin density profile distributions for all of the different nuclei analysed. For normal colorectal tissue, data are shown from epithelial, muscle cell and submucosa nuclei within these regions in normal colorectal tissue (Figure 5A). Additionally, a comparison of data from carcinoma cell nuclei (tumour region) versus normal mucosa epithelial cells are shown (Figure 5B). Distributions from Figure 5 were obtained as described in the SMLM—Binning section of Materials and Methods. The distributions are represented as a combination of violin and box plots. The *y*-axis in Figure 5 is a logarithmic scale of the number of blinking events (counts) in a 50×50 nm^2 bin. The *x*-axis quantifies the frequency of a given count number in a bin. It can be observed that, for all types of cells except for the mucosa-derived normal epithelial cells, the big majority of bins had only one event. This was more strongly observed in the carcinoma nuclei than in all of the cell types from the normal colorectal tissue. In contrast, outlier bins (black dots in Figure 5) with very high numbers of counts were detected in all of the different cell types measured. The horizontal black lines in the middle of the box plots of Figure 5 represent the median for each one of the distributions. As can be seen from the figure, the carcinoma nuclei had the lowest median value of all (value of 3), suggesting their low density chromatin areas are more abundant than for all of the normal colorectal cell types in all of the tissue regions investigated.

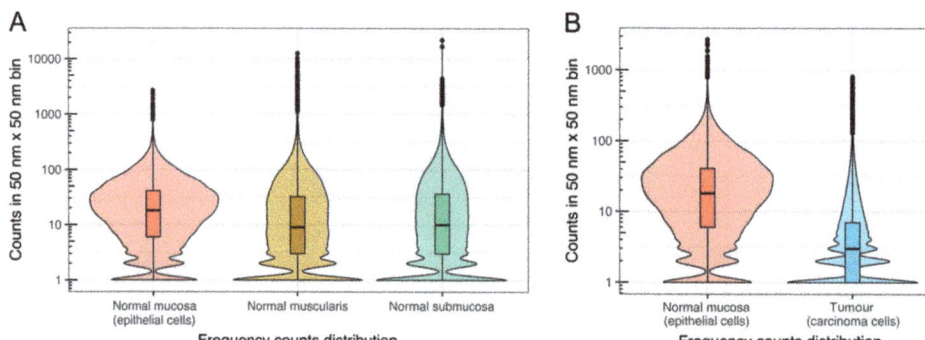

Figure 5. Violin + box plot representations of the localisation signal histograms for nuclei from different regions. A side-by-side comparison is shown between nuclei from (**A**) normal epithelial cells of the mucosa, cells of the submucosa, and of the muscularis layer, and (**B**) between normal epithelial cells of the normal mucosa, and carcinoma cells within the mucosa of a tumour sample. Binning analysis was done in the super-resolved reconstruction images, and signature chromatin density profile distributions were found for each cell type. Horizontal lines in each box plot represent the median value of each one of the distributions. Each distribution is the combination of the replicates (7 for normal submucosa, 2 for normal mucosa, 3 for normal muscularis and 4 for carcinoma cells in the tumour region) for each cell type. Plots of all the replicates from each cell type can be found in Supplementary Figure S2. The horizontal black lines in the middle of the box plots represent the median for each one of the distributions. The values are: mucosa-derived normal epithelial cells 18, muscle cells 9, submucosal cells 13, carcinoma cells 3.

Radial Chromatin Density

To further investigate the chromatin density differences between carcinoma cells and normal cells, we applied the chromatin radial density analysis. The radial density analysis allows visualizing density differences across the nucleus by measuring densities inside rings, starting from the centre of the nucleus to the periphery of the nucleus.

Figure 6 shows the box plot representation of the chromatin radial density analysis for nuclei taken from the epithelial, muscle cell, submucosa, and tumour regions (Figure 6A). Additionally, a comparison of data from carcinoma cells of the tumour region versus normal epithelial cells is shown (Figure 6B).

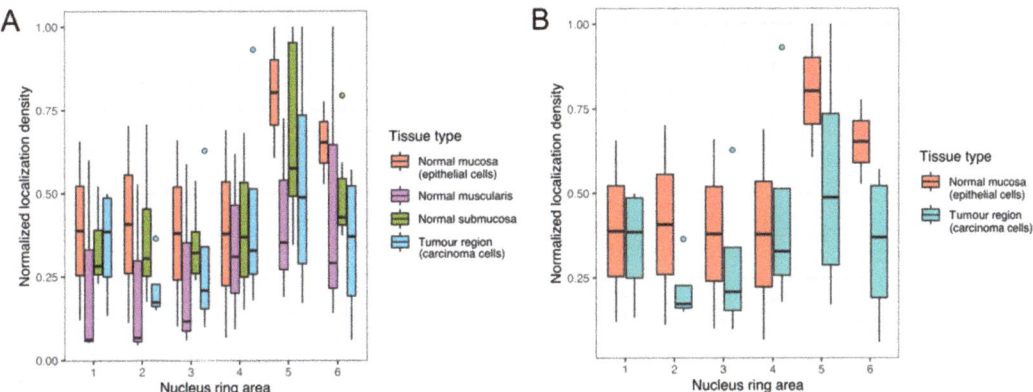

Figure 6. Box plot representations of the radial chromatin density analysis. Box plots show densities measured in rings of equal area from the nuclear centre (Nucleus ring area 1) to the nuclear periphery (Nucleus ring area 6) for cells taken from normal mucosa, normal muscularis, normal submucosa, carcinoma cells from the tumour region (**A**), and, for better comparison, from epithelial cells of normal mucosa and carcinoma cells of the tumour region (**B**). Horizontal lines in each box plot represent the median value of each one of the distributions.

It can be observed that the chromatin density shows a high variability across individual nuclei and across cell types taken from different regions. For all of the cell types, chromatin densities are highest in the outer rings, indicating a trend to higher chromatin densities close to the nuclear periphery. The centre regions show lower chromatin densities.

Compared to the normal cells, carcinoma cell nuclei taken from the tumour region show a pronounced variability. This becomes evident when looking at the number of outliers. Whereas within the normal cells, only one outlier is present for the submucosa region in the outmost ring, the carcinoma cell distribution shows multiple outliers, suggesting an increased variability within these cells.

3.2. miRNA Detection on Human Colon Tissue Sections

In the following, we present our work on the stepwise development of single cell, single molecule microRNA analysis for selective, metastatically relevant miRs to be applicable to tissue sections of human colorectal carcinomas.

3.2.1. DNA Probe Synthesis and Characterisation

After synthesis, the commercially available Cy5 dye was incorporated in all probes of interest (as described in Materials and Methods), and the resulting probes were used for the first step of confocal measurements. Probes with AF488 dye were used for single molecule measurements. Figure 7 lists all the sequences of the probes, the miRNA each one targets, and the positive and negative controls used.

probe-135b	5'—T—C—A—C—A—T—A—G—G—A—A-cU-G—A—A—A—A—G—C—C—A—T—A—3'
probe-210	5'—T—C—A—G—C—C—G—C—T—G-cU-C—A—C—A—C—G—C—A—C—A—G—3'
probe-21	5'—T—C—A—A—C—A—T—C—A—G-cU-C—T—G—A—T—A—A—G—C—T—A—3'
probe-31	5'—A—G—C—T—A—T—G—C—C—A—G—C—A-cU-C—T—T—G—C—C—T—3'
pos. Con.	5'—C—A—C—G—A—A—T—T—T—G—C—G-cU-G—T—C—A—T—C—C—T—T—3'
neg. Con.	5'—G—T—G—T—A—A—C—A—C—G-cU-C—T—A—T—A—C—G—C—C—C—A—3'

Figure 7. DNA sequences of the synthesised miRNA probes; cU = 2′-O-propargyl-uridine was modified with Cy5 (first set of probes) and AF488 (second set of probes).

Spectroscopic measurements were performed to characterise the optical properties of the synthetic single stranded DNA probes and as annealed hybrids with their target RNA sequences (of the same length, Figure S3). The excitation wavelengths for the fluorescence measurements were 647 nm for Cy5 and 488 nm for AF488, respectively, to fit the laser in the later microscopic experiments. In all cases, the variations in UV/Vis absorption and fluorescence of the DNA probes were rather small, showing that the optical properties do not significantly depend on the individual sequences around the site of fluorophore modification. The Cy5 modified probes showed a slight decrease in fluorescence due to double strand building with the complementary miRNA targets, whereas the AF488 modified probes show a small increase of the fluorescence in the double strand except for the miR-135b probe. The latter probe showed a small decrease that can be explained by the hypochromic shift in absorption.

3.2.2. miRNA Signal Detection of Human Colorectal Tissues

For every set of confocal images, the background signal was subtracted (tissue with no staining) from the images. As positive control, a U6snRNA probe was used, and a scrambled sequence probe served as negative control (Figure S4).

miRNA probes with different fluorophores were synthesised. Amongst these, the set of probes conjugated with Cy5 performed best since their emission spectrum is furthest away from the tissue autofluorescence emission, which was stronger in the 488 channel. Figure 8 shows representative confocal images of normal and carcinoma colorectal human tissues. Images were taken in the mucosa area of each of the tissue samples. Green signals correspond to the miRNA probes conjugated with Cy5, whereas purple signals represent the nuclear DNA stained with Sytox Orange.

Images from Figure 8 confirmed that the four miRNAs imaged here show a higher number of molecules in carcinoma cells of CRC cancer tissue, in contrast to a rather low or absent expression in cells of the normal tissue. This is evident for miR-21 and especially miR-31. For miR-135b, the signal intensity in the carcinoma tissue is lower, but still present in comparison with miR-21 and miR-31. For miR-210, there is some miRNA signal coming from the normal tissue in contrast to what was observed for the other miRs. Still, however, the overall miRNA signal is higher in the carcinoma tissue.

The last column from Figure 8 offers a more detailed view of the miRNA signals. In these zoomed images, miRNA signals appear to be located preferentially in the cytoplasm, close to the nuclear periphery, however, other subcellular locations such as nuclear ones cannot be excluded.

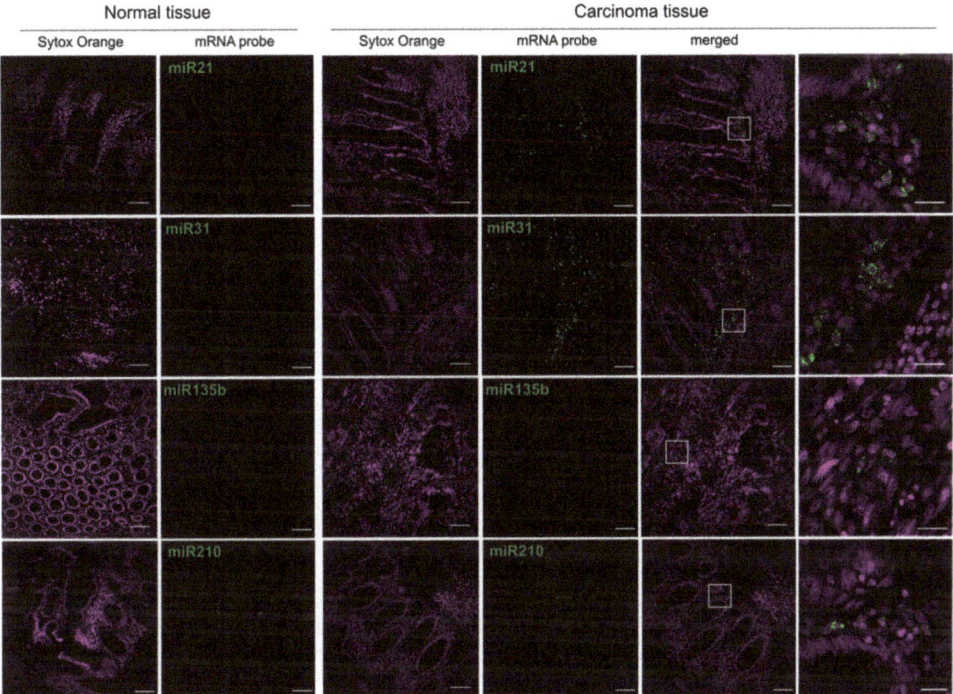

Figure 8. Representative confocal images of FISH performed at normal and carcinoma colorectal human tissue samples with various pro-metastatic miRNA probes: miR-21, miR-31, miR-135b, and miR-210. Green signals correspond to the Cy5 on the miRNA probe, and purple signals represent the nuclear stain by Sytox Orange. The last column shows magnifications of the areas delineated in white rectangles within the second last column (merged images of carcinoma tissue). The brightness range (0–255) of images with miR signals (except the last column) was re-set to 5–100 for this figure alone to enhance the contrast. Quantification of miRNA signals can be found in Figure 9. Scale bars: 100 µm. Scale bars for the last column: 20 µm.

miR Positive Cell Fractions

To have a better overview of the FISH results, Columbus Software (PerkinElmer) was used to quantify the number of miR positive (miR+) cells in a given field of view (for a description of the miR+ cells detection pipeline see Section 2 Materials and Methods and Figure S5). miR+ cells were defined here as cells with a high miRNA probe intensity signals located in their cytoplasm. High intensity was defined as an intensity value in the miR channel equal to or higher than 5. Quantification analysis using Columbus Software resulted in a list of miR+ cells with an intensity value representing how strongly a given miRNA signal was observed in each cell's cytoplasm region. This analysis included miRNA negative (miR-) cells as well, which presented a probe intensity lower than 5 which was comparable to signals detected in the background (see Section 2 Methods).

Figure 9 shows the percentage of miR+ cells according to the definition above in 20× magnification fields of view. For each analysed field of view, the total number of cells was quantified (as shown in Figure S5); this value represented 100%. A subset of these cells, the miR+ cells, is shown as a percentage for each of the four miRNAs analysed: miR-21, miR-31, miR-135b, and miR-210.

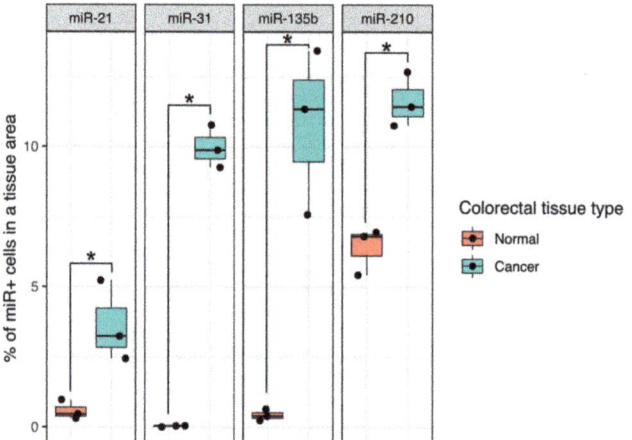

Figure 9. Quantification of the fraction of miR+ cells in normal and colorectal carcinoma human tissues in which FISH was done for four miRNAs that have been shown to be significant players in metastasis. Percentage values shown are with respect to the total cell number in a 20× magnification field of view. Unpaired one-sided Wilcoxon, * $p \leq 0.05$.

For all of the four miRNAs analysed, the miR+ cell tissue fractions were always higher in comparison to corresponding normal tissue, which matches the published literature on these miRs including our own publications [18,20,26,34]. Differences between normal and tumour tissues were significant in all four cases.

miRNA Signal Detection at the Nanoscale in Human Tissue Samples

Based on the previous confocal and FISH analysis, a first-in-field imaging attempt of miRNAs was performed at the single-cell, single-molecule level in routine colorectal cancer patient whole tissue sections. To select miR+ single cells for later SMLM, FISH with a miR-21 probe conjugated with AF488 was conducted on a colorectal carcinoma tissue sample. This fluorophore had to be chosen because of its blinking capabilities in pyranose oxidase embedding buffer, with the disadvantage that its emission coincided with the fluorescence blinking frequency in cases when colorectal tissue presented a strong level of autofluorescence. In spite of this difficulty, SMLM images were taken successfully for carcinoma tissue samples incubated with the miR-21 probe. MiR-signals, and vesicle-like structures containing miR-21 signals, tended to accumulate in the periphery of the nucleus as already shown in confocal microscopy and FISH (see above); in addition, besides some cytoplasmic signals, they also showed localisation signals that seemed to be located inside the nucleus (Figure 10).

Figure 10 shows the representative example of a single-cell nucleus of a human colorectal cancer tissue sample. Figure 10A shows the conventional widefield image of the nucleus, Figure 10B the super-resolved reconstruction image. Aggregates of considerable size of miR-21 signals were detected in the peripheral nuclear area. MiR-21 smaller signals, located in the cytosol, were detected as well (Figure 10B). The two small insets (white rectangles) where miR-21 signals were found to be located in rounded shapes are enlarged (Figure 10(Bi,Bii)). Diameters of the structures in which the miR-signal was condensed were measured along and across (140 × 110 nm for Bi and 240 × 120 nm for Bii, respectively). This visually confirms previous evidence that mature miRNAs, besides a well-described localisation in the cytoplasm and within exosomes [34,42–44] are located inside the nucleus and act, for example, like localisation signals for other biomolecules active in chromatin restructuring, nucleolar organisation or in gene silencing/gene activation, chromatin reorganisation in itself having been linked to an increase of metastatic capacity of tumour cells [13,24,45,46]. This, taken together, renders a logical link between analysing chromatin nanostructure and miR-localisation within single cells as first attempts to tackle cancer cell heterogeneity, including the putative metastatic potential of particular cells, within whole tissue sections of individual patient tumours [45].

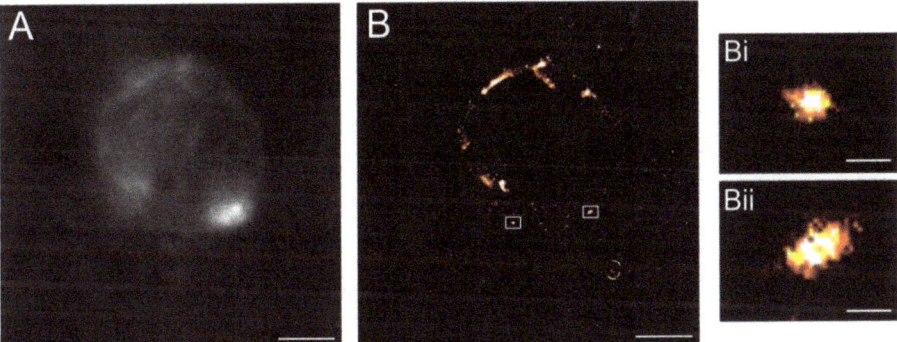

Figure 10. SMLM of miR-21 aggregates in the nuclear area of a carcinoma cell within a human colorectal cancer tissue sample. Smaller blinking events were detected in the cytosolic area as well. (**A**) Widefield and (**B**) super-resolved reconstruction images. Two ROIs are highlighted in white (**Bi,Bii**) showing miR21 aggregates. Scale bars 3 μm. Insets scale bars 200 nm.

4. Discussion

Our present study demonstrates the feasibility of our single-cell, single-molecule localisation microscopy methodology on whole, 10 μm thick routine patient tissue sections of primary colorectal tumours and corresponding normal tissue for the diagnosis of (changes of) chromatin texture and microRNA subcellular localisation at the nanoscale. We have chosen changes in chromatin nanostructure and particular microRNAs as first diagnostic targets in our attempt to transfer this technology from cell culture/monolayers to an application in human tissue sections, since both of them have been shown to be in the current focus of interest, and of functional importance, for the ability of tumour cells to metastasise [12,13,18,20,34]. Metastasis, as it is well known, is still the most frequent cause of death of cancer patients, and one of the most fundamental unsolved problems for personalised diagnosis and therapy to date is the highly limited ability to recognise specific, metastatically relevant cells or cell clones within the huge context of heterogeneity in primary tumours of patients [47–49]. Ideally, diagnostic technologies are needed that are capable of detecting metastatically relevant cells already in an individual primary tumour of a patient within the first stage of initial diagnosis, before relapse and macroscopic metastasis can arise. This also can be crucial for prospective targeted therapy planning, which then could be specifically designed to include particular molecular changes detected in suchlike individual cells.

In the present study, we used confocal and Single Molecule Localisation Microscopy (SMLM) in the fBALM (fluctuation-assisted Binding-Activated Localisation Microscopy) mode to quantitatively analyse the nuclear chromatin texture of cell nuclei in sections of human colorectal cancer tissues. Already the confocal data (Figures 1 and 2) indicated marked differences between the chromatin texture of nuclei in normal and tumour areas of the tissue sections studied. This heterogeneity, however, became much more pronounced in the super-resolved images (Figures 3–6). In this case, the local DNA density varied up to almost two orders of magnitude and revealed a large number of very small and highly compacted chromatin clusters down to the sub-resolution range, in apparent contrast to the widefield images.

Very similar results were obtained previously in SMLM-fBALM studies of single nuclei of various cell lines [16,40,50]. To our knowledge, the results reported here for the first time show that this unexpectedly larger heterogeneity in nuclear chromatin nanotexture is also a prominent feature of cells of human colorectal tissue, especially of carcinoma cells in contrast to corresponding normal epithelial cells and other cells of the colorectal tissue context.

This large heterogeneity of nuclear chromatin distribution is typically not observed in conventional resolution microscopy where a much smoother spatial DNA distribution is obtained. The nanoscale heterogeneity of chromatin texture observed by SMLM-fBALM is in striking contrast with a plethora of nuclear genome models based on sequencing approaches like Hi-C [51,52]. These models, however, are derived from biochemical DNA–DNA interaction probabilities; therefore, the maps constructed from these probability data do not necessarily reflect spatial configurations. The SMLM-fBALM results presented here show that, also in nuclei of human colorectal tissue, the spatial distribution of DNA is substantially more heterogeneous than that observed by conventional resolution microscopy: The typically relatively smooth DNA distribution changes imaged with conventional methods were resolved by SMLM into a large number of highly compacted small chromatin domains, interspersed within a large space of low DNA density.

These results are difficult to reconcile with the typical interaction map derived of models cited above, but appear to be fully compatible with the basic tenets of the ANC-INC (Active/Inactive Nuclear Compartment) model, postulating the importance of chromatin density-related accessibility constraints for transcriptional regulation [10,36,41]. In this model, silent gene domains are compacted to such a level of DNA density that the diffusion of macromolecular complexes to target sequences in their interior may be restricted or even excluded. On the other side, transcriptionally competent gene domains are characterised by a low DNA density to enhance accessibility. Previous results obtained with SMLM-fBALM in a mouse cardiomyocyte cell line (HL-1), using YoYo-1 as a DNA stain, also indicated small compacted clusters (around 50–60 nm in diameter) interspersed within a large space of low DNA density. Furthermore, transcriptionally competent small domains were almost exclusively observed within the low density compartment only [40]. The existence of small, highly compacted chromatin domains is also in line with previous observations obtained by other methods of super-resolution microscopy [17,50].

Using Fluorescence in situ hybridisation (FISH) with Oligopaint probes synthesised on the basis of sequence information, it has become possible to directly compare Hi-C data with super-resolved microscopic observations [53]. Other recent observations also favour the concept that nucleosomes are assembled in heterogeneous groups comprising a few kb of DNA, termed nucleosome clutches or clusters (NCs) [39,54]. The acetylation state determines how tightly DNA is compacted within a given NC [55]. The nucleosome cluster concept has been supported by oligo-painting combined with super-resolved fluorescence microscopy [56,57]. While Beliveau et al. [56] used SMLM/STORM with photoswitching dyes, the ORCA method (Optical Reconstruction of Chromatin Architecture) applied by Mateo et al. [57] to Drosophila embryos relied on the sequential imaging of the 3D centre positions of the diffraction limited "spots" produced by each fluorescent probe set in the nucleus; this allowed specific sections within a diffraction-limited volume to be resolved, as in SMLM/STORM, while adding sequence resolution across the domain. A related localisation approach using 3D confocal microscopy and BAC-probes for multicolour painting has previously been reported to explore the 3D nanostructure of a specific small chromatin breakpoint domain in human leukaemia cell nuclei [58]. A comparison of these results with a random walk model indicated highly significant differences between experiment and simulation.

The previous results obtained in a variety of other cell types corroborate the notion that the high nuclear chromatin nanotexture heterogeneity observed here in human colorectal sections is not restricted to individual cells in monolayers but presents a general feature of cells also in tissues. They suggest that the space-time structure of chromatin loops in mammalian cells is generally represented by the existence of small, condensed and dynamic nuclear domains and that these form the essential building blocks for all higher order chromatin structures above the nucleosome level [55]. Altogether, they argue for a DNA density controlled accessibility of macromolecular aggregates to binding sites in the interior of such small compacted chromatin domains. These might exhibit a highly dynamic nanostructure, and we consider it highly likely that such dynamics will also include, for example, significant increases in chromatin accessibility which has been observed during the promotion of metastasis [13]. As a consequence, it may be hypothesised that the accessibility conditions would accordingly fast, in such a way that the accessibility of a nucleosome in the ensemble centre is dynamically modified with a specific transition frequency, depending on the mechanical elasticity parameters of the ensemble [59]. These dynamics might be different, or enhanced, within the highly heterogeneous nuclei of carcinoma cells which we have found in the present work to be substantially different in size, nanostructure, and distribution of condensed versus relaxed chromatin areas, as compared to corresponding normal epithelia and also other cell types within colorectal tissue. Such a dynamic transition frequency might result in a corresponding modification of the binding probability of transcription factors and, hence, contribute to the fine regulation of gene expression, including genes for miRNAs, or the accessibility for miRNAs and further regulatory molecules to modify gene transcription and chromatin modification [24,45,46]. Since chromatin is an elastic structure, the mechanical properties of such nucleosome clusters might contribute to affect the micro-environmental regulation of genome programs [59,60]. These might include programs to promote migration, invasion and metastasis [5], programs to interact with, and reprogram, the tumour cell microenvironment, to increase the transcription of genes that, for example, contribute to prime metastatic niches, to initiate programs of resistance towards particularly inflicted therapeutic pressure, etc.

In this context, our present work also confirms, within an intact whole tissue setting, that we found blinking signals of particular microRNAs previously discovered to be important players in metastasis, to condense in vesicle-like shapes of the cytoplasm or also in the nucleus. This corroborates previous SMLM super-resolution work we had presented on microRNAs in single cells of cancer cell lines [34] and in which we had demonstrated miR-localisation within exosomes, using an additional exosomal marker. It also corroborates previous findings that miRs can be accumulated in exosomes which, when secreted by tumour cells, can prime metastatic niches in distant organs via systemic spread [25,47–49]. Our first-in-field SMLM imaging of microRNAs in the nucleus of a carcinoma cell within the whole tissue context of CRC patients also confirms the functional work of colleagues in recent years who have discovered several nuclear functions of microRNAs in addition to their well-studied cytoplasmic ones as translational inhibitors [24,45,46]. Towards this end, it has been shown that microRNAs can modify, for example, gene expression (activation and silencing of transcription), chromatin remodelling and epigenetics, or nucleolar reorganisation. This can happen via several modes of interaction such as, the binding to nascent RNA transcripts and interactions with promoter and enhancer/silencer regions, or acting within molecular complexes that involve Ago proteins, transcription factors, RNA polymerase II, histone methyltransferase enzymes, and others [24]. Interestingly, one of the interaction models currently postulated suggests that microRNAs might form triple-helical structures with the target DNA, altering chromatin and thus accessibility for transcription factors [24]. In this context, it is interesting to note that, a few years ago, we published a paper showing altered triplex-DNA binding in EMSA studies of colorectal carcinoma as compared to corresponding normal tissue nuclear extracts [61], and it remains to be studied in the future whether carcinoma cell nuclei, in general, show higher triplex formation phenomena as compared to normal cells, which again might be added to an arsenal of diagnostic tools at the nanoscale to tackle single cell heterogeneity.

In summary, we have shown that SMLM super-resolution microscopy is feasible in routine histopathological sections of carcinoma- and matched normal tissues of patients with colorectal cancer, and we anticipate that this will be able to be extended to other tumour types and to further molecules/molecular conditions of interest for single cell heterogeneity diagnosis at the nanoscale. Several future applications for this technological approach can be anticipated, for example, the identification of single tumour cells in the tissue context which show active particular areas of transcription, predictive features at the nanoscale to prepare to become a cancer cell, a particular molecular potential for metastasis, or accessibility to particular therapeutics. We envisage that technologies such as the ones we introduce here could be advanced to automated micro-imaging devices [62], to support and escort pathology and macro-diagnostic imaging fields for a more efficient early differential diagnosis of heterogeneity within individual tumours and patients, up to the successful prevention of cancer progression and metastasis. A highly intriguing additional application of this technology might be to improve the identification and molecular differentiation of single circulating tumour cells (CTCs) in cancer patients [63–65], after enrichment, e.g., by flow cytometry and high content conventional resolution micros-copy. On the research side, this would allow to test and image the hypothesis, at the single cell level, that the blood is a pool of nucleic acids derived from different tissue sources and tumour cell subsets with different metastatic capabilities.

5. Conclusions

We demonstrate the feasibility of our SMLM methodology on whole, 10 μm thick patient tissue sections of carcinoma patients for the differential diagnosis of heterogeneity in chromatin texture and microRNA subcellular localisation at the nanoscale, and anticipate a promising potential of this methodology to detect, for example, individual carcinoma cells with specific metastatic potential at the molecular level as early as possible in the primary tumour context. For the future, further detailed characterisation of the chromatin density profile and cluster analysis of the images detected with confocal microscopy and SMLM, combined with Oligopainting of cancer-relevant DNA and RNA sequences, is envisaged. These might allow a better understanding of the main differences of chromatin texture, microRNA distribution, and function, in various relevant cell types, in particular, cancer- and metastatically relevant cells. The continuous advancement of this technology, extending to, for example, further molecules to be imaged, to the labelling of particular genes which are active within a given chromatin location, to "multicolour" imaging of several molecular features within the same cells and tissues, and to automated diagnostic systems might open attractive chances to tackle intra-tumour heterogeneity at the earliest possible diagnostic stage. This might contribute to prevent metastatic spread, design therapeutic strategies tailored at the individual heterogeneity of individual tumours, contribute to the development of improved therapeutics with better targeting abilities, or predict the accessibility of particular tumour cell fractions for essential therapeutics.

Supplementary Materials: The following are available online at https://www.mdpi.com/article/10.3390/cancers13153692/s1, Figure S1: (A) Images of human colorectal tissue sections: Section of carcinoma tissue (left) and of the corresponding normal tissue (right). Typical histological layers are depicted side by side for comparison. Blue areas correspond to the tumour areas (drawn by a pathologist) used for further imaging analysis. (B) Enlarged H&E image of a section of carcinoma (left) and normal (right) colorectal tissue. Magnification: 10× carcinoma tissue, 4× normal tissue. A magnification of 4× was used for the latter image with the aim to provide a clear visualisation of the different colorectal layers, Figure S2: Violin + box plot representations of the localisation (SMLM) signal histograms of normal and carcinoma human colorectal tissue nuclei, Figure S3: UV/Vis absorption (A and B) and fluorescence (C and D) of the synthetic DNA probes as single strands, and annealed in hybrids, with their target miRNA sequences; 2.5 μM DNA/RNA, 50 mM Na-Pi buffer, 250 mM NaCl, pH 7, λ_{exc} = 647 nm for Cy5 probes, λ_{exc} = 488 nm for AF488 probes, Figure S4: Positive and negative controls for the FISH staining, Figure S5: Identification of miRNA positive (miR+) cells using Columbus Software (PerkinElmer).

Author Contributions: Conceptualisation, H.A., C.C., H.-A.W.; methodology, H.-A.W., C.C., M.G., A.M.; software, M.G., O.K., F.S., J.N., K.B.; validation, F.L., M.F.C.-G., M.G.; formal analysis, F.L., M.F.C.-G., M.G., C.C., H.-A.W.; investigation, F.L., M.F.C.-G., M.G., C.C., H.-A.W.; resources, H.A., H.-A.W.; patient tissues, A.M.; data curation, M.F.C.-G., F.L., M.G., C.C., O.K., F.S.; writing—original draft preparation, H.A., C.C., H.-A.W., M.F.C.-G., F.L., M.G., A.M.; writing—review and editing, all of the authors; visualisation, F.L., M.F.C.-G., M.G.; supervision, H.A., H.-A.W., C.C.; project administration, H.A., H.-A.W.; funding acquisition, H.A., H.-A.W. All authors have read and agreed to the published version of the manuscript.

Funding: This project was specifically supported by a HEiKA Grant to H.A. and H.-A.W. of the Ruprecht-Karls-University of Heidelberg and Karlsruhe Institute of Technology (KIT). K.B. is a recipient of a doctoral research grant (Etiuda 2016/20/T/NZ1/00517) and a young researcher grant from the National Science Centre (Preludium 2015/19/N/NZ1/00323). H.A. was generally supported by the Alfried Krupp von Bohlen und Halbach Foundation, Essen; the Deutsche Krebshilfe, Bonn (grant number 70112168); the Deutsche Forschungsgemeinschaft (DFG, grant number AL 465/9-1); Dr Hella-Buehler-Foundation, Heidelberg; the DKFZ-MOST Cooperation, Heidelberg (grant number CA149); the HIPO/POP-Initiative for Personalized Oncology, Heidelberg (H032/H027). C.C. was supported by the Boehringer Ingelheim Stiftung.

Institutional Review Board Statement: Approval by the institutional ethics board (Ethics board II at UMM, approval no. 2017-806R-MA), was granted to A.M., waiving the need for informed consent for this retrospective and fully anonymised analysis of archival samples.

Informed Consent Statement: Informed consent was waived by the Institutional Review Board (see above), since the analysis was done (retrospectively) at completely anonymised, archival pathological material.

Data Availability Statement: The data presented in this study are available in the manuscript and Supplementary Materials. Any further information is available from the authors.

Acknowledgments: This paper contains parts of the dissertation of first author Fabian Lang, conducted in partial fulfilment of the requirements for the "Dr. rer. nat." at the KIT, Karlsruhe, Germany.

Conflicts of Interest: The authors declare no conflict of interest.

Abbreviations

ANC-INC: Active/Inactive Nuclear Compartment. CRC: colorectal cancer. fBALM: fluctuation-assisted Binding-Activated Localisation Microscopy. FFPE: Formalin-fixed paraffin embedded. FISH: Fluorescence in situ Hybridisation. HPLC: High Performance Liquid Chromatography. miRs: microRNAs. miR+ cells: miRNA positive cells. NC: nucleosome clutches. RT: room temperature. SMLM: Single Molecule Localisation Microscopy. STORM: Stochastic Optical Reconstruction Microscopy. ROI: region of interest.

References

1. Sung, H.; Ferlay, J.; Siegel, R.L.; Laversanne, M.; Soerjomataram, I.; Jemal, A.; Bray, F. Global cancer statistics 2020: GLOBOCAN estimates of incidence and mortality worldwide for 36 cancers in 185 countries. *CA Cancer J. Clin.* **2021**, *71*, 209–249. [CrossRef]
2. Mario, L. Colorectal liver metastasis: Towards the integration of conventional and molecularly targeted therapeutic approaches. *Front. Biosci.* **2005**, *10*, 3042–3057. [CrossRef]
3. Gang, W.; Wang, J.-J.; Guan, R.; Yan, S.; Shi, F.; Zhang, J.-Y.; Li, Z.-M.; Gao, J.; Fu, X.-L. Strategy to targeting the immune resistance and novel therapy in colorectal cancer. *Cancer Med.* **2018**, *7*, 1578–1603. [CrossRef]
4. Singh, M.P.; Rai, S.; Pandey, A.; Singh, N.K.; Srivastava, S. Molecular subtypes of colorectal cancer: An emerging therapeutic opportunity for personalized medicine. *Genes Dis.* **2021**, *8*, 133–145. [CrossRef]
5. Ishaque, N.; Abba, M.L.; Hauser, C.; Patil, N.; Paramasivam, N.; Huebschmann, D.; Leupold, J.H.; Balasubramanian, G.P.; Kleinheinz, K.; Toprak, U.H.; et al. Whole genome sequencing puts forward hypotheses on metastasis evolution and therapy in colorectal cancer. *Nat. Commun.* **2018**, *9*, 4782. [CrossRef]
6. Tieng, F.Y.F.; Baharudin, R.; Abu, N.; Mohd Yunos, R.-I.; Lee, L.-H.; Ab Mutalib, N.-S. Single Cell Transcriptome in Colorectal Cancer—Current Updates on Its Application in Metastasis, Chemoresistance and the Roles of Circulating Tumor Cells. *Front. Pharmacol.* **2020**, *11*, 135. [CrossRef] [PubMed]
7. Hervieu, C.; Christou, N.; Battu, S.; Mathonnet, M. The Role of Cancer Stem Cells in Colorectal Cancer: From the Basics to Novel Clinical Trials. *Cancers* **2021**, *13*, 1092. [CrossRef] [PubMed]
8. Galindo-Pumariño, C.; Collado, M.; Herrera, M.; Peña, C. Tumor Microenvironment in Metastatic Colorectal Cancer: The Arbitrator in Patients' Outcome. *Cancers* **2021**, *13*, 1130. [CrossRef] [PubMed]
9. Jackson, D.; Hassan, A.; Errington, R.; Cook, P. Visualization of focal sites of transcription within human nuclei. *EMBO J.* **1993**, *12*, 1059–1065. [CrossRef]

10. Cremer, T.; Cremer, M.; Hübner, B.; Strickfaden, H.; Smeets, D.; Popken, J.; Sterr, M.; Markaki, Y.; Rippe, K.; Cremer, C. The 4D nucleome: Evidence for a dynamic nuclear landscape based on co-aligned active and inactive nuclear compartments. *FEBS Lett.* **2015**, *589*, 2931–2943. [CrossRef] [PubMed]
11. Zhao, L.; Wang, S.; Cao, Z.; Ouyang, W.; Zhang, Q.; Xie, L.; Zheng, R.; Guo, M.; Ma, M.; Hu, Z.; et al. Chromatin loops associated with active genes and heterochromatin shape rice genome architecture for transcriptional regulation. *Nat. Commun.* **2019**, *10*, 3640. [CrossRef] [PubMed]
12. Gupta, R.A.; Shah, N.; Wang, K.C.; Kim, J.; Horlings, H.M.; Wong, D.J.; Tsai, M.-C.; Hung, T.; Argani, P.; Rinn, J.L.; et al. Long non-coding RNA HOTAIR reprograms chromatin state to promote cancer metastasis. *Nature* **2010**, *464*, 1071–1076. [CrossRef] [PubMed]
13. Denny, S.; Yang, D.; Chuang, C.-H.; Brady, J.J.; Lim, J.S.; Grüner, B.; Chiou, S.-H.; Schep, A.N.; Baral, J.; Hamard, C.; et al. Nfib Promotes Metastasis through a Widespread Increase in Chromatin Accessibility. *Cell* **2016**, *166*, 328–342. [CrossRef]
14. Zink, D.; Fischer, A.; Nickerson, J.A. Nuclear structure in cancer cells. *Nat. Rev. Cancer* **2004**, *4*, 677–687. [CrossRef] [PubMed]
15. Lelievre, S.; Weaver, V.M.; Nickerson, J.A.; Larabell, C.A.; Bhaumik, A.; Petersen, O.W.; Bissell, M.J. Tissue phenotype depends on reciprocal interactions between the extracellular matrix and the structural organization of the nucleus. *Proc. Natl. Acad. Sci. USA* **1998**, *95*, 14711–14716. [CrossRef]
16. Szczurek, A.; Klewes, L.; Xing, J.; Gourram, A.; Birk, U.; Knecht, H.; Dobrucki, J.; Mai, S.; Cremer, C. Imaging chromatin nanostructure with binding-activated localization microscopy based on DNA structure fluctuations. *Nucleic Acids Res.* **2017**, *45*, e56. [CrossRef] [PubMed]
17. Cremer, C.; Szczurek, A.; Schock, F.; Gourram, A.; Birk, U. Super-resolution microscopy approaches to nuclear nanostructure imaging. *Methods* **2017**, *123*, 11–32. [CrossRef] [PubMed]
18. Asangani, I.; Rasheed, S.A.K.; Nikolova, D.A.; Leupold, J.H.; Colburn, N.H.; Post, S.; Allgayer, H. MicroRNA-21 (miR-21) post-transcriptionally downregulates tumor suppressor Pdcd4 and stimulates invasion, intravasation and metastasis in colorectal cancer. *Oncogene* **2007**, *27*, 2128–2136. [CrossRef]
19. Mudduluru, G.; Ceppi, P.; Kumarswamy, R.; Scagliotti, G.V.; Papotti, M.; Allgayer, H. Regulation of Axl receptor tyrosine kinase expression by miR-34a and miR-199a/b in solid cancer. *Oncogene* **2011**, *30*, 2888–2899. [CrossRef]
20. Mudduluru, G.; Abba, M.; Batliner, J.; Patil, N.; Scharp, M.; Lunavat, T.R.; Leupold, J.H.; Oleksiuk, O.; Juraeva, D.; Thiele, W.; et al. A Systematic Approach to Defining the microRNA Landscape in Metastasis. *Cancer Res.* **2015**, *75*, 3010–3019. [CrossRef]
21. Laudato, S.; Patil, N.; Abba, M.L.; Leupold, J.H.; Benner, A.; Gaiser, T.; Marx, A.; Allgayer, H. P53-induced miR-30e-5p inhibits colorectal cancer invasion and metastasis by targeting ITGA6 and ITGB1. *Int. J. Cancer* **2017**, *141*, 1879–1890. [CrossRef]
22. Wen, X.-Q.; Qian, X.-L.; Sun, H.-K.; Zheng, L.-L.; Zhu, W.-Q.; Li, T.-Y.; Hu, J.-P. MicroRNAs: Multifaceted Regulators of Colorectal Cancer Metastasis and Clinical Applications. *OncoTargets Ther.* **2020**, *13*, 10851–10866. [CrossRef] [PubMed]
23. Krol, J.; Sobczak, K.; Wilczynska, U.; Drath, M.; Jasinska, A.; Kaczynska, D.; Krzyzosiak, W.J. Structural Features of MicroRNA (miRNA) Precursors and Their Relevance to miRNA Biogenesis and Small Interfering RNA/Short Hairpin RNA Design. *J. Biol. Chem.* **2004**, *279*, 42230–42239. [CrossRef]
24. Liu, H.; Lei, C.; He, Q.; Pan, Z.; Xiao, D.; Tao, Y. Nuclear functions of mammalian MicroRNAs in gene regulation, immunity and cancer. *Mol. Cancer* **2018**, *17*, 64. [CrossRef]
25. Garzon, R.; Calin, G.A.; Croce, C.M. MicroRNAs in Cancer. *Annu. Rev. Med.* **2009**, *60*, 167–179. [CrossRef]
26. Abba, M.L.; Patil, N.; Leupold, J.H.; Moniuszko, M.; Utikal, J.; Niklinski, J.; Allgayer, H. MicroRNAs as novel targets and tools in cancer therapy. *Cancer Lett.* **2017**, *387*, 84–94. [CrossRef]
27. Guo, Y.; Ji, X.; Liu, J.; Fan, D.; Zhou, Q.; Chen, C.; Wang, W.; Wang, G.; Wang, H.; Yuan, W.; et al. Effects of exosomes on pre-metastatic niche formation in tumors. *Mol. Cancer* **2019**, *18*, 39. [CrossRef] [PubMed]
28. Kogure, A.; Kosaka, N.; Ochiya, T. Cross-talk between cancer cells and their neighbors via miRNA in extracellular vesicles: An emerging player in cancer metastasis. *J. Biomed. Sci.* **2019**, *26*, 7. [CrossRef] [PubMed]
29. Obernosterer, G.; Martinez, J.; Alenius, M. Locked nucleic acid-based in situ detection of microRNAs in mouse tissue sections. *Nat. Protoc.* **2007**, *2*, 1508–1514. [CrossRef]
30. Chen, C.; Ridzon, D.A.; Broomer, A.J.; Zhou, Z.; Lee, D.H.; Nguyen, J.T.; Barbisin, M.; Xu, N.L.; Mahuvakar, V.R.; Andersen, M.R.; et al. Real-time quantification of microRNAs by stem-loop RT-PCR. *Nucleic Acids Res.* **2005**, *33*, e179. [CrossRef] [PubMed]
31. Lagos-Quintana, M.; Rauhut, R.; Lendeckel, W.; Tuschl, T. Identification of Novel Genes Coding for Small Expressed RNAs. *Science* **2001**, *294*, 853–858. [CrossRef]
32. Thomson, J.M.; Parker, J.; Perou, C.; Hammond, S.M. A custom microarray platform for analysis of microRNA gene expression. *Nat. Methods* **2004**, *1*, 47–53. [CrossRef]
33. Cheng, Y.; Dong, L.; Zhang, J.; Zhao, Y.; Li, Z. Recent advances in microRNA detection. *Analyst* **2018**, *143*, 1758–1774. [CrossRef]
34. Oleksiuk, O.; Abba, M.; Tezcan, K.C.; Schaufler, W.; Bestvater, F.; Patil, N.; Birk, U.; Hafner, M.; Altevogt, P.; Cremer, C.; et al. Single-Molecule Localization Microscopy allows for the analysis of cancer metastasis-specific miRNA distribution on the nanoscale. *Oncotarget* **2015**, *6*, 44745–44757. [CrossRef]
35. Schwechheimer, C.; Doll, L.; Wagenknecht, H. Synthesis of Dye-Modified Oligonucleotides via Copper(I)-Catalyzed Alkyne Azide Cycloaddition Using On- and Off-Bead Approaches. *Curr. Protoc. Nucleic Acid Chem.* **2018**, *72*, 4.80.1–4.80.13. [CrossRef] [PubMed]

36. Cremer, T.; Cremer, M.; Hübner, B.; Silahtaroglu, A.; Hendzel, M.; Lanctôt, C.; Strickfaden, H.; Cremer, C. The Interchromatin Compartment Participates in the Structural and Functional Organization of the Cell Nucleus. *BioEssays* **2020**, *42*, e1900132. [CrossRef] [PubMed]
37. Rybak, P.; Hoang, A.; Bujnowicz, L.; Bernas, T.; Berniak, K.; Zarębski, M.; Darzynkiewicz, Z.; Dobrucki, J. Low level phosphorylation of histone H2AX on serine 139 (γH2AX) is not associated with DNA double-strand breaks. *Oncotarget* **2016**, *7*, 49574–49587. [CrossRef]
38. Kaufmann, R.; Lemmer, P.; Gunkel, M.; Weiland, Y.; Müller, P.; Hausmann, M.; Baddeley, D.; Amberger, R.; Cremer, C. *SPDM: Single Molecule Superresolution of Cellular Nanostructures*; Enderlein, J., Gryczynski, Z.K., Erdmann, R., Eds.; Society of Photo-Optical Instrumentation Engineers (SPIE): San Jose, CA, USA, 2009; p. 71850.
39. Ricci, M.A.; Manzo, C.; Garcia-Parajo, M.F.; Lakadamyali, M.; Cosma, M.P. Chromatin Fibers Are Formed by Heterogeneous Groups of Nucleosomes In Vivo. *Cell* **2015**, *160*, 1145–1158. [CrossRef] [PubMed]
40. Kirmes, I.; Szczurek, A.; Prakash, K.; Charapitsa, I.; Heiser, C.; Musheev, M.; Schock, F.; Fornalczyk, K.; Ma, D.; Birk, U.; et al. A transient ischemic environment induces reversible compaction of chromatin. *Genome Biol.* **2015**, *16*, 246. [CrossRef] [PubMed]
41. Cremer, T.; Cremer, M.; Cremer, C. The 4D Nucleome: Genome Compartmentalization in an Evolutionary Context. *Biochemistry* **2018**, *83*, 313–325. [CrossRef] [PubMed]
42. Roberts, T.C. The MicroRNA Biology of the Mammalian Nucleus. *Mol. Ther. Nucleic Acids* **2014**, *3*, e188. [CrossRef]
43. Fabian, M.R.; Sonenberg, N.; Filipowicz, W. Regulation of mRNA Translation and Stability by microRNAs. *Annu. Rev. Biochem.* **2010**, *79*, 351–379. [CrossRef]
44. Leung, A.K.L.; Sharp, P.A. Quantifying Argonaute Proteins In and Out of GW/P-Bodies: Implications in microRNA Activities. *Adv. Exp. Med. Biol.* **2012**, *768*, 165–182. [CrossRef]
45. Singh, I.; Contreras, A.; Cordero, J.; Rubio, K.; Dobersch, S.; Günther, S.; Jeratsch, S.; Mehta, A.; Krüger, M.; Graumann, J.; et al. MiCEE is a ncRNA-protein complex that mediates epigenetic silencing and nucleolar organization. *Nat. Genet.* **2018**, *50*, 990–1001. [CrossRef]
46. Leung, A.K.L. The Whereabouts of microRNA Actions: Cytoplasm and Beyond. *Trends Cell Biol.* **2015**, *25*, 601–610. [CrossRef]
47. Sleeman, J.P.; Christofori, G.; Fodde, R.; Collard, J.G.; Berx, G.; Decraene, C.; Rüegg, C. Concepts of metastasis in flux: The stromal progression model. *Semin. Cancer Biol.* **2012**, *22*, 174–186. [CrossRef]
48. Oskarsson, T.; Batlle, E.; Massagué, J. Metastatic Stem Cells: Sources, Niches, and Vital Pathways. *Cell Stem Cell* **2014**, *14*, 306–321. [CrossRef]
49. Allgayer, H.; Leupold, J.H.; Patil, N. Defining the "Metastasome": Perspectives from the genome and molecular landscape in colorectal cancer for metastasis evolution and clinical consequences. *Semin. Cancer Biol.* **2020**, *60*, 1–13. [CrossRef] [PubMed]
50. Hübner, B.; Lomiento, M.; Mammoli, F.; Illner, D.; Markaki, Y.; Ferrari, S.; Cremer, M.; Cremer, T. Remodeling of nuclear landscapes during human myelopoietic cell differentiation maintains co-aligned active and inactive nuclear compartments. *Epigenet. Chromatin* **2015**, *8*, 47. [CrossRef] [PubMed]
51. Lieberman-Aiden, E.; Van Berkum, N.L.; Williams, L.; Imakaev, M.; Ragoczy, T.; Telling, A.; Amit, I.; Lajoie, B.R.; Sabo, P.J.; Dorschner, M.O.; et al. Comprehensive Mapping of Long-Range Interactions Reveals Folding Principles of the Human Genome. *Science* **2009**, *326*, 289–293. [CrossRef] [PubMed]
52. Dekker, J.; Mirny, L. The 3D Genome as Moderator of Chromosomal Communication. *Cell* **2016**, *164*, 1110–1121. [CrossRef]
53. Bintu, B.; Mateo, L.J.; Su, J.-H.; Sinnott-Armstrong, N.A.; Parker, M.; Kinrot, S.; Yamaya, K.; Boettiger, A.N.; Zhuang, X. Super-resolution chromatin tracing reveals domains and cooperative interactions in single cells. *Science* **2018**, *362*, eaau1783. [CrossRef]
54. Szabo, Q.; Jost, D.; Chang, J.-M.; Cattoni, D.I.; Papadopoulos, G.L.; Bonev, B.; Sexton, T.; Gurgo, J.; Jacquier, C.; Nollmann, M.; et al. TADs are 3D structural units of higher-order chromosome organization inDrosophila. *Sci. Adv.* **2018**, *4*, eaar8082. [CrossRef] [PubMed]
55. Otterstrom, J.; Castells-Garcia, A.; Vicario, C.; García, P.A.G.; Cosma, M.P.; Lakadamyali, M. Super-resolution microscopy reveals how histone tail acetylation affects DNA compaction within nucleosomes in vivo. *Nucleic Acids Res.* **2019**, *47*, 8470–8484. [CrossRef]
56. Beliveau, B.J.; Boettiger, A.N.; Avendaño, M.S.; Jungmann, R.; McCole, R.B.; Joyce, E.F.; Kim-Kiselak, C.; Bantignies, F.; Fonseka, C.Y.; Erceg, J.; et al. Single-molecule super-resolution imaging of chromosomes and in situ haplotype visualization using Oligopaint FISH probes. *Nat. Commun.* **2015**, *6*, 7147. [CrossRef]
57. Mateo, L.; Murphy, S.E.; Hafner, A.; Cinquini, I.S.; Walker, C.A.; Boettiger, A.N. Visualizing DNA folding and RNA in embryos at single-cell resolution. *Nat. Cell Biol.* **2019**, *568*, 49–54. [CrossRef]
58. Esa, A.; Edelmann, P.; Kreth, G.; Trakhtenbrot, L.; Amariglio, N.; Rechavi, G.; Hausmann, M.; Cremer, C. Three-dimensional spectral precision distance microscopy of chromatin nanostructures after triple-colour DNA labelling: A study of the BCR region on chromosome 22 and the Philadelphia chromosome. *J. Microsc.* **2000**, *199*, 96–105. [CrossRef] [PubMed]
59. Shivashankar, G. Mechanical regulation of genome architecture and cell-fate decisions. *Curr. Opin. Cell Biol.* **2019**, *56*, 115–121. [CrossRef] [PubMed]
60. Dreger, M.; Madrazo, E.; Hurlstone, A.; Redondo-Muñoz, J. Novel contribution of epigenetic changes to nuclear dynamics. *Nucleus* **2019**, *10*, 42–47. [CrossRef]

61. Nelson, L.D.; Bender, C.; Mannsperger, H.; Buergy, D.; Kambakamba, P.; Mudduluru, G.; Korf, U.; Hughes, D.; Van Dyke, M.W.; Allgayer, H. Triplex DNA-binding proteins are associated with clinical outcomes revealed by proteomic measurements in patients with colorectal cancer. *Mol. Cancer* **2012**, *11*, 38. [CrossRef] [PubMed]
62. Diederich, B.; Helle, Ø.; Then, P.; Carravilla, P.; Schink, K.O.; Hornung, F.; Deinhardt-Emmer, S.; Eggeling, C.; Ahluwalia, B.S.; Heintzmann, R. Nanoscopy on the Chea(i)p. *bioRxiv* **2020**. [CrossRef]
63. Alix-Panabières, C.; Pantel, K. Liquid Biopsy: From Discovery to Clinical Application. *Cancer Discov.* **2021**, *11*, 858–873. [CrossRef] [PubMed]
64. Keller, L.; Pantel, K. Unravelling tumour heterogeneity by single-cell profiling of circulating tumour cells. *Nat. Rev. Cancer* **2019**, *19*, 553–567. [CrossRef] [PubMed]
65. Anfossi, S.; Babayan, A.; Pantel, K.; Calin, G.A. Clinical utility of circulating non-coding RNAs—An update. *Nat. Rev. Clin. Oncol.* **2018**, *15*, 541–563. [CrossRef] [PubMed]

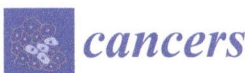

Review

Clinical Applications of Circulating Tumor Cells and Circulating Tumor DNA as a Liquid Biopsy Marker in Colorectal Cancer

Isabel Heidrich [1], Thaer S. A. Abdalla [2], Matthias Reeh [2] and Klaus Pantel [1,*]

1. Center of Experimental Medicine, Department of Tumor Biology, University Medical Center Hamburg-Eppendorf, 20246 Hamburg, Germany; i.heidrich@uke.de
2. Department for Operative Medicine University, University Medical Center Hamburg-Eppendorf, 20246 Hamburg, Germany; thaer.abdalla@uksh.de (T.S.A.A.); m.reeh@uke.de (M.R.)
* Correspondence: pantel@uke.de

Simple Summary: Colorectal cancer is one of the most frequent malignant tumors worldwide and the spread of tumor cells through the blood circulation followed by the colonization of distant organs ("metastases") is the main cause of cancer-related death. The blood is, therefore, an important fluid that can be explored for diagnostic purposes. Liquid biopsy is a new diagnostic concept defined as the analysis of circulating tumor cells or cellular products such as cell-free DNA in the blood or other body fluids of cancer patients. In this review, we summarize and discuss the latest findings using circulating tumor cells and cell-free DNA derived from tumor lesions in the blood of patients with colorectal cancer. Clinical applications include early detection of cancer, identification of patients with a high risk for disease progression after curative surgery, monitoring for disease progression in the context of cancer therapies, and discovery of mechanisms of resistance to therapy.

Abstract: Colorectal cancer (CRC) is the third most commonly diagnosed cancer worldwide. It is a heterogeneous tumor with a wide genomic instability, leading to tumor recurrence, distant metastasis, and therapy resistance. Therefore, adjunct non-invasive tools are urgently needed to help the current classical staging systems for more accurate prognostication and guiding personalized therapy. In recent decades, there has been an increasing interest in the diagnostic, prognostic, and predictive value of circulating cancer-derived material in CRC. Liquid biopsies provide direct non-invasive access to tumor material, which is shed into the circulation; this enables the analysis of circulating tumor cells (CTC) and genomic components such as circulating free DNA (cfDNA), which could provide the key for personalized therapy. Liquid biopsy (LB) allows for the identification of patients with a high risk for disease progression after curative surgery, as well as longitudinal monitoring for disease progression and therapy response. Here, we will review the most recent studies on CRC, demonstrating the clinical potential and utility of CTCs and ctDNA. We will discuss some of the advantages and limitations of LBs and the future perspectives in the field of CRC management.

Keywords: colorectal cancer; liquid biopsy; biomarker

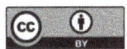

1. Introduction

Colorectal cancer (CRC) is the 4th leading cause of cancer-related death worldwide [1]. It is expected that the global burden of CRC will increase by 60% by 2030 making CRC a major global health problem [2].

In recent decades, there has been remarkable progress in the management of CRC. Starting with the implementation of national screening programs for the early detection of CRC [3], as well as the improvement of the surgical technique with the introduction of total mesorectal excision for rectal cancer and complete mesocolic excision for colon cancer, where sharp dissection along the embryological planes increases lymph node yields, subsequently improving staging and survival [4,5]. In addition, different neoadjuvant and adjuvant biological, chemotherapeutic, and radiotherapeutic strategies have been developed in the last two decades to improve survival and overall outcome in patients with CRC. The goal of these strategies is not only to reach resectability but also to increase local and systemic tumor control [6]. However, the overall outcome is still limited; currently, the overall 5-year survival is 65% [1,7]. Tumor recurrence or formation of distant metastases still occurs in 20% of the patients despite proper treatment and is the leading cause of death in these patients [8].

It is well known that the prognosis of CRC is dependent on the tumor stage at diagnosis. The most common used system for tumor classification is the AJCC TNM staging system, which uses anatomical parameters to discriminate patients into different groups with variable survival outcomes [9]. However, CRC is a very heterogeneous disease in respect to the clinical and tumor-related features, resulting in overwhelming differences in the course of disease and treatment responses. These differences in CRC complicate prognostication and guidance for optimal timing and treatment selection at an individual level [10]. Therefore, new non-invasive biomarkers are needed to personalize therapies and to prevent both under and overtreatment of CRC patients.

More than 10 years ago, the term liquid biopsy (LB) has been introduced by Pantel and Alix-Panabieres [11] as a minimally invasive way for tissue sampling, which allows for analysis of tumor cells or tumor cell products (e.g., cell-free circulating nucleic acids (ctDNA, cfRNA), extracellular vesicles, or proteins) released from primary or metastatic tumor lesions into blood or other body fluids [12]. Here, we discuss recently published reports on CTCs and ctDNA (within the last five years) because these are the most prominent LB markers [12], and we restricted our review to studies in patients with colorectal carcinoma as one of the most common solid tumors worldwide [13]. Following a brief introduction of CTC and ctDNA technologies, we will focus on the current clinical applications of these biomarkers, including early detection, risk assessment, and monitoring of cancer therapies.

2. Technologies for CTC and ctDNA Analyses

Before discussing the clinical applications, we would like to give a brief overview of the methods used for the enumeration and characterization of CTCs and ctDNA.

2.1. CTCs

Working with CTCs includes the following three analytical steps: enrichment, detection, and analysis. Enrichment includes label-dependent approaches based on antibodies used for positive or negative enrichment of CTCs as well as label-independent technologies (e.g., size exclusion by microfiltration, in which blood is passed through filters with small pores or microfluidic chips calibrated to capture CTCs). Effective enrichment exploits differences between tumor cells and normal blood cells, such as differential expression of tumor-associated cell surface proteins (e.g., EpCAM, mucin-1, HER2, or epithelial growth factor receptor (EGFR)) or distinct physical properties (e.g., larger size or reduced deformability) of tumor cells [14]. In contrast, negative enrichment approaches enrich CTCs by the depletion of normal blood cells that are removed by antibodies against antigens expressed on leukocytes or circulating endothelial cells [15]. Besides the capture of single tumor cells, CTC clusters have attracted recent attention [13,16].

CTCs can be identified by the use of specific tumor-associated or tissue-specific proteins such as keratins in patients with carcinomas. However, keratins (and other epithelial markers) can be downregulated or lost during an epithelial-mesenchymal transition (EMT) of the tumor cells, which can lead to false-negative findings [17]. Therefore, new markers are being sought out that are neither downregulated during EMT nor expressed on normal blood cells.

In the last decade, individual CTCs or CTC clusters could be analyzed downstream at the DNA, RNA, or protein level. Separation of individual CTCs can be achieved by manual micromanipulation or automated DEP array technology, but usually, a sufficiently high initial CTC concentration is required [18]. The whole genome amplification (WGA) method has been used to perform DNA analysis on a single cell level to generate a sufficient amount of DNA for subsequent sequencing analysis. However, WGA causes bias; thus, new methods avoiding WGA are currently being developed. In addition to RNA sequencing, multiplex real-time polymerase chain reaction can already provide some insights into the heterogeneity of CTCs [19]. In addition to protein-level analysis using immunostaining, new multiplex proteomics approaches are under development.

In addition to descriptive methods, there are functional CTC analyses, such as epithelial immune SPOT, which is based on the measurement of secreted proteins by live CTCs after short-term culture. In patients with extremely high numbers of CTCs (usually > 100/mL of blood), the functional properties of CTCs can be further investigated by establishing long-term cell cultures/cell lines or CTC-derived xenograft models [20,21]. These models provide unique insights into the functional properties of CTCs but the success rate of establishing these models needs to be improved to use them for drug screening in clinical trials or decision making for individual patients in advanced disease stages.

2.2. ctDNA

Circulating free DNA (cfDNA) is released by both normal and tumor cells to the blood circulation mainly through cellular necrosis and apoptosis but active secretion through EVs may also play a role [22]. cfDNA consists mostly of 166 bp, which is consistent with the length of a DNA fragment wrapped around a nucleosome. In cancer patients, a small portion of cfDNA (usually 0.01–5%) is shed into the blood by tumor cells; this is called ctDNA (ctDNA, which is shed from tumor cells, represents a small portion of cfDNA (usually 0.01–5%)) [14]. ctDNA is cleared soon after entering the circulation due to its short half-life of two hours, allowing for non-invasive real-time tumor monitoring [23,24]. The molecular biological analysis allows for the identification and characterization of ctDNA. The following paragraph briefly delineates the types of ctDNA analyses depending on the objective of the planned investigation.

Plasma DNA can be analyzed by approaches targeting specific tumor-associated genes (e.g., mutations in the EGFR gene in non-small cell lung carcinoma (NSCLC)) or non-targeted screening approaches such as array CGH, whole-genome sequencing, or exome sequencing) [25,26]. In general, targeted approaches have higher analytical sensitivity than non-targeted approaches, but there are strong efforts to improve the detection limits of non-targeted approaches [27,28]. Ultrasensitive methods have been developed for the detection of minute amounts of 0.01% or less ctDNA in blood plasma (e.g., DELPHI, BEAMing Safe-SeqS, TamSeq, CAPP-Seq, and digital PCR) [12,29]. In addition to mutation analysis, reliable assays for assessing epigenetic changes such as DNA methylation have been developed in recent years for blood testing in several types of solid tumors including CRC [30–32].

3. Clinical Applications of Circulating Tumor Cells (CTCs)

CTCs have the potential to extravasate and seed metastases in distant organs, which is the most common reason for cancer-related death in CRC and other solid tumors. CTC analysis has the potential to be used as a biomarker for tumor detection, prognostication, therapy monitoring, and to tailor appropriate individualized treatments (Figure 1). The following chapter illustrates the latest developments of CTC-based clinical studies in CRC [33].

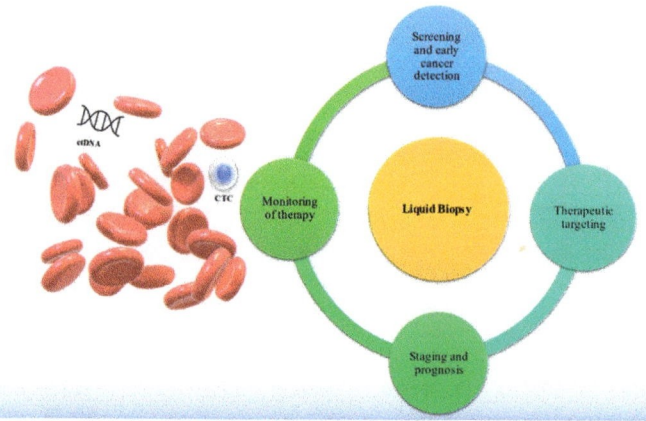

Figure 1. Clinical applications of liquid biopsies. Clinical hallmark applications of liquid biopsy (LB): (1) screening and early cancer detection, (2) therapeutic targeting, (3) staging and prognosis, and (4) monitoring of therapy. LB allows for the portrayal of the entire disease by using blood-based tumor-specific biomarkers, such as circulating tumor cells (CTCs) and circulating tumor DNA (ctDNA) released from all metastatic or primary tumor sites to provide comprehensive and real-time information on tumor cell evolution, therapeutic targets, and mechanisms of resistance to therapy.

3.1. Early Detection of Cancer

The ideal screening tool should be reproducible and efficient with high sensitivity and specificity. The detection of CTCs in CRC is still infrequent and limited. According to Bork et al., the detection of CTCs in nodal negative CRC (UICC stage I–II) is as low as 9% [34,35]. In another study, the detection of CTCs using Cellsearch® in CRC (UICC stage I–IV) was 45% [26]. Therefore, the utility of CTC-based screening using Cellsearch® is still rather challenging and still not applicable (Table 1).

Table 1. Overview of relevant studies for the detection of CTC in CRC using different isolation methods and their outcome. OS, overall survival. PFS, progression-free survival. HR, Hazard Ratio. CI, Confidence Interval.

Author Country (Year) [Reference]	Tumor Stage (UICC)	Number of Patients and Detection Rate n, (Percentage%)	Method	Sampling Time	Clinical Outcome
Abdalla et al. Germany 2021 [26]	I–IV data	68, 31 (45%) preoperatively	Cellsearch® data	pre- and postoperative	Multivariate analyses showed that only preoperative detection of ≥1 CTCs/7.5 mL is an independent prognostic indicator for OS (HR 3.14; CI 1.18–8.32; p = 0.021).
Silva et al. Brazil 2021 [36]	IV	75, 45 (60%)	ISET®	pretherapeutic	In multivariate analysis, presence of ≥1.5 CTCs/mL was associated with worse OS (HR 2.34, CI 1.11–4.9, p = 0.025).
Kust et al. Croatia 2016 [37]	I–III	82, 69 (72.6%) preoperatively 74 (77.9%) postoperatively	RT-PCR	preoperative and postoperative	PFS was significantly shorter in patients with CK20-positive CTCs postoperatively in comparison to patients negative for CK20 postoperatively (p = 0.01, log-rank test). CTC detection was not significant in multivariate analysis outcome.
Sotelo et al. Spain 2015 [38]	I–III	519, 166 (35%)	Cellsearch®	postoperative and pretherapeutic	≥1 CTCs/7.5 mL was not associated with worse PFS (HR 0.97, CI 0.68–1.38, p = 0.85) or OS (HR 1.03, CI 0.66–1.59, p = 0.89).
Bork et al. Germany 2015 [34]	I–IV	287, 30 (10.5%)	Cellsearch®	pre- and postoperative	Multivariate analysis showed that preoperative detection ≥ 1 CTCs/7.5 mL was associated with worse OS (HR 5.5; CI 2.3–13.6; p = 0.001) and PFS (HR 12.7; CI 5.2–31.1; p = 0.001) in stage I–III CRC as well as worse OS (HR 5.6; CI 2.6–12.0; p = 0.001) and PFS (HR 7.8; CI 3.9–15.5; p = 0.001) in stages I–IV.
Seeberg et al. Norway 2015 [39]	IV	194, 37 (19.6%)	Cellsearch®	preoperative	In multivariate analysis, the presence of ≥2 CTCs/7.5 mL at baseline was associated with worse PFS (HR 2.32, CI 1.26–4.27, p = 0.007) and OS (HR 2.48, CI 1.40–4.38, p = 0.002)
Yokobori et al. Japan 2013 [40]	I–IV	711, 179 (33.6%)	RT-PCR	preoperative	Multivariate analysis showed that PLS3-positive CTCs are associated with poor OS (HR 2.17; CI 1.38–3.40) and PFS (HR 2.32, CI 1.42–3.74).
Cohen et al. US, Netherlands, and UK 2008 [41]	IV	430, ≥1 CTCs, 198 (48%). ≥3 CTCs, 108 (26%)	Cellsearch®	Pre- and post-therapeutic	In multivariate analyses, patients with ≥3 CTCs/7.5 mL at baseline had shorter PFS (HR 1.74, CI 1.33–2.26, p ≤ 0.001), and OS (HR 2.45, CI 1.77–3.39, p ≤ 0.001).

In 2018, Tsai et al. reported for the first time that CTCs could be used for early cancer detection. This prospective study was conducted on 620 subjects including 438 with precancerous lesions or CRC (UICC stage I–IV) and 182 healthy controls. CTC detection was performed using the Cellmax platform, which uses a microfluidic anti-EpCAM-antibody-coated biochip. In precancerous lesions, CTCs showed a sensitivity of 76.6%, a specificity of 97.3%, and an area under the curve (AUC) of 0.84. In patients with CRC, CTC showed a sensitivity of 86.9%, specificity of 97.3%, and AUC of 0.88 [42]. Despite the promising results, larger validation studies are needed before the implementation of CTC-based screening using Cellmax in CRC.

3.2. Prediction of Treatment Response and Survival

Mesenteric venous blood compartments of patients with CRC harbor more CTCs than the peripheral blood, which might be explained by the fact that viable CTCs can home to the liver, frequently leading to liver metastasis in CRC [43]. In advanced CRC, several studies have shown that CTC count before and during treatment predicts PFS and OS and provides additional information beyond CT imaging [44–46], whereas surgical resection of metastases immediately lowers CTC levels [47]. Patients with elevated CTC count, even when classified as responders by CT imaging, showed significantly shorter survival (Table 1) [35].

In patients who underwent curative resection (stage III) followed by FOLFOX chemotherapy, CTC count predicted relapse after chemotherapy [48]. In nonmetastatic CRC, preoperative CTC detection is an independent prognostic marker [34], and CTC count correlated with reduced DFS [49]. Thus, CTC detection could help select high-risk stage II CRC candidates for adjuvant chemotherapy [50,51]. Interventional studies are now needed to assess whether stage II patients with CTCs benefit from chemotherapy. Recently, Aranda et al. evaluated whether CTC counts may be a useful non-invasive biomarker to assist with the selection of patients for intensive therapy with FOLFOXIRI-bevacizumab. This combination is more effective than FOLOFOX plus bevacizumab but is not widely used because of concerns about toxicity and so far a lack of predictive biomarkers. In their phase III study in patients with previously untreated, unresectable metastatic CRC, Aranda et al. found that first-line FOLFOXIRI-bevacizumab significantly improved PFS compared with FOLFOX-bevacizumab in patients with metastatic CRC who presented with ≥ 3 CTCs at baseline [52].

Thus, CTC enumeration can contribute to the identification of a high-risk group of CRC patients who might profit from more intense therapy.

3.3. Molecular and Functional Characterization of CTCs

KRAS, BRAF, and PIK3CA mutations are important determinants of CRC patients' response to targeted therapies. For example, blocking EGFR signaling by an antibody therapy in CRC is inefficient in patients with mutated KRAS tumors, which provide a stimulatory signal downstream of EGFR. In-depth analysis of individual CTCs from patients with CRC revealed the striking heterogeneity of KRAS status within and between patients [53,54], and the occurrence and concordance of these mutations in metastatic CRC may vary between primary tumors, CTCs, and metastatic tumors [54–56]. When KRAS mutations in CTCs from patients with metastatic CRC were examined throughout disease progression and compared with their corresponding primary tumors, CTCs had different KRAS mutations during treatment [57]. Thus, CTCs are promising markers for evaluating and predicting treatment response in patients with rectal cancer superior to carcinoembryonic antigen [58]. Liquid biopsy analyses might also lead to the discovery of new targets. For example, the comparative analyses of blood from healthy controls, patients with polyps and adenomas, and cancer patients revealed that lncRNA SNHG11 might serve as a novel therapeutic target in CRC [59].

Among cancer therapies, the new era of immunotherapy has opened new avenues for the treatment of cancer patients; although, the benefits for CRC patients are still limited, which might—among other reasons—result also from a lack of appropriate predictive markers. Changes in the composition of immune cells in the tumor lesion may also affect the release of CTC into the blood. Microsatellite instability in CRC is a marker of immunogenicity and is associated with an increased abundance of tumor-infiltrating lymphocytes. Recently, Toh et al. found that microsatellite instability was associated with an increase in CTC numbers intra-operatively and post-operatively when combining data for all stage I–III CRC patients [60].

Functional CTC analysis using cell lines and xenograft models may also help to find appropriate targets or pathways for therapeutic intervention. Recent study results by Smit et al. showed that the PI3K/AKT/mTOR signaling pathway plays a key role in the proliferation of metastatic CRC [61]. They investigated a functional role of this pathway in a metastatic CRC cell line called CTC-MCC-41 and suggested that therapies targeting AKT and mTOR could be beneficial for targeting CTCs in CRC and possibly other tumor types [61]. Functional CRC models also provide a unique opportunity to study the biology of CTCs. In CRC, hierarchical organization is maintained during disease progression, and functional cancer stem cells are marked by Lgr5 expression. Fumagalli et al. aimed to investigate the cell of origin of metastases in CRC by using a mouse model of CRC and human tumor xenografts. Given that most disseminating cells were Lgr5− and could initiate metastatic growth, this leads to the assumption that the majority of metastases are seeded by Lgr5− cancer cells. Furthermore, the appearance of Lgr5+ CSCs is indispensable for the outgrowth of metastases founded by Lgr5− cancer cells. Their data indicate that besides targeting CSC and the CSC inducing niche, there is also a need to co-target endogenous cellular plasticity to inactivate any potential seeds of metastasis [62].

4. Clinical Applications of Circulating Cell-Free DNA

The quantity of ctDNA varies among individual patients and depends on the type and location of the primary or metastatic tumor lesion and the stage of the disease. The implementation of ctDNA in clinical practice holds great potential for early detection and personalized medicine in CRC [33,59]. The following chapter illustrates the latest clinical developments of using ctDNA as a biomarker in patients with CRC.

4.1. Early Detection of Cancer

ctDNA measurements hold promise for early detection in CRC and offer the possibility to address the heterogeneity of the tumor (Figure 1).

To encompass tumor heterogeneity, a complex blood test based on the detection of more than 1000 mutations in 16 cancer genes was combined with the measurement of eight tumor-associated blood plasma proteins. The so-called CancerSEEK-Test can detect CRC through assessment of the levels of circulating proteins and mutations in cell-free DNA and reached a sensitivity of more than 60% for CRC detection. The advantages of this test are the non-invasive screening by blood sampling (versus colonoscopy) and the low cost compared to the approved tests [63].

There is also a potential use of ctDNA methylation markers for early diagnosis of CRC. Luo et al. determine that a single ctDNA methylation marker, cg10673833, could yield high sensitivity (89.7%) and specificity (86.8%) for the detection of CRC and precancerous lesions in a high-risk population of 1493 participants in a prospective cohort study, which underlines the value of ctDNA methylation markers in the diagnosis, surveillance, and prognosis of CRC [31].

Future large-scale studies have to demonstrate that the ctDNA blood tests will add important information or easier acceptance by the individuals at risk than the established CRC screening tests including improved stool tests for occult blood and colonoscopy.

4.2. Assessment of Tumor Evolution towards Resistance to Therapy

The development of individualized treatment strategies might also profit from ctDNA analyses, in particular with regard to a better molecular understanding of resistance to therapy through ctDNA monitoring [64]. Despite a high degree of concordance between the mutational status of KRAS in tumor tissue and ctDNA [65,66], ctDNA can sometimes harbor KRAS mutations that are not detected in the primary lesion [25]. Sequential ctDNA analysis during EGFR inhibition has shown that KRAS and NRAS mutations can emerge rapidly due to the selective pressure exerted by targeted therapy [67]. Interestingly, the emerging population of KRAS-mutated subclones was able to decline after discontinuation of anti-EGFR therapy [67], indicating the potential to guide "cyclic therapy" characterized by sequential discontinuation and reintroduction of EGFR inhibitors based on ctDNA analyses. Patient-specific ctDNA assays can be developed through mutational analyses of primary tumors [68]. In addition, ctDNA analyses also helped to distinguish recurrent CRC from a second primary tumor [68].

ctDNA blood analysis can be complemented by tissue DNA analysis in case of a LB-negative result, which saves LB-positive patients from the unnecessary side effects of needle biopsies, and this strategy also appears to be a cost saving, in particular in the context of monitoring resistance to anti-EGFR-targeted therapies [69]. ctDNA genotyping has the potential to accelerate innovation in precision medicine and its delivery to individual patients. By evaluating the utility of ctDNA genotyping, Nakamura et al. enrolled 1687 patients with advanced gastrointestinal cancer and showed a significant shorter screening duration for patients undergoing ctDNA genotyping, which had a positive effect on trial enrollment without negative effects on treatment efficacy compared to tissue genotyping. Moreover, new candidates for potential clinical development were discovered through in-depth analysis of the ctDNA profiles [70].

4.3. Early Detection of Molecular Relapse by ctDNA Surveillance

Surveillance of ctDNA concentrations by sequential blood testing following the initial treatment (e.g., surgery, radiation, or (neo)adjuvant therapy) is another important clinical application of LB [71]. LB in early-stage, non-metastatic CRC must be sensitive enough to detect extremely low ctDNA levels. This challenge has been met by combining next-generation sequencing (NGS) and digital PCR (dPCR) to detect ctDNAs in non-metastatic CRC patients ($n = 39$); the NGS/dPCR test reached a sensitivity of 63.6% when combined with circulating carcinoembryonic antigen protein measurements [72]. ctDNA responders could be identified by monitoring ctDNA levels before and during chemotherapy including 1046 plasma samples from 230 patients with stage II colon cancer [73]. ctDNA analyzed by NGS was revealed post-surgery in 14 (7.9%) of 178 patients who did not receive adjuvant chemotherapy. Twenty-seven months later, ctDNA-positive patients had higher recurrence rates than ctDNA-negative patients, and a similar prognostic value was observed after completion of adjuvant chemotherapy [73].

Furthermore, ctDNA also identified patients at risk of developing metastases during neoadjuvant therapy and post-surgery. In the study of Khakoo et al., ctDNA detection rates were 74% ($n = 35/47$) before treatment, 21% ($n = 10/47$) at mid chemoradiotherapy (CRT), 21% ($n = 10/47$) after completing CRT, and 13% ($n = 3/23$) after surgery. Following 26.4 months of observation, ctDNA-positive patients had an unfavorable metastases-free survival [HR 7.1; 95% confidence interval (CI), 2.4–21.5; $p < 0.001$], as compared to ctDNA-negative patients [74]. In addition, a prospective multicenter trial that recruited 106 patients with locally advanced rectal cancer for treatment with nCRT followed by surgery ctDNA suggested that the median variant allele frequency of baseline ctDNA and ctDNA positivity at all four time points (baseline, during neoadjuvant CRT, pre-surgery, and post-surgery) is also a strong independent predictor of metastasis-free survival ($p < 0.05$) [75].

Taken together, these findings lead to the conclusion that ctDNA monitoring identified patients at risk of developing metastases during the neoadjuvant period and after surgery in CRC patients.

5. Conclusions and Perspectives

This review illustrates the latest developments in clinical applications of CTC and ctDNA as LB markers in CRC. LB enables the development of new methods for the early detection of primary cancer or minimal residual disease (MRD), monitoring the efficacy of cancer therapies, and determining therapeutic targets and resistance mechanisms to tailor therapy to the specific needs of an individual patient. Significant progress has been made in developing technologies to detect blood-based tumor-specific biomarkers, such as CTCs and ctDNA, and in developing downstream analyses of CTCs and ctDNA to provide new information about natural or therapy-induced tumor evolution in cancer patients. In addition, new members of the LB marker family include extracellular vesicles (EVs) [76], microRNAs [77], and tumor-derived platelets [78]. The newest findings have shown that miRNAs play an important role in many signal pathways. Dysregulated expression of several miRNA expressions is associated with a higher malignant potential and poor clinical response to therapy, and analysis of specific miRNA expression patterns can be used to predict chemotherapy efficacy [79–81]. miRNAs can also be detected in CTCs and contribute to a better understanding of the biology and clinical value of these cells [82]. Besides miRNA, increasing evidence has confirmed that EVs play a significant role in intercellular communication in CRC. EVs enable tumor communication and manipulation between tumor cells and the host immune system or the tumor microenvironment and can be induced by various cell signals such as hypoxia [83,84]. Both EVs and circulating miRNAs have great potential as biomarkers in cancer patients including CRC [77,78]. Besides tumor-derived cells and products, the peripheral blood is also a pool of host-derived cells (e.g., circulating immune cells, endothelial cells or fibroblasts) and cellular products (e.g., EVs from immune cells that may affect the immune response) [83]. Future studies on the interaction between CTCs and host cells might provide further insights into tumor biology with potential implications for the discovery of new prognostic and predictive biomarkers.

Immune checkpoint inhibition therapy has opened a new therapeutic avenue in oncology. However, only a fraction of patients will benefit so far from harnessing the immune response through the application of antibodies to inhibition checkpoint such as PDL1 or PD1, but the discovery of new checkpoints such as TGIT will offer new opportunities [85]. The utility of liquid biomarkers such as CTCs and ctDNA as prognostic and in particular predictive markers in the context of immunotherapies in solid tumors including gastrointestinal cancers have been recently reviewed in detail [86]. While ctDNA offers the possibility to determine the tumor mutational burden as potential (but still debated) predictive factor, CTC analysis can enlarge the spectrum by the detection of proteins relevant for the immune response such as MHC antigens or PDL1 on tumor cells responsible for the recognition or activation of T cells [87]. Interestingly, the expression of carcinoembryonic antigen and telomerase reverse transcriptase in CTCs predicted an unfavorable response to nivolumab, a PD1 inhibiting antibody [87].

To implement LB into clinical practice, harmonized protocols need to be developed. In this context, the EU-based CANCER-ID consortium has recently validated pre-analytical and analytical conditions of LB assays for CTCs [88], ctDNA [82], and microRNAs [83]. The activities of CANCER-ID are sustained by the new consortium designated European Society for LB (ELBS, www.elbs.eu, accessed on 4 September 2021), which is part of the International Alliance for LB Standardization [84].

Most importantly, the clinical utility of standardized LB assays needs to be proven in future interventional clinical trials. Previous studies have shown that CTC and ctDNA detection at the time of CRC diagnosis defines a subgroup of stage II patients at higher risk to develop relapse; however, it remains to be seen if these patients will benefit from more aggressive therapy. As another example, postoperative LB surveillance has been shown to be able to detect early molecular relapse many months before radiological imaging, but the key question is whether an earlier intervention based on the LB result leads to a survival benefit for CRC patients. Clinical trials addressing these (and other) relevant questions will open new avenues for introducing LB into future guidelines for the personalized treatment of CRC patients.

Author Contributions: Design, data analysis, and manuscript writing: I.H., T.S.A.A., M.R., K.P. All authors have read and agreed to the published version of the manuscript.

Funding: This work was supported by the ERC Advanced Investigator Grant INJURMET (K.P., No. 834974).

Conflicts of Interest: The authors declare no conflict of interest.

Abbreviations

cfDNA	circulating free DNA
CI	confidence interval
ctDNA	circulating tumor-derived DNA
CTC	circulating tumor cell
CRC	colorectal cancer
CRT	chemoradiotherapy
DEP	dielectrophoresis
DFS	disease-free survival
EGFR	epithelial growth factor receptor
EMT	epithelial-mesenchymal transition
EpCAM	epithelial cell adhesion molecule
EPISPOT	epithelial immune SPOT
EV	extracellular vesicle
FOLFOX	folinic acid, fluorouracil and oxaliplatin
FOLFOXIRI	fluorouracil, folinate, oxaliplatin, and irinotecan
HR	hazard ratio
HER2	human epidermal growth factor receptor 2
LB	liquid biopsy
MRD	minimal residual disease
mRNA	messenger RNA mRNA
NGS	next generation sequencing NSCLC, non-small cell lung carcinoma
OS	overall survival
PFS	progression-free survival
rtPCR	real-time polymerase chain reaction
tDNA	tumor DNAs
WGA	whole genome amplification

References

1. Sung, H.; Ferlay, J.; Siegel, R.L.; Laversanne, M.; Soerjomataram, I.; Jemal, A.; Bray, F. Global Cancer Statistics 2020: GLO-BOCAN Estimates of Incidence and Mortality Worldwide for 36 Cancers in 185 Countries. *CA-Cancer J. Clin.* **2021**, *71*, 209–249. [CrossRef]
2. Arnold, M.; Sierra, M.S.; Laversanne, M.; Soerjomataram, I.; Jemal, A.; Bray, F. Global Patterns and Trends in Colorectal Cancer Incidence and Mortality. *Gut* **2017**, *66*, 683–691. [CrossRef]
3. Kaminski, M.F.; Robertson, D.J.; Senore, C.; Rex, D.K. Optimizing the Quality of Colorectal Cancer Screening Worldwide. *Gastroenterology* **2020**, *158*, 404–417. [CrossRef]
4. Hohenberger, W.; Weber, K.; Matzel, K.; Papadopoulos, T.; Merkel, S. Standardized Surgery for Colonic Cancer: Complete Mesocolic Excision and Central Ligation—Technical Notes and Outcome. *Colorectal Dis.* **2009**, *11*, 354–364. [CrossRef]
5. Heald, R.J.; Santiago, I.; Pares, O.; Carvalho, C.; Figueiredo, N. The Perfect Total Mesorectal Excision Obviates the Need for Anything Else in the Management of Most Rectal Cancers. *Clin. Colon. Rectal. Surg.* **2017**, *30*, 324–332. [CrossRef]
6. Franke, A.J.; Skelton, W.P.; Starr, J.S.; Parekh, H.; Lee, J.J.; Overman, M.J.; Allegra, C.; George, T.J. Immunotherapy for Colo-rectal Cancer: A Review of Current and Novel Therapeutic Approaches. *J. Natl. Cancer Inst.* **2019**, *111*, 1131–1141. [CrossRef] [PubMed]
7. Surveillance, Epidemiology, and End Results (SEER) Program. SEER*Stat Database: North American Association of Central Cancer Registries (NAACCR) Incidence–CiNA Analytic File, 1995–2016, for NHIAv2 Origin, Custom File with County, ACS Facts and Figures projection Project. NAACCR. 2019. Available online: cancer.gov (accessed on 4 September 2021).
8. Siegel, R.L.; Miller, K.D.; Goding Sauer, A.; Fedewa, S.A.; Butterly, L.F.; Anderson, J.C.; Cercek, A.; Smith, R.A.; Jemal, A. Colorectal cancer statistics. *CA A Cancer J. Clin.* **2020**, *70*, 145–164. [CrossRef]
9. AJCC Cancer Staging Manual; Edge, S.B. *American Joint Committee on Cancer*, 7th ed.; Springer: New York, NY, USA, 2010; ISBN 978-0-387-88440-0.

10. Punt, C.J.A.; Koopman, M.; Vermeulen, L. From Tumour Heterogeneity to Advances in Precision Treatment of Colorectal Cancer. *Nat. Rev. Clin. Oncol.* **2017**, *14*, 235–246. [CrossRef] [PubMed]
11. Pantel, K.; Alix-Panabières, C. Circulating Tumour Cells in Cancer Patients: Challenges and Perspectives. *Trends Mol. Med.* **2010**, *16*, 398–406. [CrossRef] [PubMed]
12. Alix-Panabières, C.; Pantel, K. Liquid Biopsy: From Discovery to Clinical Application. *Cancer Discov.* **2021**, *11*, 858–873. [CrossRef] [PubMed]
13. Donato, C.; Kunz, L.; Castro-Giner, F.; Paasinen-Sohns, A.; Strittmatter, K.; Szczerba, B.M.; Scherrer, R.; Di Maggio, N.; Heusermann, W.; Biehlmaier, O.; et al. Hypoxia Triggers the Intravasation of Clustered Circulating Tumor Cells. *Cell Rep.* **2020**, *32*, 108105. [CrossRef]
14. Pantel, K.; Alix-Panabières, C. Liquid Biopsy and Minimal Residual Disease-Latest Advances and Implications for Cure. *Nat. Rev. Clin. Oncol.* **2019**, *16*, 409–424. [CrossRef] [PubMed]
15. Keller, L.; Pantel, K. Unravelling Tumour Heterogeneity by Single-Cell Profiling of Circulating Tumour Cells. *Nat. Rev. Cancer* **2019**, *19*, 553–567. [CrossRef] [PubMed]
16. Szczerba, B.M.; Castro-Giner, F.; Vetter, M.; Krol, I.; Gkountela, S.; Landin, J.; Scheidmann, M.C.; Donato, C.; Scherrer, R.; Singer, J.; et al. Neutrophils Escort Circulating Tumour Cells to Enable Cell Cycle Progression. *Nature* **2019**, *566*, 553–557. [CrossRef]
17. Alix-Panabières, C.; Mader, S.; Pantel, K. Epithelial-mesenchymal plasticity in circulating tumor cells. *J. Mol. Med.* **2017**, *95*, 133–142. [CrossRef] [PubMed]
18. Joosse, S.A.; Gorges, T.M.; Pantel, K. Biology, Detection, and Clinical Implications of Circulating Tumor Cells. *EMBO Mol. Med.* **2015**, *7*, 1–11. [CrossRef] [PubMed]
19. Gorges, T.M.; Kuske, A.; Röck, K.; Mauermann, O.; Müller, V.; Peine, S.; Verpoort, K.; Novosadova, V.; Kubista, M.; Riethdorf, S.; et al. Accession of Tumor Heterogeneity by Multiplex Transcriptome Profiling of Single Circulating Tumor Cells. *Clin. Chem.* **2016**, *62*, 1504–1515. [CrossRef] [PubMed]
20. Soler, A.; Cayrefourcq, L.; Mazard, T.; Babayan, A.; Lamy, P.-J.; Assou, S.; Assenat, E.; Pantel, K.; Alix-Panabières, C. Autol-ogous Cell Lines from Circulating Colon Cancer Cells Captured from Sequential Liquid Biopsies as Model to Study Therapy-Driven Tumor Changes. *Sci. Rep.* **2018**, *8*, 15931. [CrossRef]
21. Koch, C.; Kuske, A.; Joosse, S.A.; Yigit, G.; Sflomos, G.; Thaler, S.; Smit, D.J.; Werner, S.; Borgmann, K.; Gärtner, S.; et al. Characterization of Circulating Breast Cancer Cells with Tumorigenic and Metastatic Capacity. *EMBO Mol. Med.* **2020**, *12*, e11908. [CrossRef]
22. Lo, Y.M.D.; Han, D.S.C.; Jiang, P.; Chiu, R.W.K. Epigenetics, Fragmentomics, and Topology of Cell-Free DNA in Liquid Biopsies. *Science* **2021**, *372*, eaaw3616. [CrossRef]
23. Diehl, F.; Schmidt, K.; Choti, M.A.; Romans, K.; Goodman, S.; Li, M.; Thornton, K.; Agrawal, N.; Sokoll, L.; Szabo, S.A.; et al. Circulating Mutant DNA to Assess Tumor Dynamics. *Nat. Med.* **2008**, *14*, 985–990. [CrossRef]
24. Naidoo, M.; Gibbs, P.; Tie, J. CtDNA and Adjuvant Therapy for Colorectal Cancer: Time to Re-Invent Our Treatment Paradigm. *Cancers* **2021**, *13*, 346. [CrossRef] [PubMed]
25. Heitzer, E.; Ulz, P.; Geigl, J.B. Circulating Tumor DNA as a Liquid Biopsy for Cancer. *Clin. Chem.* **2015**, *61*, 112–123. [CrossRef] [PubMed]
26. Abdalla, T.S.A.; Meiners, J.; Riethdorf, S.; König, A.; Melling, N.; Gorges, T.; Karstens, K.-F.; Izbicki, J.R.; Pantel, K.; Reeh, M. Prognostic Value of Preoperative Circulating Tumour Cells Counts in Patients with UICC Stage I-IV Colorectal Cancer. *PLoS ONE* **2021**, *16*, e0252897. [CrossRef] [PubMed]
27. Wan, J.C.M.; Heider, K.; Gale, D.; Murphy, S.; Fisher, E.; Mouliere, F.; Ruiz-Valdepenas, A.; Santonja, A.; Morris, J.; Chandrananda, D.; et al. CtDNA Monitoring Using Patient-Specific Sequencing and Integration of Variant Reads. *Sci. Transl. Med.* **2020**, *12*, eaaz8084. [CrossRef]
28. Cristiano, S.; Leal, A.; Phallen, J.; Fiksel, J.; Adleff, V.; Bruhm, D.C.; Jensen, S.Ø.; Medina, J.E.; Hruban, C.; White, J.R.; et al. Genome-Wide Cell-Free DNA Fragmentation in Patients with Cancer. *Nature* **2019**, *570*, 385–389. [CrossRef] [PubMed]
29. Heitzer, E.; Haque, I.S.; Roberts, C.E.S.; Speicher, M.R. Current and Future Perspectives of Liquid Biopsies in Genomics-Driven Oncology. *Nat. Rev. Genet.* **2019**, *20*, 71–88. [CrossRef] [PubMed]
30. Liu, M.C.; Oxnard, G.R.; Klein, E.A.; Swanton, C.; Seiden, M.V. CCGA Consortium Sensitive and Specific Multi-Cancer Detection and Localization Using Methylation Signatures in Cell-Free DNA. *Ann. Oncol.* **2020**, *31*, 745–759. [CrossRef] [PubMed]
31. Luo, H.; Zhao, Q.; Wei, W.; Zheng, L.; Yi, S.; Li, G.; Wang, W.; Sheng, H.; Pu, H.; Mo, H.; et al. Circulating Tumor DNA Methylation Profiles Enable Early Diagnosis, Prognosis Prediction, and Screening for Colorectal Cancer. *Sci. Transl. Med.* **2020**, *12*, eaax7533. [CrossRef] [PubMed]
32. Keller, L.; Belloum, Y.; Wikman, H.; Pantel, K. Clinical Relevance of Blood-Based CtDNA Analysis: Mutation Detection and Beyond. *Br. J. Canc.* **2021**, *124*, 345–358. [CrossRef]
33. Bardelli, A.; Pantel, K. Liquid Biopsies, What We Do Not Know (Yet). *Cancer Cell* **2017**, *31*, 172–179. [CrossRef] [PubMed]
34. Bork, U.; Rahbari, N.N.; Schölch, S.; Reissfelder, C.; Kahlert, C.; Büchler, M.W.; Weitz, J.; Koch, M. Circulating Tumour Cells and Outcome in Non-Metastatic Colorectal Cancer: A Prospective Study. *Br. J. Cancer* **2015**, *112*, 1306–1313. [CrossRef] [PubMed]
35. Barbazán, J.; Muinelo-Romay, L.; Vieito, M.; Candamio, S.; Díaz-López, A.; Cano, A.; Gómez-Tato, A.; de los Ángeles Casares de Cal, M.; Abal, M.; López-López, R. A Multimarker Panel for Circulating Tumor Cells Detection Predicts Patient Outcome and Therapy Response in Metastatic Colorectal Cancer. *Int. J. Cancer* **2014**, *135*, 2633–2643. [CrossRef]

36. Silva, V.S.E.; Abdallah, E.A.; de Brito, A.B.C.; Braun, A.C.; Tariki, M.S.; de Mello, C.A.L.; Calsavara, V.F.; Riechelmann, R.; Chinen, L.T.D. Baseline and Kinetic Circulating Tumor Cell Counts Are Prognostic Factors in a Prospective Study of Meta-static Colorectal Cancer. *Diagnostics* **2021**, *11*, 502. [CrossRef]
37. Kust, D.; Šamija, I.; Kirac, I.; Radić, J.; Kovačević, D.; Kusić, Z. Cytokeratin 20 Positive Cells in Blood of Colorectal Cancer Patients as an Unfavorable Prognostic Marker. *Acta Clin. Belg.* **2016**, *71*, 235–243. [CrossRef]
38. Sotelo, M.J.; Sastre, J.; Maestro, M.L.; Veganzones, S.; Viéitez, J.M.; Alonso, V.; Grávalos, C.; Escudero, P.; Vera, R.; Aranda, E.; et al. Role of Circulating Tumor Cells as Prognostic Marker in Resected Stage III Colorectal Cancer. *Ann. Oncol.* **2015**, *26*, 535–541. [CrossRef]
39. Seeberg, L.T.; Waage, A.; Brunborg, C.; Hugenschmidt, H.; Renolen, A.; Stav, I.; Bjørnbeth, B.A.; Brudvik, K.W.; Borgen, E.F.; Naume, B.; et al. Circulating Tumor Cells in Patients with Colorectal Liver Metastasis Predict Impaired Survival. *Ann. Surg.* **2015**, *261*, 164–171. [CrossRef]
40. Yokobori, T.; Iinuma, H.; Shimamura, T.; Imoto, S.; Sugimachi, K.; Ishii, H.; Iwatsuki, M.; Ota, D.; Ohkuma, M.; Iwaya, T.; et al. Plastin3 Is a Novel Marker for Circulating Tumor Cells Undergoing the Epithelial-Mesenchymal Transition and Is Associ-ated with Colorectal Cancer Prognosis. *Cancer Res.* **2013**, *73*, 2059–2069. [CrossRef] [PubMed]
41. Cohen, S.J.; Punt, C.J.A.; Iannotti, N.; Saidman, B.H.; Sabbath, K.D.; Gabrail, N.Y.; Picus, J.; Morse, M.; Mitchell, E.; Miller, M.C.; et al. Relationship of Circulating Tumor Cells to Tumor Response, Progression-Free Survival, and Overall Survival in Patients with Metastatic Colorectal Cancer. *J. Clin. Oncol.* **2008**, *26*, 3213–3221. [CrossRef]
42. Tsai, W.-S.; Nimgaonkar, A.; Segurado, O.; Chang, Y.; Hsieh, B.; Shao, H.-J.; Wu, J.; Lai, J.-M.; Javey, M.; Watson, D.; et al. Prospective Clinical Study of Circulating Tumor Cells for Colorectal Cancer Screening. *JCO* **2018**, *36*, 556. [CrossRef]
43. Heidrich, I.; Ačkar, L.; Mohammadi, P.M.; Pantel, K. Liquid Biopsies: Potential and Challenges. *Int. J. Cancer* **2021**, *148*, 528–545. [CrossRef]
44. Matsusaka, S.; Suenaga, M.; Mishima, Y.; Takagi, K.; Terui, Y.; Mizunuma, N.; Hatake, K. Circulating Endothelial Cells Predict for Response to Bevacizumab-Based Chemotherapy in Metastatic Colorectal Cancer. *Cancer Chemother. Pharmacol.* **2011**, *68*, 763–768. [CrossRef]
45. Zhao, R.; Cai, Z.; Li, S.; Cheng, Y.; Gao, H.; Liu, F.; Wu, S.; Liu, S.; Dong, Y.; Zheng, L.; et al. Expression and clinical relevance of epithelial and mesenchymal markers in circulating tumor cells from colorectal cancer. *Oncotarget* **2017**, *8*, 9293. [CrossRef] [PubMed]
46. Schøler, L.V.; Reinert, T.; Ørntoft, M.-B.W.; Kassentoft, C.G.; Árnadóttir, S.; Vang, S.; Nordentoft, I.K.; Knudsen, M.; Lamy, P.; Andreasen, D.; et al. Clinical implications of monitoring circulating tumor DNA in patients with colorectal cancer. *Clin. Cancer Res.* **2017**, *23*, 5437–5445. [CrossRef] [PubMed]
47. Chou, W.-C.; Wu, M.-H.; Chang, P.-H.; Hsu, H.-C.; Chang, G.-J.; Huang, W.-K.; Wu, C.-E.; Hsieh, J.C.-H. A Prognostic Model Based on Circulating Tumour Cells is Useful for Identifying the Poorest Survival Outcome in Patients with Metastatic Colorectal Cancer. *Int. J. Biol. Sci.* **2018**, *14*, 137–146. [CrossRef]
48. Murray, N.P.; Aedo, S.; Villalon, R.; López, M.A.; Minzer, S.; Muñoz, L.; Orrego, S.; Contreras, L.; Arzeno, L.; Guzman, E. Effect of FOLFOX on minimal residual disease in Stage III colon cancer and risk of relapse. *Ecancermedicalscience* **2019**, *13*, 935. [CrossRef] [PubMed]
49. Tsai, W.-S.; Chen, J.-S.; Shao, H.-J.; Wu, J.-C.; Lai, J.-M.; Lu, S.-H.; Hung, T.-F.; Chiu, Y.-C.; You, J.-F.; Hsieh, P.-S.; et al. Circulating Tumor Cell Count Correlates with Colorectal Neoplasm Progression and Is a Prognostic Marker for Distant Metastasis in Non-Metastatic Patients. *Sci. Rep.* **2016**, *6*, 24517. [CrossRef]
50. Gazzaniga, P.; Gianni, W.; Raimondi, C.; Gradilone, A.; Lo Russo, G.; Longo, F.; Gandini, O.; Tomao, S.; Frati, L. Circulating Tumor Cells in High-Risk Nonmetastatic Colorectal Cancer. *Tumor. Biol.* **2013**, *34*, 2507–2509. [CrossRef] [PubMed]
51. Lu, Y.-J.; Wang, P.; Peng, J.; Wang, X.; Zhu, Y.-W.; Shen, N. Meta-analysis Reveals the Prognostic Value of Circulating Tumour Cells Detected in the Peripheral Blood in Patients with Non-Metastatic Colorectal Cancer. *Sci. Rep.* **2017**, *7*, 905. [CrossRef] [PubMed]
52. Aranda, E.; Viéitez, J.M.; Gómez-España, A.; Gil Calle, S.; Salud-Salvia, A.; Graña, B.; Garcia-Alfonso, P.; Rivera, F.; Quintero-Aldana, G.A.; Reina-Zoilo, J.J.; et al. Spanish Cooperative Group for the Treatment of Digestive Tumors (TTD). FOLFOXIRI plus bevacizumab versus FOLFOX plus bevacizumab for patients with metastatic colorectal cancer and ≥3 circulating tumour cells: The randomised phase III VISNÚ-1 trial. *ESMO Open* **2020**, *5*, e000944. [CrossRef]
53. Vivancos, A.; Aranda, E.; Benavides, M.; Elez, E.; Gómez-España, M.A.; Toledano, M.; Alvarez, M.; Parrado, M.R.C.; García-Barberán, V.; Diaz-Rubio, E. Comparison of the Clinical Sensitivity of the Idylla Platform and the OncoBEAM RAS CRC Assay for KRAS Mutation Detection in Liquid Biopsy Samples. *Sci. Rep.* **2019**, *9*, 8976. [CrossRef]
54. László, L.; Kurilla, A.; Takács, T.; Kudlik, G.; Koprivanacz, K.; Buday, L.; Vas, V. Recent Updates on the Significance of KRAS Mutations in Colorectal Cancer Biology. *Cells* **2021**, *10*, 667. [CrossRef]
55. Mohamed Suhaimi, N.-A.; Foong, Y.M.; Lee, D.Y.S.; Phyo, W.M.; Cima, I.; Lee, E.X.W.; Goh, W.L.; Lim, W.-Y.; Chia, K.S.; Kong, S.L.; et al. Non-invasive Sensitive Detection of KRAS and BRAF Mutation in Circulating Tumor Cells of Colorectal Cancer Patients. *Mol. Oncol.* **2015**, *9*, 850–860. [CrossRef]
56. Jung, H.R.; Oh, Y.; Na, D.; Min, S.; Kang, J.; Jang, D.; Shin, S.; Kim, J.; Lee, S.E.; Jeong, E.M.; et al. CRISPR screens identify a novel combination treatment targeting BCL-XL and WNT signaling for KRAS/BRAF-mutated colorectal cancers. *Oncogene* **2021**, *40*, 3287–3302. [CrossRef]

57. Kalikaki, A.; Politaki, H.; Souglakos, J.; Apostolaki, S.; Papadimitraki, E.; Georgoulia, N.; Tzardi, M.; Mavroudis, D.; Geor-goulias, V.; Voutsina, A. KRAS Genotypic Changes of Circulating Tumor Cells during Treatment of Patients with Metastatic Colorectal Cancer. *PLoS ONE* **2014**, *9*, e104902. [CrossRef]
58. Luo, H.; Shen, K.; Li, B.; Li, R.; Wang, Z.; Xie, Z. Clinical significance and diagnostic value of serum NSE, CEA, CA19-9, CA125 and CA242 levels in colorectal cancer. *Oncol. Lett.* **2020**, *20*, 742–750. [CrossRef] [PubMed]
59. Xu, W.; Zhou, G.; Wang, H.; Liu, Y.; Chen, B.; Chen, W.; Lin, C.; Wu, S.; Gong, A.; Xu, M. Circulating LncRNA SNHG11 as a Novel Biomarker for Early Diagnosis and Prognosis of Colorectal Cancer. *Int. J. Cancer* **2020**, *146*, 2901–2912. [CrossRef] [PubMed]
60. Toh, J.W.T.; Lim, S.H.; MacKenzie, S.; de Souza, P.; Bokey, L.; Chapuis, P.; Spring, K.J. Association between Microsatellite Instability Status and Peri-Operative Release of Circulating Tumour Cells in Colorectal Cancer. *Cells* **2020**, *9*, 425. [CrossRef] [PubMed]
61. Smit, D.J.; Cayrefourcq, L.; Haider, M.-T.; Hinz, N.; Pantel, K.; Alix-Panabières, C.; Jücker, M. High Sensitivity of Circulating Tumor Cells Derived from a Colorectal Cancer Patient for Dual Inhibition with AKT and MTOR Inhibitors. *Cells* **2020**, *9*, 2129. [CrossRef]
62. Fumagalli, A.; Oost, K.C.; Kester, L.; Morgner, J.; Bornes, L.; Bruens, L.; Spaargaren, L.; Azkanaz, M.; Schelfhorst, T.; Beer-ling, E.; et al. Plasticity of Lgr5-Negative Cancer Cells Drives Metastasis in Colorectal Cancer. *Cell Stem Cell* **2020**, *26*, 569–578.e7. [CrossRef]
63. Cohen, J.D.; Li, L.; Wang, Y.; Thoburn, C.; Afsari, B.; Danilova, L.; Douville, C.; Javed, A.A.; Wong, F.; Mattox, A.; et al. Detection and Localization of Surgically Resectable Cancers with a Multi-Analyte Blood Test. *Science* **2018**, *359*, 926–930. [CrossRef]
64. Cao, H.; Liu, X.; Chen, Y.; Yang, P.; Huang, T.; Song, L.; Xu, R. Circulating Tumor DNA Is Capable of Monitoring the Therapeutic Response and Resistance in Advanced Colorectal Cancer Patients Undergoing Combined Target and Chemotherapy. *Front. Oncol.* **2020**, *10*, 466. [CrossRef]
65. Siravegna, G.; Marsoni, S.; Siena, S.; Bardelli, A. Integrating Liquid Biopsies into the Management of Cancer. *Nat. Rev. Clin. Oncol.* **2017**, *14*, 531–548. [CrossRef]
66. Lastraioli, E.; Antonuzzo, L.; Fantechi, B.; Di Cerbo, L.; Di Costanzo, A.; Lavacchi, D.; Armenio, M.; Arcangeli, A.; Castiglione, F.; Messerini, L.; et al. KRAS and NRAS mutation detection in circulating DNA from patients with metastatic colorectal cancer using BEAMing assay: Concordance with standard biopsy and clinical evaluation. *Oncol. Lett.* **2021**, *21*, 15. [CrossRef] [PubMed]
67. Siravegna, G.; Mussolin, B.; Buscarino, M.; Corti, G.; Cassingena, A.; Crisafulli, G.; Ponzetti, A.; Cremolini, C.; Amatu, A.; Lauricella, C.; et al. Monitoring Clonal Evolution and Resistance to EGFR Blockade in the Blood of Metastatic Colorectal Cancer Patients. *Nat. Med.* **2015**, *21*, 795–801. [CrossRef] [PubMed]
68. Ng, S.B.; Chua, C.; Ng, M.; Gan, A.; Poon, P.S.; Teo, M.; Fu, C.; Leow, W.Q.; Lim, K.H.; Chung, A.; et al. Individualised Mul-tiplexed Circulating Tumour DNA Assays for Monitoring of Tumour Presence in Patients after Colorectal Cancer Surgery. *Sci. Rep.* **2017**, *7*, 40737. [CrossRef]
69. Erve, I.; Greuter, M.J.E.; Bolhuis, K.; Vessies, D.C.L.; Leal, A.; Vink, G.R.; van den Broek, D.; Velculescu, V.E.; Punt, C.J.A.; Meijer, G.A.; et al. Diagnostic Strategies toward Clinical Implementation of Liquid Biopsy RAS/BRAF Circulating Tumor DNA Analyses in Patients with Metastatic Colorectal Cancer. *J. Mol. Diagn.* **2020**, *22*, 1430–1437. [CrossRef] [PubMed]
70. Nakamura, Y.; Taniguchi, H.; Ikeda, M.; Bando, H.; Kato, K.; Morizane, C.; Esaki, T.; Komatsu, Y.; Kawamoto, Y.; Takahashi, N.; et al. Clinical Utility of Circulating Tumor DNA Sequencing in Advanced Gastrointestinal Cancer: SCRUM-Japan GI-SCREEN and GOZILA Studies. *Nat. Med.* **2020**, *26*, 1859–1864. [CrossRef] [PubMed]
71. Garlan, F.; Laurent-Puig, P.; Sefrioui, D.; Siauve, N.; Didelot, A.; Sarafan-Vasseur, N.; Michel, P.; Perkins, G.; Mulot, C.; Blons, H.; et al. Early Evaluation of Circulating Tumor DNA as Marker of Therapeutic Efficacy in Metastatic Colorectal Cancer Patients (PLACOL Study). *Clin. Cancer Res.* **2017**, *23*, 5416–5425. [CrossRef]
72. Allegretti, M.; Cottone, G.; Carboni, F.; Cotroneo, E.; Casini, B.; Giordani, E.; Amoreo, C.A.; Buglioni, S.; Diodoro, M.; Pescarmona, E.; et al. Cross-Sectional Analysis of Circulating Tumor DNA in Primary Colorectal Cancer at Surgery and during Post-Surgery Follow-up by Liquid Biopsy. *J. Exp. Clin. Cancer Res.* **2020**, *39*, 69. [CrossRef]
73. Tie, J.; Wang, Y.; Tomasetti, C.; Li, L.; Springer, S.; Kinde, I.; Silliman, N.; Tacey, M.; Wong, H.-L.; Christie, M.; et al. Circulating Tumor DNA Analysis Detects Minimal Residual Disease and Predicts Recurrence in Patients with Stage II Colon Cancer. *Sci. Transl. Med.* **2016**, *8*, 346ra92. [CrossRef]
74. Khakoo, S.; Carter, P.D.; Brown, G.; Valeri, N.; Picchia, S.; Bali, M.A.; Shaikh, R.; Jones, T.; Begum, R.; Rana, I.; et al. MRI Tumor Regression Grade and Circulating Tumor DNA as Complementary Tools to Assess Response and Guide Therapy Adaptation in Rectal Cancer. *Clin. Cancer Res.* **2020**, *26*, 183–192. [CrossRef]
75. Zhou, J.; Wang, C.; Lin, G.; Xiao, Y.; Jia, W.; Xiao, G.; Liu, Q.; Wu, B.; Wu, A.; Qiu, H.; et al. Serial Circulating Tumor DNA in Predicting and Monitoring the Effect of Neoadjuvant Chemoradiotherapy in Patients with Rectal Cancer: A Prospective Multicenter Study. *Clin. Cancer Res.* **2021**, *27*, 301–310. [CrossRef]
76. Kalluri, R.; LeBleu, V.S. The Biology, Function, and Biomedical Applications of Exosomes. *Science* **2020**, *367*, eaau6977. [CrossRef] [PubMed]
77. Anfossi, S.; Fu, X.; Nagvekar, R.; Calin, G.A. MicroRNAs, Regulatory Messengers Inside and Outside Cancer Cells. *Adv. Exp. Med. Biol.* **2018**, *1056*, 87–108. [CrossRef] [PubMed]
78. Best, M.G.; Wesseling, P.; Wurdinger, T. Tumor-Educated Platelets as a Noninvasive Biomarker Source for Cancer Detection and Progression Monitoring. *Cancer Res.* **2018**, *78*, 3407–3412. [CrossRef]

79. Jamali, L.; Tofigh, R.; Tutunchi, S.; Panahi, G.; Borhani, F.; Akhavan, S.; Nourmohammadi, P.; Ghaderian, S.M.H.; Rasouli, M.; Mirzaei, H. Circulating microRNAs as diagnostic and therapeutic biomarkers in gastric and esophageal cancers. *J. Cell Physiol.* **2018**, *233*, 8538–8550. [CrossRef] [PubMed]
80. Moridikia, A.; Mirzaei, H.; Sahebkar, A.; Salimian, J. MicroRNAs: Potential candidates for diagnosis and treatment of colorectal cancer. *J. Cell Physiol.* **2018**, *233*, 901–913. [CrossRef] [PubMed]
81. Gasparello, J.; Papi, C.; Allegretti, M.; Giordani, E.; Carboni, F.; Zazza, S.; Pescarmona, E.; Romania, P.; Giacomini, P.; Scapoli, C.; et al. A Distinctive microRNA (miRNA) Signature in the Blood of Colorectal Cancer (CRC) Patients at Surgery. *Cancers* **2020**, *12*, 2410. [CrossRef] [PubMed]
82. Tsukamoto, M.; Iinuma, H.; Yagi, T.; Matsuda, K.; Hashiguchi, Y. Circulating Exosomal MicroRNA-21 as a Biomarker in Each Tumor Stage of Colorectal Cancer. *Oncology* **2017**, *92*, 360–370. [CrossRef]
83. Zhou, J.; Li, X.L.; Chen, Z.R.; Chng, W.J. Tumor-derived exosomes in colorectal cancer progression and their clinical applications. *Oncotarget* **2017**, *8*, 100781–100790. [CrossRef] [PubMed]
84. Hu, X.; Mu, Y.; Liu, J.; Mu, X.; Gao, F.; Chen, L.; Wu, H.; Wu, H.; Liu, W.; Zhao, Y. Exosomes Derived from Hypoxic Colorectal Cancer Cells Transfer miR-410-3p to Regulate Tumor Progression. *J. Cancer* **2020**, *1*, 4724–4735. [CrossRef]
85. Freed-Pastor, W.A.; Lambert, L.J.; Ely, Z.A.; Pattada, N.B.; Bhutkar, A.; Eng, G.; Mercer, K.L.; Garcia, A.P.; Lin, L.; Rideout, W.M.; et al. The CD155/TIGIT axis promotes and maintains immune evasion in neoantigen-expressing pancreatic cancer. *Cancer Cell* **2021**. [CrossRef]
86. Leone, K.; Poggiana, C.; Zamarchi, R. The Interplay between Circulating Tumor Cells and the Immune System: From Immune Escape to Cancer Immunotherapy. *Diagnostics* **2018**, *30*, 59. [CrossRef]
87. Mohme, M.; Riethdorf, S.; Pantel, K. Circulating and disseminated tumour cells-mechanisms of immune surveillance and escape. *Nat. Rev. Clin. Oncol.* **2017**, *14*, 155–167. [CrossRef]
88. Kloten, V.; Neumann, M.H.D.; Di Pasquale, F.; Sprenger-Haussels, M.; Shaffer, J.M.; Schlumpberger, M.; Herdean, A.; Bet-sou, F.; Ammerlaan, W.; Af Hällström, T.; et al. Multicenter Evaluation of Circulating Plasma MicroRNA Extraction Technologies for the Development of Clinically Feasible Reverse Transcription Quantitative PCR and Next-Generation Sequencing Analytical Work Flows. *Clin. Chem.* **2019**, *65*, 1132–1140. [CrossRef]

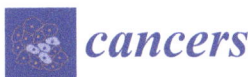

Article

Clinical Relevance of Viable Circulating Tumor Cells in Patients with Metastatic Colorectal Cancer: The COLOSPOT Prospective Study

Thibault Mazard [1,2,*], Laure Cayrefourcq [3,4], Françoise Perriard [5], Hélène Senellart [6], Benjamin Linot [7], Christelle de la Fouchardière [8], Eric Terrebonne [9], Eric François [10], Stéphane Obled [11], Rosine Guimbaud [12], Laurent Mineur [13], Marianne Fonck [14], Jean-Pierre Daurès [5], Marc Ychou [1], Eric Assenat [2] and Catherine Alix-Panabières [3,4,*]

1. IRCM, Inserm, University of Montpellier, ICM, 34000 Montpellier, France; marc.ychou@icm.unicancer.fr
2. Department of Medical Oncology, University Medical Center of Montpellier, St. Eloi Hospital, 34295 Montpellier, France; e-assenat@chu-montpellier.fr
3. Laboratory of Rare Human Circulating Cells, University Medical Center of Montpellier, University of Montpellier, 34093 Montpellier, France; l-cayrefourcq@chu-montpellier.fr
4. CREEC, MIVEGEC, University of Montpellier, CNRS, IRD, 34000 Montpellier, France
5. Biostatistiques, Nouvelles Technologies, AESIO Santé, 34394 Montpellier, France; f.perriard@languedoc-mutualite.fr (F.P.); jp.daures@languedoc-mutualite.fr (J.-P.D.)
6. Department of Medical Oncology, Institut de Cancérologie de l'Ouest, 44800 Saint Herblain, France; helene.senellart@ico.unicancer.fr
7. Department of Oncology, Institut de Cancérologie de l'Ouest, 49100 Nantes-Angers, France; benjamin.linot@groupeconfluent.fr
8. Department of Medical Oncology, Centre Léon Bérard, 69008 Lyon, France; christelle.delafouchardiere@lyon.unicancer.fr
9. Department of Gastroenterology, CHU Haut-Lévêque, 33600 Pessac, France; eric.terrebonne@chu-bordeaux.fr
10. CLCC Antoine Lacassagne, 06100 Nice, France; eric.francois@nice.unicancer.fr
11. Department of Gastroenterology, University of Montpellier-Nîmes, Carémeau Hospital, 30900 Nîmes, France; stephane.obled@chu-nimes.fr
12. Department of Oncology, Toulouse-Rangueil University Hospital, 31059 Toulouse, France; guimbaud.r@chu-toulouse.fr
13. Oncology, Radiothérapy, Sainte-Catherine Institut, 84918 Avignon, France; l.mineur@isc84.org
14. Department of Medical Oncology, Institut Bergonié, 33000 Bordeaux, France; m.fonck@bordeaux.unicancer.fr
* Correspondence: thibault.mazard@icm.unicancer.fr (T.M.); c-panabieres@chu-montpellier.fr (C.A.-P.); Tel.: +33-4-67-61-30-29 (T.M.); +33-4-11-75-99-31 (C.A.-P.); Fax: +33-4-67-61-23-47 (T.M.); +33-4-67-33-52-81 (C.A.-P.)

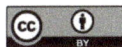

Simple Summary: The analysis of circulating tumor cells (CTCs) as a "real-time liquid biopsy" in epithelial tumors for personalized medicine has received tremendous attention over the past years, with important clinical implications. In metastatic colorectal cancer (mCRC), the CellSearch® system has already demonstrated its prognostic value and interest in monitoring treatment response, but the number of recovered CTCs remains low. In this article, we evaluate the early prognostic and predictive value of viable CTCs in patients with mCRC treated with FOLFIRI–bevacizumab with an alternative approach, the functional EPISPOT assay. This study shows that viable CTCs can be detected in patients with mCRC before and during FOLFIRI–bevacizumab treatment and that CTC detection at D_{28} and the D_0–D_{28} CTC kinetics evaluated with the EPISPOT assay are associated with response to treatment.

Abstract: Background: Circulating tumor cells (CTCs) allow the real-time monitoring of tumor course and treatment response. This prospective multicenter study evaluates and compares the early predictive value of CTC enumeration with EPISPOT, a functional assay that detects only viable CTCs, and with the CellSearch® system in patients with metastatic colorectal cancer (mCRC). Methods: Treatment-naive patients with mCRC and measurable disease (RECIST criteria 1.1) received FOLFIRI–bevacizumab until progression or unacceptable toxicity. CTCs in peripheral blood were enumerated at D_0, D_{14}, D_{28}, D_{42}, and D_{56} (EPISPOT assay) and at D_0 and D_{28} (CellSearch® system). Progression-free survival (PFS) and overall survival (OS) were assessed with the Kaplan–Meier method and log-rank test. Results: With the EPISPOT assay, at least 1 viable CTC was detected in 21% (D_0), 15% (D_{14}), 12% (D_{28}), 10% (D_{42}), and 12% (D_{56}) of 155 patients. PFS and OS were shorter in patients who remained positive, with viable CTCs between D_0 and D_{28} compared with the other patients (PFS = 7.36 vs. 9.43 months, p = 0.0161 and OS = 25.99 vs. 13.83 months, p = 0.0178). The prognostic and predictive values of ≥ 3 CTCs (CellSearch® system) were confirmed. Conclusions: CTC detection at D_{28} and the D_0–D_{28} CTC dynamics evaluated with the EPISPOT assay were associated with outcomes and may predict response to treatment.

Keywords: circulating tumor cells; colorectal cancer; EPISPOT assay; CellSearch® system; predictive value

1. Introduction

In western countries, colorectal cancer (CRC) is one of the most frequently diagnosed cancers and a leading cause of cancer death. In Europe, an estimated 499,700 new cases occurred in 2018, and 242,500 patients died of CRC in the same year [1].

CRC's high mortality rate is due to the development of distant unresectable metastases in more than 50% of patients at some point during the disease course [2]. In this setting, the current guidelines recommend the use of cytotoxic chemotherapy regimens that combine fluoropyrimidine with oxaliplatin or irinotecan and a targeted agent (bevacizumab or cetuximab/panitumumab) as first-line standard-of-care therapy, [3–5]. Although the RAS oncogene's mutational status is an unquestionable marker to select patients who are unlikely to benefit from EGFR antibody therapy [6,7], robust biomarkers for predicting outcome and early treatment response are still lacking, especially for bevacizumab-based regimens [8].

The "liquid biopsy" has been introduced for the analysis of circulating tumor cells (CTCs) in the blood of patients with solid cancers, and many clinical trials have focused on this new approach for precision medicine over the past decade [9]. Specifically, the most aggressive tumor cells are actively released by the tumor and/or metastases in body fluids [10]. They can be isolated from peripheral blood and were the first "liquid biopsy" component investigated as a biomarker in many cancer types [9]. In metastatic CRC, the CTC prognostic value has been clinically validated using the FDA-cleared CellSearch® system (www.cellsearchctc.com, accessed on 21 May 2021). Briefly, three large prospective studies demonstrated that patients with ≥ 3 CTCs before chemotherapy have shorter progression-free (PFS) and overall survival (OS) [10–12]. They also found that the CTC number remains a strong prognostic factor after a few treatment cycles and might also help monitor the treatment response. In these studies, most patients received the fluoropyrimidine–oxaliplatin combination and bevacizumab as first-line treatment. With the CellSearch® system, CTC capture is based on immunoselection using antibodies against the epithelial cell surface adhesion molecule (EpCAM) [13]. However, CTCs are phenotypically heterogeneous, and some may not express epithelial markers anymore or weakly, especially if they have undergone an epithelial-to-mesenchymal transition [14,15]. Consequently, these subpopulations might not be detected by the CellSearch® system, underlining the need to develop alternative approaches to improve CTC enrichment.

In this context, we developed a functional assay called the Epithelial ImmunoSPOT assay (EPISPOT) that selects viable CTCs based on the detection of specific secreted tumor-associated proteins. Therefore, EPISPOT enumerates only viable CTCs, irrespective of EpCAM expression, because this innovative technology is always combined with depletion of leukocytes [16]. Using cytokeratin-19 (CK19) as the released protein to detect CTCs in the bloodstream, we have already validated the prognostic value of functional CTCs in a prospective study with more than 250 patients with metastatic breast cancer. We found that functional CTCs are correlated with OS and could be used in combination with the CTCs detected by the CellSearch® system to refine the prognostic stratification of these patients [17]. Moreover, in non-metastatic CRC, the CK19-EPISPOT assay detected more CTCs than the CellSearch® system in peripheral and mesenteric blood samples from patients with treatment-naïve tumors [18].

Therefore, we carried out a prospective study, called COLOSPOT, on patients with untreated metastatic CRC, about to receive FOLFIRI (folinic acid, fluorouracil, and irinotecan) and bevacizumab as first-line therapy, to further investigate the clinical utility of viable CTCs detected with the CK19-EPISPOT assay. The objectives were to assess the prognostic and early predictive values of viable CTC enumeration and their dynamics during treatment using the CK19-EPISPOT assay and to compare the CTC detection of the CK19-EPISPOT assay and the CellSearch® system (the gold standard).

2. Materials and Methods

2.1. Study Design

We carried out a multicenter prospective study named "COLOSPOT" (ClinicalTrials.gov: NCT01596790) in 11 medical centers in France. The human investigations were performed after approval by the human investigation committee Sud Méditerranée III (Ref: 2011.11.01). Patients with untreated metastatic colorectal adenocarcinoma, with measurable disease according to Response Evaluation Criteria in Solid Tumors (RECIST) 1.1, who started first-line systemic therapy with FOLFIRI–bevacizumab were eligible. Other inclusion criteria were: patients older than 18 years and an Eastern Cooperative Oncology Group (ECOG) performance status (PS) score of 0 to 2. Chemotherapy was continued until disease progression, unacceptable toxicity, or patient/investigator's decision. Tumor response was assessed every 8 weeks during the first year of treatment and every 3 months thereafter until disease progression or for a maximum period of 2 years. Tumor response was evaluated using contrast-enhanced chest–abdomen–pelvis computed tomography images and the RECIST 1.1 criteria. All patients gave their written informed consent before inclusion.

For CTC enumeration, peripheral blood samples were drawn just before and during therapy, as follows: for the EPISPOT assay, 15 mL of blood was collected in EDTA tubes at baseline (D_0) and at day 14 (D_{14}), day 28 (D_{28}), day 42 (D_{42}) and day 56 (D_{56}) after treatment initiation. For the CellSearch system, 10 mL of peripheral blood was collected in CellSave tubes (Silicon Biosystems-Menarini) at D_0 and D_{28}, based on the data previously reported by Cohen et al., showing that the conversion of baseline unfavorable ($\geq$3 CTCs/7.5 mL of blood) to favorable (<3 CTCs/7.5 mL of blood) CTC profiles at 3–5 weeks is associated with significantly longer PFS and OS [10]. All blood samples were sent to LCCRH–Montpellier, where all the CTC detection experiments were processed.

2.2. CTC Isolation and Enumeration

All CK19-EPISPOT assays were performed at LCCRH–Montpellier. The detailed procedure of the EPISPOT assay has been previously described [16]. Briefly, within 24 h after blood collection, leukocytes were depleted with RosetteSep CTC enrichment cocktails (#15167) from Stemcell Technologies. Then, the enriched fraction was frozen in liquid nitrogen (90% fetal calf serum + 10% DMSO) and unfrozen when all samples from the same patient were obtained. The idea was to run a single CK19-EPISPOT experiment per patient, avoiding inter-assay variation during the follow-up. Enriched cells were cultured in 96-well plates (MAIPN4550, Milipore, Darmstadt, Germany), precoated with an anti-CK19 antibody (Ks19.1, Progen, Heidelberg, Germany), to capture CK19-releasing CTCs. After 48 h, wells were washed to remove cells, and CK19 molecules captured by the coating antibody were detected with a second anti-CK19 antibody (Ks19.2, Progen) conjugated to the AlexaFluor 555 fluorochrome. Single fluorescent CK19 immunospots were counted under a fluorescent microscope equipped with a camera and computer-assisted analysis

(KS ELISPOT, Carl Zeiss Vision, Oberkochen, Germany). Results were expressed as the number of cells per 15 mL of blood.

All CellSearch® analyses were performed within 96 h after blood collection using the CellSearch® CTC kit (7900001, Silicon Biosystem, Menarini, Bologna, Italy), according to the manufacturer's instructions. This method enriches CTCs via positive selection with magnetic beads coated with anti-EpCAM antibodies, followed by immunofluorescence-based detection. CTCs are Pan-CK$^{(+)}$, DAPI$^{(+)}$, and CD45$^{(-)}$. Results are expressed as the number of cells per 7.5 mL of blood.

2.3. Statistical Analyses

Data were summarized with medians and ranges for continuous variables and frequency for categorical variables. Fischer's exact test was used to study the correlation between CTC detection and clinical–pathological characteristics. Concordance between technologies was assessed at D_0 and D_{28} by calculating the intraclass correlation coefficient.

PFS and OS were analyzed with the Kaplan–Meier method. Survival curves were compared with the non-parametric log-rank test ($p \leq 0.05$ was considered significant). PFS was defined as the elapsed time from blood collection to disease progression or death from any cause. Patients who began a second-line treatment without disease progression were censored at the date of treatment switch. OS was defined as the elapsed time from blood collection to death from any cause.

Univariate and multivariate Cox proportional hazards regression models were used to obtain the unadjusted and fully adjusted hazard ratios (HRs) and 95% confidence intervals (CIs).

Statistical analyses were performed with SAS version 9.4 (SAS Institute, Cary, NC, USA).

3. Results

3.1. Clinical and Tumor Characteristics

Between April 2012 and September 2016, 168 patients were enrolled in the study, among whom 155 met the inclusion and exclusion criteria and were assessable. The number of patients included at each stage of the analysis and the reasons for exclusion are summarized in the study flowchart (Figure 1).

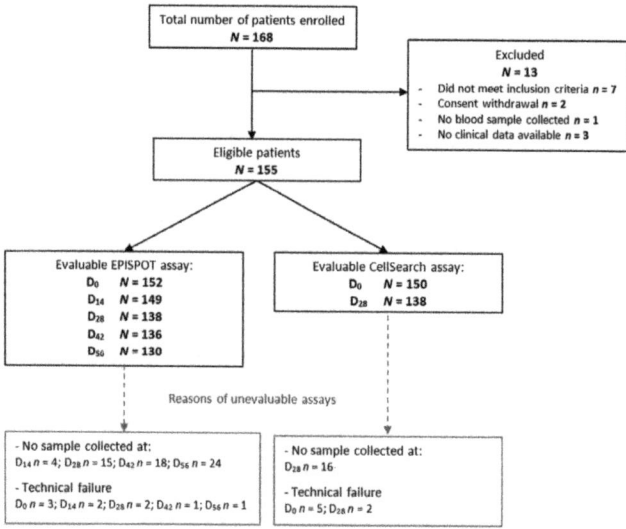

Figure 1. Study flowchart showing the number of included patients and the number of patients in whom CTCs could be assessed in peripheral blood samples at different time points before (D_0) and during treatment (EPISPOT: D_{14}, D_{28}, D_{42}, D_{56}; CellSearch®: D_{28}). Abbreviations: N, number; D, day.

The patient and tumor characteristics are summarized in Table S1. At the time of the final analysis (July 2019), the median follow-up was 24.5 months (range, 0.99–75.04 months), and the median PFS and OS were 9.4 (95% CI, 8.1–10.2 months) and 26.2 months (95% CI, 21.3–29.8 months), respectively.

3.2. CTC Prevalence at Different Time Points and Correlation with Baseline Characteristics

Table S2 summarizes the results obtained with the CK19-EPISPOT and CellSearch® assays at different time points. With the EPISPOT assay, 32/152 (21%) patients had ≥1 CTC/sample and 18/152 had ≥2 CTCs/sample (11.8%) at D_0. During treatment, the number of patients with at least 1 CTC decreased to 15.4% at D_{14}, 12.3% at D_{28}, 9.6% at D_{42}, and 11.5% at D_{56}. According to the CellSearch® assay, 59/150 (39.3%) and 13/138 (9.4%) patients had ≥3 CTCs/sample at D_0 and D_{28}, respectively.

The concordance between methods was low, as indicated by the Cohen K coefficient of 0.23 ($p = 0.002$) and 0.34 ($p \leq 0.0001$) at D_0 and D_{28}, respectively.

Only CTCs detected with the CellSearch® system at D_0 (≥3) correlated significantly with some biological and clinical characteristics. Baseline performance status was worse and more patients had synchronous metastases, liver involvement, and abnormal CEA levels in the group with ≥3 CTCs/sample than in the group with <3 CTCs/sample at D_0 (Table 1).

Table 1. Patient characteristics and correlation with CTC number. CTCs were detected with two methods: CK19-EPISPOT and CellSearch®.

Parameters	EPISPOT (n = 152)			CellSearch® (n = 150)		
	≥1	<1	p-Value (Fisher)	≥3	<3	p-Value (Fisher)
Age						
<70 years	21 (66%)	77 (64%)	1	42 (71%)	55 (61%)	0.22
≥70 years	11 (34%)	43 (36%)		17 (29%)	36 (39%)	
Sex						
Men	23 (72%)	73 (61%)	0.31	35 (59%)	58 (64%)	0.61
Women	9 (28%)	47 (39%)		24 (41%)	33 (36%)	
Baseline ECOG PS score						
0	15 (47%)	67 (57%)	0.32	22 (39%)	59 (66%)	0.0021
1–2	17 (53%)	50 (43%)		35 (61%)	31 (34%)	
CRC localization						
Right	11 (37%)	39 (32%)	0.67	21 (37%)	29 (32%)	0.59
Left	19 (63%)	81 (68%)		36 (63%)	62 (68%)	
Metastases						
Synchronous	23 (74%)	77 (65%)	0.40	48 (83%)	50 (57%)	0.0012
Metachronous	8 (26%)	41 (35%)		10 (17%)	38 (43%)	
Nb of organs with metastases						
1	14 (45%)	47 (39%)	0.55	21 (36%)	39 (43%)	0.49
>1	17 (55%)	73 (61%)		37 (64%)	51 (57%)	
Liver metastases						
Yes	26 (84%)	97 (81%)	0.80	54 (93%)	66 (73%)	0.0025
No	5 (16%)	23 (19%)		4 (7%)	24 (27%)	
RAS status						
Wild type	10 (38%)	30 (31%)	0.49	13 (29%)	26 (34%)	0.69
Mutant	16 (62%)	66 (69%)		32 (71%)	50 (66%)	
B-RAF status						
Wild type	28 (97%)	92 (92%)	0.68	46 (92%)	74 (95%)	0.71
Mutant	1 (3%)	8 (8%)		4 (8%)	4 (5%)	
CEA value						
Normal	8 (25%)	36 (31%)	0.66	7 (12%)	37 (42%)	0.0001
>normal	24 (75%)	81 (69%)		51 (88%)	52 (58%)	

Abbreviations: M, men; W, women; CRC, colorectal cancer; PS, performance status.

3.3. CTC Presence Correlates with PFS and OS in Patients with Metastatic CRC

Considering the CTC data obtained with the CK19-EPISPOT assay, the number of viable CTCs at D_{28}, but not at D_0, was significant correlated with PFS and OS (Figure 2A,B). PFS and OS were shorter in patients with ≥ 2 CTCs than in patients without or with only 1 CTC (median PFS = 5.82 months, 95% CI (0.92–6.37 months) vs. 8.28 months, 95% CI (7.20–9.17 months); p = 0.0082 and median OS = 10.28 months, 95% CI (4.63–14.26 months) vs. 24.84 months, 95% CI (20.11–28.45 months); p = 0.0003). Similar results were obtained for CTCs at D_{42} and OS. No prognostic correlation was observed using 1 CTC as cut-off, regardless of the sampling time (Table S3).

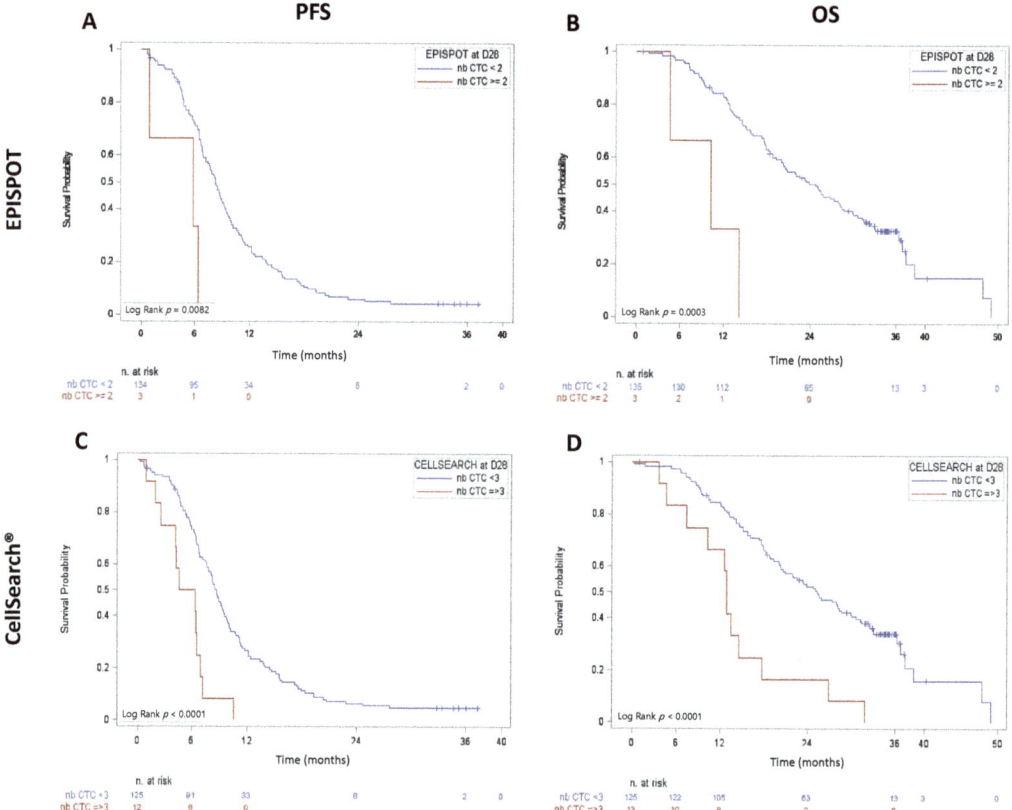

Figure 2. PFS and OS in patients with metastatic CRC at D_{28}. CTCs were enumerated after the first two chemotherapy cycles (D_{28}) with the (**A**,**B**) CK19-EPISPOT (≥ 2 vs. <2) and (**C**,**D**) CellSearch® (≥ 3 vs. <3) assays.

With the CellSearch® system, at D_0, OS was shorter in patients with ≥ 3 CTCs than in those with <3 CTCs (median OS = 19.1 months, 95% CI (15.57–21.59 months) vs. 37.3 months, 95% CI (26.81–44.58 months); p < 0.0001). Conversely, PFS was not significantly different (data not shown). At D_{28}, ≥ 3 CTCs was associated with shorter PFS and OS compared with <3 CTCs (median PFS = 5.50 months, 95% CI (1.90–6.93 months) vs. 8.64 months, 95% CI (7.67–9.56 months); p < 0.0001 and median OS = 12.91 months, 95% CI (4.63–17.77 months) vs. 25.27 months, 95% CI (20.40–30.10 months); p < 0.0001 respectively) (Figure 2C,D).

3.4. CTC Kinetics between D_0 and D_{28} Correlates with PFS and OS

To study the CTC kinetics between D_0 and D_{28}, patients were divided in two groups: (1) CTC-positive at D_0 and D_{28}, and (2) CTC-negative at D_0 and D_{28} or CTC-positive only at D_0 or D_{28}. PFS and OS were significant shorter in patients in the first group, with both the CK19-EPISPOT method (median PFS = 7.36 months, 95% CI (1.84–8.97 months) vs. 9.43 months, 95% CI (8.08–10.25 months); p = 0.0161 and median OS = 13.83 months, 95% CI (5.55–31.63 months) vs. 25.99 months, 95% CI (20.99–29.17 months); p = 0.0176) and the CellSearch® method (median PFS = 6.6 months, 95% CI (1.84–7.85 months) vs. 9.46 months, 95% CI (8.54–10.31 months); p = 0.0018 and median OS = 14.13 months, 95% CI (5.55–18.69 months) vs. 26.18 months, 95% CI (21.29–29.83 months); p = 0.0010) (Figure 3).

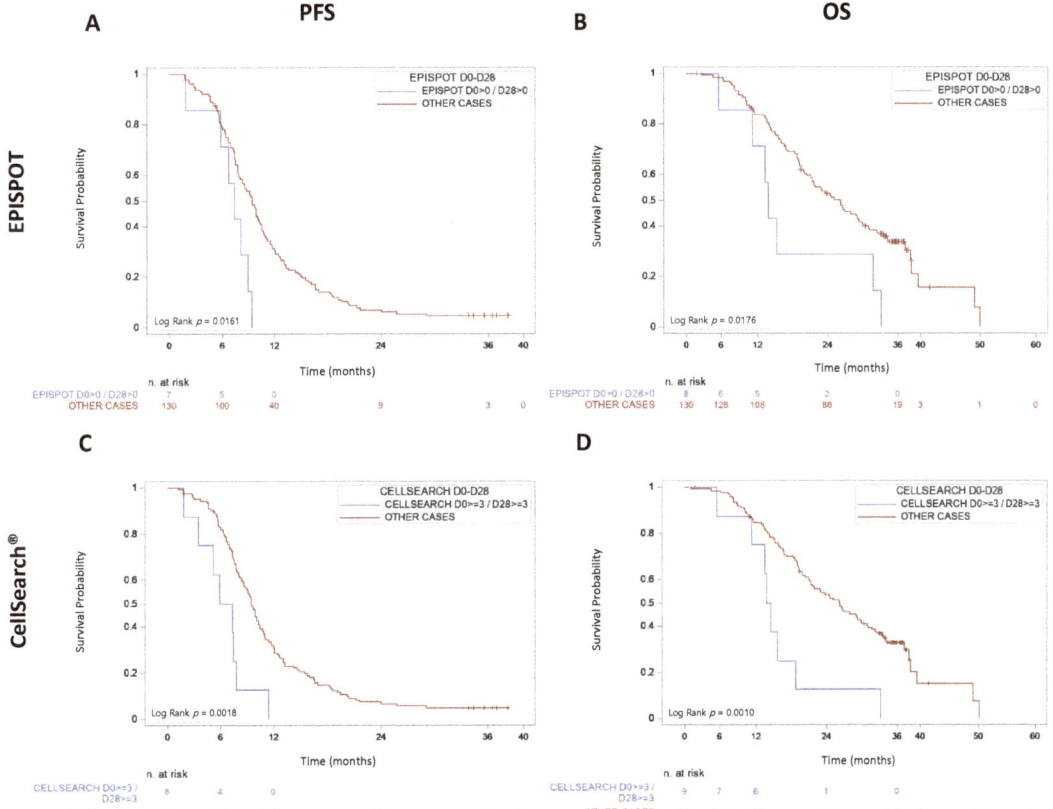

Figure 3. PFS and OS in metastatic CRCs according to the D_0–D_{28} CTC kinetics. Patients were divided into two groups in the function of CTC enumeration at D_0 and D_{28}, using the (**A**,**B**) CK19-EPISPOT and (**C**,**D**) CellSearch® assays.

Univariate analysis confirmed that the early CTC dynamics (both assays), ECOG PS at D_0, and BRAF mutational status were predictors of PFS and OS. A primary tumor localized to the right colon also significantly correlated with worse OS (Table 2).

Table 2. Univariate Cox regression analysis for PFS and OS prediction.

Parameters	PFS			OS		
	HR	95% CI	p-Value	HR	95% CI	p-Value
Age: ≥70 vs. <70 years	1.04	0.74–1.46	0.84	1.08	0.72–1.62	0.71
Sex: W vs. M	0.84	0.6–1.19	0.32	1.28	0.86–1.89	0.22
ECOG PS: 1–2 vs. 0	1.46	1.05–2.05	0.0259	2.66	1.77–3.99	<0.0001
Right vs. left colon	1.07	0.75–1.51	0.72	1.54	1.03–2.31	0.04
Synchronous vs. metachronous mets	0.78	0.55–1.11	0.17	1.24	0.81–1.88	0.32
N of organs with mets: >1 vs. 1	1.21	0.86–1.69	0.27	1.34	0.9–2	0.15
Liver mets vs. no-liver mets	0.9	0.59–1.37	0.62	1.53	0.87–2.69	0.14
CEA: >nal vs. nal	1.04	0.71–1.5	0.85	1.46	0.92–2.32	0.11
RAS: MT vs. WT	0.76	0.51–1.12	0.16	0.71	0.45–1.12	0.14
B-RAF: MT vs. WT	3.27	1.61–6.64	0.001	7.39	3.36–16.25	<0.0001
D_0-D_{28} CTC kinetics (EPISPOT): Positive at both time points (≥1) vs. other cases	2.52	1.15–5.52	0.0204	2.48	1.14–5.37	0.0219
D_0-D_{28} CTC kinetics (CellSearch®): Positive at both time points (≥3) vs. other cases	3.02	1.45–6.3	0.0031	3.22	1.54–6.74	0.0019

Abbreviations: M, men; W, women; HR, hazard ratio; vs., versus; PS, performance status; nal, normal; mets, metastases; CEA, carcinoembryonic antigen; MT, mutated; WT, wild type; D, day; PFS, progression-free survival; OS, overall survival; CI, confidence interval.

In multivariate analysis, D_0–D_{28} CTC kinetics according to the CK19-EPISPOT assay (HR 2.445, 95% CI (1.04–5.78), $p = 0.0414$) and the CellSearch® system (HR 2.461, 95% CI (1.06–5.74), $p = 0.037$) remained significant predictors of PFS but not of OS (Table 3).

Table 3. Multivariate Cox regression analysis for PFS and OS prediction.

Parameters	PFS			OS		
	HR	95% CI	p-Value	HR	95% CI	p-Value
ECOG PS: 1–2 vs. 0				2.48	1.51–4.07	0.0003
B-RAF: MT vs. WT	3.046	1.43–6.5	0.0043	5.34	2.23–12.79	0.0002
D_0–D_{28} CTC kinetics (EPISPOT): Positive at both time points (≥1) vs. other cases	2.445	1.04–5.78	0.0414			
D_0–D_{28} CTC kinetics (CellSearch®): Positive at both time points (≥3) vs. other cases	2.461	1.06–5.74	0.037			

Abbreviations: HR, hazard ratio; vs., versus; PS, performance status; MT, mutated; WT, wild type; D, day; PFS, progression-free survival; OS, overall survival; CI, confidence interval.

4. Discussion

More than a decade ago, it was shown that CTC enumeration is a prognostic factor in metastatic breast, prostate, and colorectal cancer [10,19,20]. In this field of expertise, it was then important to show the clinical validity of CTCs with meta-analyses of thousands of cancer patients [21] and, especially, to demonstrate their clinical utility for introducing them in daily clinical practice [22]. CTC clinical validity and utility have been reported for metastatic breast cancer; conversely, in CRCs, many key questions are still unanswered.

To determine whether viable CTCs are clinically relevant in patients with metastatic CRC as an early criterion of response to FOLFIRI–bevacizumab treatment, we performed a prospective multicenter study in which peripheral blood samples were tested before and during treatment, with two different CTC detection technologies: (i) the EPISPOT assay to detect viable CTCs, and (ii) the FDA-cleared CellSearch® system. We then determined whether the subpopulation of viable CTCs detected with the EPISPOT assay is clinically relevant for the prognosis and as an early biomarker to predict clinical outcomes after treatment initiation. We assessed the CTC count at different time points and different CTC cut-offs for the EPISPOT assay because this system is still under study. Conversely, on the basis of the work by Cohen et al., with the CellSearch® system, we only tested CTCs at D_0 and D_{28} and considered only the cut-off of $\geq$3 CTCs [10].

The studied population is representative because their OS (26.2 months) and PFS (9.4 months) are consistent with previously reported data on unselected patients with metastatic CRC treated with FOLFIRI and bevacizumab [23]. The detection of viable CTCs could be assessed in most patients during their routine follow-up at 11 centers in France, demonstrating the feasibility of this technique in clinical practice. During treatment, we found significant correlations between survival and the presence of viable CTCs (threshold: $\geq$2 CTCs) at D_{28} (PFS and OS) and D_{42} (only OS). Moreover, the D_0–D_{28} CTC kinetics predicted both PFS and OS and was an independent factor of PFS by multivariate analysis. This finding confirms the clinical interest of the CTC kinetic previously assessed with ISET technology [24] or other assays [25] for early detection of poor outcomes in patients with metastatic CRC under treatment. During the last decade, the EPISPOT assay's prognostic value has already been demonstrated in advanced breast, prostate, and head and neck cancer as well as in melanoma and non-metastatic CRC [18,26–28]. The prognostic value of the early kinetics of viable CTCs has already been reported in recurrent and metastatic head and neck squamous cell carcinoma [28].

According to the CellSearch® system, 40% of patients had $\geq$3 CTCs, in line with previous studies (24–52% of untreated patients with metastatic CRC) [10–12,29,30]. We then confirmed that the CellSearch® system, using the conventional cut-off of 3 CTCs, provides prognostic information before and early after initiation of the first line of treatment. PFS and OS were significantly shorter in patients who became or remained positive ($\geq$3 CTCs) after 4 weeks of chemotherapy (D_{28}), demonstrating that they did not benefit from therapy.

Considering the detection of viable CTCs (EPISPOT), the number of positive patients was lower at baseline compared with the CellSearch® system, and it decreased during treatment. Thus, the low number of patients with unfavorable CTC evolution according to the EPISPOT assay is a limitation of our study. As already shown in previous studies [17,26–28], the concordance between EPISPOT and CellSearch® technologies for CTC detection was low at baseline and during treatment. This could be explained by the fact that the EPISPOT assay detects only CK19-releasing viable CTCs and not the others (e.g., apoptotic CTCs). Moreover, the enrichment and detection steps are different. The CellSearch® system uses positive selection based on EpCAMs to enrich CTCs, whereas the EPISPOT assay is combined with negative selection by leukocyte depletion. In the CellSearch® system, detection is based on Pan CK, DAPI, and CD45 staining of fixed CTCs. Conversely, the EPISPOT assay detects only CK19-releasing CTCs in culture. Despite this low agreement, the dynamic CTC count, which changes with both methods, remained significantly correlated with PFS in multivariate analysis, suggesting that these assays are complementary for predicting clinical outcomes during treatment. Interestingly, CTC positivity ($\geq$3 cells) by CellSearch® is correlated with surrogate markers of tumor burden ([30,31] and the present study), but not the presence of viable CTCs. This might suggest that their predictive value is not directly linked to the tumor mass changes but more to the identification of an aggressive chemotherapy-resistant subpopulation of tumor cells that are certainly at the origin of cancer progression.

Currently, we are developing a new version of the EPISPOT assay, named EPIDROP (EPIspot in a DROP), that combines EPISPOT and CellSearch® strategies and might represent an ideal liquid biopsy tool. Indeed, with this new technology, we can detect the total amount of CTCs by immunostaining, as done by the CellSearch® system, and also the subset of viable CTCs on the basis of their ability to secrete, shed, or release some proteins. EPIDROP might also allow the use of a larger panel of CTC biomarkers, such as VEGF monitoring during bevacizumab therapy. This innovative technology should open new avenues to detect CTCs that are relevant as prognostic and early predictive information in metastatic CRC with high specificity and sensitivity.

5. Conclusions

The CK19-EPISPOT assay detects viable CTCs in metastatic CRC. This prospective study shows that real-time liquid biopsy for CTC analysis could be clinically relevant in this setting, particularly to monitor the early response to FOLFIRI–bevacizumab.

Supplementary Materials: The following are available online at https://www.mdpi.com/article/10.3390/cancers13122966/s1, Table S1: Patient and tumor characteristics (n = 155), Table S2: CTC detection at each time point, Table S3: Prognostic value of CTCs according to the CK19-EPISPOT assay.

Author Contributions: Conceptualization, C.A.-P. and T.M.; Methodology, J.-P.D.; Validation, L.C., C.A.-P. and T.M.; Formal analysis, L.C. and F.P.; Data curation, L.C., T.M. and F.P.; Resources, H.S., B.L., C.d.l.F., E.T., E.F., S.O., R.G., L.M., M.F., M.Y., E.A. and T.M.; Writing—original draft preparation, L.C., C.A.-P. and T.M.; Writing—review and editing, L.C., E.A., H.S., B.L., C.d.l.F., E.T., E.F., S.O., R.G., L.M., M.F., M.Y., C.A.-P. and T.M.; Supervision, C.A.-P. and T.M.; Funding acquisition, C.A.-P. and T.M. All authors have read and agreed to the published version of the manuscript.

Funding: This work was supported by the National Cancer Institute (INCa) "Recherche Translationnelle-Projet Libre 2011" and the General Direction for Caregiving (DGOS) for patient recruitment and analyses in the COLOSPOT study (NCT01596790). We also received financial support from F Hoffmann-La Roche Ltd., Basel, Switzerland. The LCCRH was also supported by a SIRIC Montpellier Cancer Grant (INCa_Inserm_DGOS_12553) for staff salary.

Institutional Review Board Statement: The study was conducted according to the guidelines of the Declaration of Helsinki and approved by the Ethics Committee Sud Méditerranée III (Ref: 2011.11.01).

Informed Consent Statement: Informed consent was obtained from all subjects involved in the study.

Data Availability Statement: The data presented in this study are available in the main article and its supplementary material.

Acknowledgments: The authors express their gratitude to the patients who participated in this trial. They thank all the participating physicians, the supporting staff, especially Julie Duval and Anne Cadène, and Elisabetta Andermarcher for assistance with her comments and proofreading, which greatly improved the manuscript.

Conflicts of Interest: C.A.P. has received an honorarium from Menarini. T.M. discloses research funding from ROCHE and AMGEN; an honorarium from AMGEN, SANOFI, BMS, SANDOZ, and AAA; and travel, accommodations, and expenses paid by AMGEN. The other authors declare no conflict of interest.

References

1. Ferlay, J.; Colombet, M.; Soerjomataram, I.; Dyba, T.; Randi, G.; Bettio, M.; Gavin, A.; Visser, O.; Bray, F. Cancer incidence and mortality patterns in Europe: Estimates for 40 countries and 25 major cancers in 2018. *Eur. J. Cancer* **2018**, *103*, 356–387. [CrossRef]
2. Siegel, R.L.; Miller, K.D.; Fedewa, S.A.; Ahnen, D.J.; Meester, R.G.S.; Barzi, A.; Jemal, A. Colorectal cancer statistics, 2017. *CA Cancer J. Clin.* **2017**, *67*, 177–193. [CrossRef]
3. Benson, A.B.; Venook, A.P.; Al-Hawary, M.M.; Arain, M.A.; Chen, Y.J.; Ciombor, K.K.; Cohen, S.; Cooper, H.S.; Deming, D.; Farkas, L.; et al. Colon Cancer, Version 2.2021, NCCN Clinical Practice Guidelines in Oncology. *J. Natl. Compr. Cancer Netw.* **2021**, *19*, 329–359. [CrossRef]
4. Van Cutsem, E.; Cervantes, A.; Adam, R.; Sobrero, A.; van Krieken, J.; Aderka, D.; Aguilar, E.A.; Bardelli, A.; Benson, A.; Bodoky, G.; et al. ESMO consensus guidelines for the management of patients with metastatic colorectal cancer. *Ann. Oncol.* **2016**, *27*, 1386–1422. [CrossRef]
5. Phelip, J.M.; Tougeron, D.; Léonard, D.; Benhaim, L.; Desolneux, G.; Dupré, A.; Michel, P.; Penna, C.; Tournigand, C.; Louvet, C.; et al. Metastatic colorectal cancer (mCRC): French intergroup clinical practice guidelines for diagnosis, treatments and follow-up (SNFGE, FFCD, GERCOR, UNICANCER, SFCD, SFED, SFRO, SFR). *Dig. Liver Dis.* **2019**, *51*, 1357–1363. [CrossRef] [PubMed]
6. Loupakis, F.; Ruzzo, A.; Cremolini, C.; Vincenzi, B.; Salvatore, L.; Santini, D.; Masi, G.; Stasi, I.; Canestrari, E.; Rulli, E.; et al. KRAS codon 61, 146 and BRAF mutations predict resistance to cetuximab plus irinotecan in KRAS codon 12 and 13 wild-type metastatic colorectal cancer. *Br. J. Cancer* **2009**, *101*, 715–721. [CrossRef]
7. Douillard, J.-Y.; Oliner, K.S.; Siena, S.; Tabernero, J.; Burkes, R.; Barugel, M.; Humblet, Y.; Bodoky, G.; Cunningham, D.; Jassem, J.; et al. Panitumumab–FOLFOX4 Treatment and RAS Mutations in Colorectal Cancer. *N. Engl. J. Med.* **2013**, *369*, 1023–1034. [CrossRef] [PubMed]

8. Cidon, E.U.; Alonso, P.; Masters, B. Markers of Response to Antiangiogenic Therapies in Colorectal Cancer: Where are We Now and What should be Next? *Clin. Med. Insights Oncol.* **2016**, *10*, CMO.S34542. [CrossRef] [PubMed]
9. Pantel, K.; Alix-Panabières, C. Circulating tumour cells in cancer patients: Challenges and perspectives. *Trends Mol. Med.* **2010**, *16*, 398–406. [CrossRef] [PubMed]
10. Cohen, S.J.; Punt, C.J.A.; Iannotti, N.; Saidman, B.H.; Sabbath, K.D.; Gabrail, N.Y.; Picus, J.; Morse, M.; Mitchell, E.; Miller, M.C.; et al. Relationship of Circulating Tumor Cells to Tumor Response, Progression-Free Survival, and Overall Survival in Patients With Metastatic Colorectal Cancer. *J. Clin. Oncol.* **2008**, *26*, 3213–3221. [CrossRef]
11. Tol, J.; Koopman, M.; Miller, M.C.; Tibbe, A.; Cats, A.; Creemers, G.J.M.; Vos, A.H.; Nagtegaal, I.; Terstappen, L.W.M.M.; Punt, C.J.A. Circulating tumour cells early predict progression-free and overall survival in advanced colorectal cancer patients treated with chemotherapy and targeted agents. *Ann. Oncol.* **2010**, *21*, 1006–1012. [CrossRef] [PubMed]
12. Sastre, J.; Maestro, M.L.; Gómez-España, A.; Rivera, F.; Valladares, M.; Massuti, B.; Benavides, M.; Gallen, M.; Marcuello, E.; Abad, A.; et al. Circulating Tumor Cell Count Is a Prognostic Factor in Metastatic Colorectal Cancer Patients Receiving First-Line Chemotherapy Plus Bevacizumab: A Spanish Cooperative Group for the Treatment of Digestive Tumors Study. *Oncologist* **2012**, *17*, 947–955. [CrossRef] [PubMed]
13. Riethdorf, S.; Fritsche, H.; Müller, V.; Rau, T.; Schindlbeck, C.; Rack, B.; Janni, W.; Coith, C.; Beck, K.; Jänicke, F.; et al. Detection of Circulating Tumor Cells in Peripheral Blood of Patients with Metastatic Breast Cancer: A Validation Study of the CellSearch System. *Clin. Cancer Res.* **2007**, *13*, 920–928. [CrossRef] [PubMed]
14. Mikolajczyk, S.D.; Millar, L.S.; Tsinberg, P.; Coutts, S.M.; Zomorrodi, M.; Pham, T.; Bischoff, F.Z.; Pircher, T.J. Detection of EpCAM-Negative and Cytokeratin-Negative Circulating Tumor Cells in Peripheral Blood. *J. Oncol.* **2011**, *2011*, 252361. [CrossRef] [PubMed]
15. Serrano, M.J.; Ortega, F.G.; Cubero, M.J.A.; Nadal, R.; Sánchez, F.G.O.; Salido, M.; Rodríguez, M.; García-Puche, J.L.; Delgado-Rodriguez, M.; Solé, F.; et al. EMT and EGFR in CTCs cytokeratin negative non-metastatic breast cancer. *Oncotarget* **2014**, *5*, 7486–7497. [CrossRef]
16. Soler, A.; Cayrefourcq, L.; Mazel, M.; Alix-Panabières, C. EpCAM-Independent Enrichment and Detection of Viable Circulating Tumor Cells Using the EPISPOT Assay. In *Circulating Tumor Cells*; Magbanua, M.J.M., Park, J.W., Eds.; Springer: New York, NY, USA, 2017; Volume 1634, pp. 263–276. [CrossRef]
17. Ramirez, J.-M.; Fehm, T.; Orsini, M.; Cayrefourcq, L.; Maudelonde, T.; Pantel, K.; Alix-Panabières, C. Prognostic Relevance of Viable Circulating Tumor Cells Detected by EPISPOT in Metastatic Breast Cancer Patients. *Clin. Chem.* **2014**, *60*, 214–221. [CrossRef]
18. DeNeve, E.; Riethdorf, S.; Ramos, J.; Nocca, D.; Coffy, A.; Daurès, J.-P.; Maudelonde, T.; Fabre, J.-M.; Pantel, K.; Alix-Panabières, C. Capture of Viable Circulating Tumor Cells in the Liver of Colorectal Cancer Patients. *Clin. Chem.* **2013**, *59*, 1384–1392. [CrossRef]
19. Cristofanilli, M.; Budd, G.T.; Ellis, M.J.; Stopeck, A.; Matera, J.; Miller, M.C.; Reuben, J.M.; Doyle, G.V.; Allard, W.J.; Terstappen, L.W.; et al. Circulating Tumor Cells, Disease Progression, and Survival in Metastatic Breast Cancer. *N. Engl. J. Med.* **2004**, *351*, 781–791. [CrossRef]
20. De Bono, J.S.; Scher, H.I.; Montgomery, R.B.; Parker, C.; Miller, M.C.; Tissing, H.; Doyle, G.V.; Terstappen, L.W.; Pienta, K.; Raghavan, D. Circulating Tumor Cells Predict Survival Benefit from Treatment in Metastatic Castration-Resistant Prostate Cancer. *Clin. Cancer Res.* **2008**, *14*, 6302–6309. [CrossRef]
21. Bidard, F.-C.; Peeters, D.J.; Fehm, T.; Nolé, F.; Gisbert-Criado, R.; Mavroudis, D.; Grisanti, S.; Generali, D.; Garcia-Saenz, J.A.; Stebbing, J.; et al. Clinical validity of circulating tumour cells in patients with metastatic breast cancer: A pooled analysis of individual patient data. *Lancet Oncol.* **2014**, *15*, 406–414. [CrossRef]
22. Bidard, F.-C.; Jacot, W.; Kiavue, N.; Dureau, S.; Kadi, A.; Brain, E.; Bachelot, T.; Bourgeois, H.; Gonçalves, A.; Ladoire, S.; et al. Efficacy of Circulating Tumor Cell Count–Driven vs Clinician-Driven First-line Therapy Choice in Hormone Receptor–Positive, ERBB2-Negative Metastatic Breast Cancer. *JAMA Oncol.* **2021**, *7*, 34–41. [CrossRef] [PubMed]
23. Cremolini, C.; Loupakis, F.; Antoniotti, C.; Lupi, C.; Sensi, E.; Lonardi, S.; Mezi, S.; Tomasello, G.; Ronzoni, M.; Zaniboni, A.; et al. FOLFOXIRI plus bevacizumab versus FOLFIRI plus bevacizumab as first-line treatment of patients with metastatic colorectal cancer: Updated overall sur-vival and molecular subgroup analyses of the open-label, phase 3 TRIBE study. *Lancet Oncol.* **2015**, *16*, 1306–1315. [CrossRef]
24. E Silva, V.S.; Chinen, L.; Abdallah, E.A.; Damascena, A.; Paludo, J.; Chojniak, R.; Dettino, A.; Mello, C.A.L.; Alves, V.S.; Fanelli, M.F. Early detection of poor outcome in patients with metastatic colorectal cancer: Tumor kinetics evaluated by circulating tumor cells. *OncoTargets Ther.* **2016**, *9*, 7503–7513. [CrossRef] [PubMed]
25. Yang, C.; Chen, F.; Wang, S.; Xiong, B. Circulating Tumor Cells in Gastrointestinal Cancers: Current Status and Future Perspectives. *Front. Oncol.* **2019**, *9*, 1427. [CrossRef] [PubMed]
26. Kuske, A.; Gorges, T.M.; Tennstedt, P.; Tiebel, A.-K.; Pompe, R.S.; Preißer, F.; Prues, S.; Mazel, M.; Markou, A.; Lianidou, E.; et al. Improved detection of circulating tumor cells in non-metastatic high-risk prostate cancer patients. *Sci. Rep.* **2016**, *6*, 39736. [CrossRef] [PubMed]
27. Cayrefourcq, L.; De Roeck, A.; Garcia, C.; Stoebner, P.-E.; Fichel, F.; Garima, F.; Perriard, F.; Daures, J.-P.; Meunier, L.; Alix-Panabières, C. S100-EPISPOT: A New Tool to Detect Viable Circulating Melanoma Cells. *Cells* **2019**, *8*, 755. [CrossRef]

28. Garrel, R.; Mazel, M.; Perriard, F.; Vinches, M.; Cayrefourcq, L.; Guigay, J.; Digue, L.; Aubry, K.; Alfonsi, M.; Delord, J.-P.; et al. Circulating Tumor Cells as a Prognostic Factor in Recurrent or Metastatic Head and Neck Squamous Cell Carcinoma: The CIRCUTEC Prospective Study. *Clin. Chem.* **2019**, *65*, 1267–1275. [CrossRef]
29. Krebs, M.; Renehan, A.; Backen, A.; Gollins, S.; Chau, I.; Hasan, J.; Valle, J.W.; Morris, K.; Beech, J.; Ashcroft, L.; et al. Circulating Tumor Cell Enumeration in a Phase II Trial of a Four-Drug Regimen in Advanced Colorectal Cancer. *Clin. Color. Cancer* **2015**, *14*, 115–122.e2. [CrossRef] [PubMed]
30. Sastre, J.; de la Orden, V.; Martínez, A.; Bando, I.; Balbín, M.; Bellosillo, B.; Palanca, S.; Gomez, M.I.P.; Mediero, B.; Llovet, P.; et al. Association Between Baseline Circulating Tumor Cells, Molecular Tumor Profiling, and Clinical Characteristics in a Large Cohort of Chemo-naïve Metastatic Colorectal Cancer Patients Prospectively Collected. *Clin. Color. Cancer* **2020**, *19*, e110–e116. [CrossRef]
31. Kaifi, J.T.; Kunkel, M.; Dicker, D.T.; Joude, J.; E Allen, J.; Das, A.; Zhu, J.; Yang, Z.; E Sarwani, N.; Li, G.; et al. Circulating tumor cell levels are elevated in colorectal cancer patients with high tumor burden in the liver. *Cancer Biol. Ther.* **2015**, *16*, 690–698. [CrossRef]

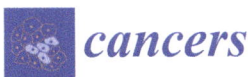

Article

Clinical Characteristics and Outcomes of Colorectal Cancer in the ColoCare Study: Differences by Age of Onset

Caroline Himbert [1,2], Jane C. Figueiredo [3], David Shibata [4], Jennifer Ose [1,2], Tengda Lin [1,2], Lyen C. Huang [1,2], Anita R. Peoples [1,2], Courtney L. Scaife [1], Bartley Pickron [1], Laura Lambert [1], Jessica N. Cohan [1], Mary Bronner [1], Seth Felder [5], Julian Sanchez [5], Sophie Dessureault [5], Domenico Coppola [5], David M. Hoffman [3], Yosef F. Nasseri [3], Robert W. Decker [3], Karen Zaghiyan [3], Zuri A. Murrell [3], Andrew Hendifar [3], Jun Gong [3], Eiman Firoozmand [3], Alexandra Gangi [3], Beth A. Moore [3], Kyle G. Cologne [3], Maryliza S. El-Masry [3], Nathan Hinkle [4], Justin Monroe [4], Matthew Mutch [6], Cory Bernadt [6], Deyali Chatterjee [6], Mika Sinanan [7,8], Stacey A. Cohen [7,8], Ulrike Wallin [7], William M. Grady [7], Paul D. Lampe [7], Deepti Reddi [7,8], Mukta Krane [7,8], Alessandro Fichera [9], Ravi Moonka [7], Esther Herpel [10], Peter Schirmacher [10], Matthias Kloor [10], Magnus von Knebel-Doeberitz [10], Johanna Nattenmueller [10], Hans-Ulrich Kauczor [10], Eric Swanson [1], Jolanta Jedrzkiewicz [1,2], Stephanie L. Schmit [5], Biljana Gigic [10], Alexis B. Ulrich [10], Adetunji T. Toriola [6], Erin M. Siegel [5], Christopher I. Li [7], Cornelia M. Ulrich [1,2,†] and Sheetal Hardikar [1,2,7,*,†]

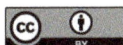

Citation: Himbert, C.; Figueiredo, J.C.; Shibata, D.; Ose, J.; Lin, T.; Huang, L.C.; Peoples, A.R.; Scaife, C.L.; Pickron, B.; Lambert, L.; et al. Clinical Characteristics and Outcomes of Colorectal Cancer in the ColoCare Study: Differences by Age of Onset. Cancers **2021**, 13, 3817. https://doi.org/10.3390/cancers13153817

Academic Editor: Heike Allgayer

Received: 18 May 2021
Accepted: 6 July 2021
Published: 29 July 2021

Publisher's Note: MDPI stays neutral with regard to jurisdictional claims in published maps and institutional affiliations.

Copyright: © 2021 by the authors. Licensee MDPI, Basel, Switzerland. This article is an open access article distributed under the terms and conditions of the Creative Commons Attribution (CC BY) license (https://creativecommons.org/licenses/by/4.0/).

1. Huntsman Cancer Institute, Salt Lake City, UT 84112, USA; caroline.himbert@hci.utah.edu (C.H.); jennifer.ose@hci.utah.edu (J.O.); tengda.lin@hci.utah.edu (T.L.); lyen.huang@hsc.utah.edu (L.C.H.); Anita.peoples@hci.utah.edu (A.R.P.); courtney.scaife@hci.utah.edu (C.L.S.); Bartley.Pickron@hsc.utah.edu (B.P.); Laura.Lambert@hci.utah.edu (L.L.); jessica.cohan@hsc.utah.edu (J.N.C.); mary.bronner@aruplab.com (M.B.); Swanson.Eric@scrippshealth.org (E.S.); Jolanta.Jedrzkiewicz@hsc.utah.edu (J.J.); Neli.ulrich@hci.utah.edu (C.M.U.)
2. Department of Population Health Sciences, University of Utah, Salt Lake City, UT 84112, USA
3. Cedars-Sinai Center, Los Angeles, CA 90048, USA; jane.figueiredo@cshs.org (J.C.F.); hoffmand@toweroncology.com (D.M.H.); Yosef.Nasseri@cshs.org (Y.F.N.); deckerr@toweroncology.com (R.W.D.); Karen.zaghiyan@cshs.org (K.Z.); Zuri.murrell@cshs.org (Z.A.M.); andrew.hendifar@cshs.org (A.H.); jun.gong@cshs.org (J.G.); efiroozmand@yahoo.com (E.F.); alexandra.gangi@cshs.org (A.G.); Beth.Moore@cshs.org (B.A.M.); kyle.cologne@med.usc.edu (K.G.C.); maryliza.el-masry@csmns.org (M.S.E.-M.)
4. Department of Surgery, University of Tennessee Health Science Center, Memphis, TN 37996, USA; dshibata@uthsc.edu (D.S.); natehinkle27@gmail.com (N.H.); jmonroe1@uthsc.edu (J.M.)
5. H. Lee Moffitt Cancer Center and Research Institute, Tampa, FL 33612, USA; seth.felder@moffitt.org (S.F.); Julian.sanchez@moffitt.org (J.S.); sophie.dessureault@moffitt.org (S.D.); domenico.coppola@fdhs.org (D.C.); Stephanie.Schmit@moffitt.org (S.L.S.); Erin.Siegel@moffitt.org (E.M.S.)
6. Department of Surgery, Washington University St. Louis, St. Louis, MO 63130, USA; mutchm@wustl.edu (M.M.); cbernadt@wustl.edu (C.B.); deyali@wustl.edu (D.C.); a.toriola@wustl.edu (A.T.T.)
7. Fred Hutchinson Cancer Research Center, Seattle, WA 98109, USA; mssurg@uw.edu (M.S.); shiovitz@uw.edu (S.A.C.); ulrik.wallin@polyclinic.com (U.W.); wgrady@fredhutch.org (W.M.G.); plampe@fredhutch.org (P.D.L.); dreddi@uw.edu (D.R.); mkrane@uw.edu (M.K.); Ravi.Moonka@vmmc.org (R.M.); cili@fredhutch.org (C.I.L.)
8. Department of Laboratory Medicine and Pathology, University of Washington, Seattle, WA 98195, USA
9. Baylor Scott & White Health, Dallas, TX 76712, USA; Alessandro.Fichera@BSWHealth.org
10. Pathologisches Institut, University Hospital Heidelberg, 69120 Heidelberg, Germany; Esther.Herpel@med.uni-heidelberg.de (E.H.); Peter.Schirmacher@med.uni-heidelberg.de (P.S.); matthias.kloor@med.uni-heidelberg.de (M.K.); magnus.knebel-doeberitz@med.uni-heidelberg.de (M.v.K.-D.); johanna.nattenmueller@med.uni-heidelberg.de (J.N.); hans-ulrich.kauczor@med.uni-heidelberg.de (H.-U.K.); Biljana.Gigic@med.uni-heidelberg.de (B.G.); aulrich@lukasneuss.de (A.B.U.)
* Correspondence: sheetal.hardikar@hci.utah.edu; Tel.: +1-(801)-213-6238
† These authors contributed equally.

Simple Summary: The number of new colorectal cancer cases continues to increase in individuals under 50 years of age in the Western world. Underlying reasons for this observation remain unclear. Here, we compare demographic, clinical, and lifestyle characteristics by age at diagnosis in a large cohort of newly diagnosed colorectal cancer patients. We aim to identify potential risk factors and clinical characteristics of colorectal cancer patients diagnosed under the age of 50 years, compared to those over 50. The results of this study will help elucidate factors related to colorectal cancer in younger patients, and may help guide future research on colorectal cancer in younger patients.

Abstract: Early-onset colorectal cancer has been on the rise in Western populations. Here, we compare patient characteristics between those with early- (<50 years) vs. late-onset ($\geq$50 years) disease in a large multinational cohort of colorectal cancer patients (n = 2193). We calculated descriptive statistics and assessed associations of clinicodemographic factors with age of onset using mutually-adjusted logistic regression models. Patients were on average 60 years old, with BMI of 29 kg/m^2, 52% colon cancers, 21% early-onset, and presented with stage II or III (60%) disease. Early-onset patients presented with more advanced disease (stages III–IV: 63% vs. 51%, respectively), and received more neo and adjuvant treatment compared to late-onset patients, after controlling for stage (odds ratio (OR) (95% confidence interval (CI)) = 2.30 (1.82–3.83) and 2.00 (1.43–2.81), respectively). Early-onset rectal cancer patients across all stages more commonly received neoadjuvant treatment, even when not indicated as the standard of care, e.g., during stage I disease. The odds of early-onset disease were higher among never smokers and lower among overweight patients (1.55 (1.21–1.98) and 0.56 (0.41–0.76), respectively). Patients with early-onset colorectal cancer were more likely to be diagnosed with advanced stage disease, to have received systemic treatments regardless of stage at diagnosis, and were less likely to be ever smokers or overweight.

Keywords: early onset; colorectal cancer; cohort; epidemiology

1. Introduction

An emerging concern in colorectal cancer is the rapidly rising incidence among those under the age of 50 years (early-onset patients) [1–3]. Since 1990, early-onset colorectal cancer has significantly increased globally and the number of new cases is expected to increase by 140% by the end of 2030 [4,5]. In response, the American Cancer Society and the United States Preventive Services Task Force (USPSTF) guidelines have been recently updated to advocate for initiating colorectal cancer screening at the age of 45 years [6,7]. Drivers of the recent increase in early-onset colorectal cancer have yet to be identified, although established modifiable risk factors for late-onset colorectal cancer including diet, obesity, low physical activity, and smoking are potential key players [8–11].

Accumulating evidence suggests that distinct biological characteristics and mechanisms underlie the development of early-onset colorectal cancer as compared to colorectal cancer diagnosed among individuals over 50 years old [12]. Genetic profiles of patients with early-onset colorectal cancer still remain unclear [12]. About 30% of early-onset cases can be attributed to family history and hereditary conditions, although these are not hypothesized to drive the increasing incidence in this population [12]. Early-onset colorectal cancers are more likely to be microsatellite stable, and investigators continue to discover chromosomal abnormalities specific to early-onset disease [12]. Recently, our team has discovered deregulated redox homeostasis as one molecular phenotype of early-onset colorectal cancer patients [13]. Dysbiosis of the gut microbiome is another hypothesized molecular driver of the early-onset colorectal cancer burden [12]. External (e.g., stress, antibiotics, diet, etc.) and internal (e.g., inflammation) elements throughout life can alter gut microbiome health and may affect the risk of developing colorectal cancer in early years [12]. Key pathways within these hypothesized biological mechanisms that are associated with early-onset disease have yet to be discovered [12].

To date, clinical recommendations for colorectal cancer treatment do not differ by age of onset [14]. Yet, prior studies have observed that a more aggressive treatment regimen is generally adopted for early-onset patients as compared to late-onset patients [15–18]; in particular, an increased use of systemic treatments, including neoadjuvant and adjuvant therapy, are reported. Regardless of tumor stage and treatment regimens, survival among the early-onset patient population seems to be superior to the older population [19]. Hence, whether or not early-onset patients experience a greater benefit and less side effects from these systemic treatments remains unclear [15–18].

Here, we describe demographic (age, sex, race, ethnicity), clinical (stage at diagnosis, site, treatment), and lifestyle (smoking status, body mass index (BMI)) characteristics of a large international cohort of prospectively followed patients with colorectal cancer, with the goal of identifying potential risk factors and clinical correlates of early-onset colorectal cancer.

2. Materials and Methods

2.1. Study Population

The design and population of the ColoCare Study (www.clinicaltrials.gov (accessed on 19 July 2021), Identifier: NCT02328677) have previously been described [20–24]. Briefly, the ColoCare Study is a multicenter international prospective cohort recruiting patients with newly diagnosed colorectal cancer at any stage (International Classification of Diseases, 10th edition, C18–C20). Patients are recruited at multiple sites in the United States [Fred Hutchinson Cancer Research Center (FHCRC, Seattle, WA, USA); H. Lee Moffitt Cancer Center and Research Institute (Moffitt, Tampa, FL, USA); University of Tennessee Health Science Center (UTHSC, Memphis, TN, USA); Washington University School of Medicine (WUSM, St. Louis, MO, USA); Huntsman Cancer Institute (HCI, Salt Lake City, UT, USA); Cedars-Sinai Medical Center (Cedars, Los Angeles, CA, USA)] and in Germany (University of Heidelberg(HBG, Heidelberg, Germany)).

In the current analysis, we report data on $n = 2193$ men and women recruited in the ColoCare Study cohort from December 2009 through to March 2020, with detailed data from questionnaires and medical chart abstractions. The study was approved by the Institutional Review Boards of the respective recruitment sites, and all patients provided written informed consent.

2.2. Data Collection

Questionnaires administered at study enrollment (baseline) assessed demographic (age at diagnosis, sex, race/ethnicity) and behavioral (smoking, BMI) characteristics. Clinical characteristics including stage at diagnosis and primary tumor site, recurrence, vital status, and adjuvant and neoadjuvant treatment were abstracted from medical records.

2.3. Data Elements

Demographic characteristics: Patients were categorized by age of onset (<50 and ≥50 years) at the time of diagnosis, ethnicity (Hispanic and non-Hispanic) and race (White, African American, and other, which includes Asians, Native Hawaiians, Native Americans, and patients reporting belonging to more than one race).

Tumor and clinical characteristics: Patients were grouped by stage at diagnosis (0, I, II, III, IV—before receipt of any neoadjuvant treatment), tumor site based on ICD-10 codes (colon = C18.0–C18.9; rectum = C19.9, C20.9, C21.8), recurrence status at 2 years after surgery ("yes" = had recurrence, "no" = no recurrence), vital status ("alive", "deceased"), and neo (rectal cancers only) and/or adjuvant treatment ("yes" = received neo/adjuvant treatment, "no" = did not receive neo/adjuvant treatment).

Behavioral characteristics: Patients were categorized by their smoking behavior (current, former, never smoker). BMI was computed using anthropometric measurements (kg/m^2). BMI categories were computed following the World Health Organization (WHO) categorization (underweight: $\leq 18.5\ kg/m^2$, normal weight: >18.5 to $<25\ kg/m^2$, overweight: $\geq 25\ kg/m^2$ to $<30\ kg/m^2$, obese: $\geq 30\ kg/m^2$).

2.4. Statistical Analyses

Mean and standard deviation (SD) values were calculated for continuous variables (age, BMI). Frequencies and percentages were calculated for categorical variables (age of onset, sex, race, ethnicity, tumor stage, tumor site, recurrence, vital status, neoadjuvant and adjuvant treatment, smoking, BMI categories). Clinical characteristics were compared by age of onset (early- vs. late-onset) and tumor site. Furthermore, we also compared the clinical characteristics by tumor site within age groups. We have currently modeled all missing data as a separate category in our statistical models.

Multivariate logistic regression models (odds ratio (OR) and 95% confidence interval (95% CI)) were computed to assess the independent associations of stage at diagnosis, tumor treatment (neoadjuvant (rectal cancer patients only) and adjuvant), smoking, and BMI categories with age of onset. The primary outcome was early-onset colorectal cancer in each model. ORs and 95% CI were computed for three models: (1) adjusted for sex and race; (2) adjusted for sex, race, tumor site, and stage at diagnosis; and (3) adjusted for sex, race, tumor site, stage at diagnosis, smoking, BMI, and study site, respectively. These variables were parameterized as outlined above. Some studies have suggested a varying risk for intermediate onset colorectal cancers [25]; therefore, subgroup analyses were conducted categorizing patients into early- (<50 years), intermediate (50–55 years), and late-onset (>55 years). All statistical analyses were performed using SAS (Version 9.4, SAS, Cary, NC, USA) software.

3. Results

Patient characteristics, overall and by age of onset, are summarized in Table 1. Overall, 82% of patients were recruited at one of the American sites, while 18% were recruited in Germany. Fifty-seven percent were male, and the mean age was 60 years (SD ± 13 years). The majority of the cohort reported being non-Hispanic (93%) and White (87%). Of note, the initial recruitment into the ColoCare Study occurred in Germany, and the entire 18% of our German cohort was European White, impacting the overall racial/ethnic distribution. Overall, there were approximately equal numbers of colon and rectal cancers (52% vs. 47%, respectively). Study participants were diagnosed predominantly with stage II or III (60%) colorectal cancers. In a subset with detailed treatment information abstracted (75% of the cohort), 34% and 43% of the study population received neoadjuvant and/or adjuvant treatments, respectively. At the time of this analysis, 20% were deceased, and 15% had experienced a colorectal cancer recurrence. A larger proportion of patients were never smokers (40%), and overweight or obese (60%); the mean BMI of the cohort was 28.6 kg/m^2 (±6 kg/m^2).

Twenty-one percent (n = 459) of patients were diagnosed with early-onset colorectal cancer (Table 1). Early-onset colorectal cancer patients were more likely to be of Hispanic ethnicity compared to late-onset patients (8% vs. 4%), with no differences by race or sex. Early-onset patients were more likely to be diagnosed at a more advanced stage (III or IV) (early-onset: stage III: 40%, stage IV: 23%; late-onset: stage III: 34%, stage IV: 17%). They were also more likely to receive adjuvant and/or neoadjuvant treatment (neoadjuvant: 84% vs. 68%, adjuvant: 50% vs. 41% in early-onset compared to late-onset patients, respectively). A lower proportion of early-onset cancers were deceased at the time of the current analyses (14% vs. 21% early- vs. late-onset patients, respectively), while the proportion of recurrence was about 15% in both groups. Early-onset patients were less likely to be overweight (25%) or obese (28%) as compared to late-onset patients (36% and 32%, respectively), while the proportion of underweight patients was higher in early- vs. late-onset cancers (16% vs. 7%). Patients diagnosed with early-onset cancers were more likely to be never smokers (45%) in comparison with late-onset colorectal cancers (39%).

Table 2 summarizes patient characteristics comparing early- and late-onset patients by tumor site. When further categorized by tumor site, the cohort consisted of 18% early-onset and 82% late-onset colon cancers, and 21% early-onset and 79% late-onset rectal cancer patients. Forty-nine percent of early-onset patients were diagnosed with colon cancers as compared to 54% of late-onset patients, while 51% of early-onset patients were rectal cancers as compared to 46% of late-onset patients. The proportion of women was slightly higher among early-onset (51%) compared to late-onset colon cancer patients (47%). Early-onset rectal cancer patients had a slightly lower proportion of deceased patients compared to late-onset rectal cancer patients (11% vs. 20%). Among early-onset patients, the proportion of current and former smokers was higher among patients with rectal cancer compared to those with colon cancer (42% vs. 29%).

Table 1. Demographic, tumor, treatment, and behavior characteristics of the ColoCare Study cohort by age of onset [A].

		Early-Onset Colorectal Cancer (<50 Years) (n = 459)		Late-Onset Colorectal Cancer (≥50 Years) (n = 1734)		Total (n = 2193)	
		n	21%	n	79%	n	%
		Demographic Characteristics					
Sex	Male	252	55	1000	58	1293	57
	Female	207	45	734	42	941	43
Ethnicity	Hispanic	35	8	63	4	98	4
	Non-Hispanic	409	89	1649	95	2058	94
Race	White	386	84	1528	88	1914	87
	African American	28	6	114	7	142	6
	Other *	36	8	80	5	66	6
		Tumor and Clinical Characteristics					
Stage at diagnosis	0	7	2	61	4	68	3
	I	50	11	322	19	372	17
	II	93	20	436	25	529	24
	III	185	40	597	34	782	36
	IV	107	23	291	17	398	18
Tumor site	Colon	209	45	933	54	1142	52
	Rectum	219	48	799	46	1018	47
Recurrence	Yes	67	14	252	15	320	15
	No	261	57	1134	65	1395	63
Vital status	Alive	392	85	1365	79	428	20
	Deceased	64	14	364	21	1757	80
Neoadjuvant Treatment (rectal only)	Yes—Total	159	84	437	68	596	72
	No	30	16	201	32	231	28
Adjuvant treatment	Yes—Total	232	50	704	41	936	43
	No	94	21	577	33	671	31
		Behavioral Characteristics					
Smoking	Current	64	14	208	12	272	12
	Former	95	21	638	37	733	33
	Never	207	45	679	39	886	40
BMI, mean (SD)		28 (7)		29 (6)		29 (6)	
BMI categories	Underweight	62	13	95	5	195	9
	Normal weight	142	31	434	25	576	26
	Overweight	116	25	617	36	733	33
	Obese	128	28	561	32	689	31

* "Other" includes Asians, Native Hawaiians, Native Americans, and patients reporting belonging to more than one race. [A] Data has not yet been abstracted on $n = 37$ (2%) for ethnicity, $n = 21$ (1%) for race, $n = 56$ (3%) for tumor stage, $n = 44$ (2%) for tumor site, $n = 478$ (22%) for recurrence, $n = 8$ (0.3%) for vital status, $n = 621$ (27%) for receipt of neoadjuvant treatment, $n = 585$ (26%) for receipt of adjuvant treatment, $n = 302$ (14%) for smoking, and $n = 157$ (7%) for BMI.

Table 2. Frequencies and percentages of patient, tumor, and behavior characteristics by tumor site and age of onset [A].

		Colon Cancer (n = 1142)				Rectal Cancer (n = 1018)			
		Early-Onset (n = 209)		Late-Onset (n = 933)		Early-Onset (n = 219)		Late-Onset (n = 799)	
		n	%	n	%	n	%	n	%
		Demographic Characteristics							
Sex	Male	103	49	434	47	132	60	500	63
	Female	106	51	499	53	87	40	299	37
Ethnicity	Hispanic	15	7	36	4	19	9	27	3
	Non-Hispanic	190	91	882	94	193	88	765	96
Race	White	167	80	804	86	189	86	722	90
	African American	18	9	80	9	10	5	34	4
	Other *	19	7	43	5	16	7	37	5
		Tumor and Clinical Characteristics							
Stage at diagnosis	0	5	2	31	4	2	1	30	4
	I	27	13	191	20	18	8	130	16
	II	42	20	255	27	45	21	181	23
	III	65	31	259	28	113	52	228	42
	IV	65	31	183	20	38	17	108	14
Recurrence	Yes	34	16	626	67	33	15	507	63
	No	119	57	134	14	142	65	119	15
Vital status	Alive	171	82	721	77	193	88	642	80
	Deceased	38	18	207	22	25	11	157	20
Neoadjuvant treatment (rectal only)	Yes	-	-	-	-	159	84	437	68
	No	-	-	-	-	30	16	201	32
Adjuvant treatment *	Yes	108	52	362	39	124	57	342	43
	No	47	22	333	36	47	22	242	30
		Behavioral Characteristics							
Smoking	Current	21	10	91	10	39	18	117	15
	Former	40	19	342	37	52	24	296	37
	Never	104	50	372	40	95	43	307	38
BMI, mean (SD)		29 (8)		29 (6)		28 (6)		28 (6)	
BMI categories	Underweight	2	1	15	2	8	4	12	2
	Normal weight	72	34	231	25	68	31	203	25
	Overweight	48	23	316	34	63	29	301	38
	Obese	62	30	327	35	63	29	233	29

* "Other" includes Asians, Native Hawaiians, Native Americans, and patients reporting belonging to more than one race. [A] Data has not yet been abstracted on n = 37 (2%) for ethnicity, n = 21 (1%) for race, n = 44 (0.2%) for tumor stage, n = 478 (22%) for recurrence, n = 8 (0.3%) for vital status, n = 191 (19%) for neoadjuvant treatment, n = 585 (26%) for adjuvant treatment, n = 302 (14%) for smoking, and n = 50 (6%) for BMI.

Regardless of tumor site, early-onset patients were more likely to receive neoadjuvant and/or adjuvant treatments. Table 3 compares proportions of early- vs. late-onset colon cancer patients receiving adjuvant treatment by stage at diagnosis. A higher proportion of stage II and III early-onset colon cancer patients received adjuvant treatment (45% and 90%, respectively) as compared to late-onset colon cancer patients (27% and 85%, respectively). Table 4 compares proportions of early- vs. late-onset rectal cancer patients receiving neoadjuvant and adjuvant treatment by stage at diagnosis. A slightly higher proportion of early-onset stage I rectal cancer patients received neoadjuvant treatment (40% vs. 32%). Overall, a higher proportion of early-onset rectal cancer patients tend to receive neoadjuvant treatment as compared to late-onset rectal cancer patients (stage I: 40% vs. 32%, stage II: 82% vs. 71%, stage III: 91% vs. 79%, stage IV: 85% vs. 76%), even when such treatment may not be clinically indicated, e.g., for stage I rectal cancer patients where neoadjuvant treatment is not the standard of care. Similar observations were observed for adjuvant treatment among rectal cancer patients.

Table 3. Proportion of early- and late-onset colon cancer patients receiving adjuvant treatment by stage at diagnosis.

	Early-Onset Rectal Cancer			Late-Onset Rectal Cancer		
Stage at Diagnosis	Total *n*	Received Neoadjuvant Treatment	% Received Neoadjuvant Treatment	Total *n*	Received Neoadjuvant Treatment	% Received Neoadjuvant Treatment
Stage I	13	1	1	118	5	0.4
Stage II	31	14	45	179	49	27
Stage III	60	54	90	233	195	85
Stage IV	49	39	80	154	112	73

Table 4. Proportion of early- and late-onset rectal cancer patients receiving neoadjuvant and adjuvant treatment by stage at diagnosis (i.e., before the receipt of any neoadjuvant treatment).

	Early-Onset Rectal Cancer			Late-Onset Rectal Cancer		
Stage at Diagnosis	Total *n*	Received Neoadjuvant Treatment	% Received Neoadjuvant Treatment	Total *n*	Received Neoadjuvant Treatment	% Received Neoadjuvant Treatment
Stage I	10	4	40	81	26	32
Stage II	39	32	82	153	109	71
Stage III	101	92	91	297	230	79
Stage IV	34	29	85	90	68	76
	Total *n*	Received adjuvant treatment	% Received adjuvant treatment	Total *n*	Received adjuvant treatment	% received adjuvant treatment
Stage I	9	2	22	77	16	21
Stage II	36	28	78	136	77	57
Stage III	94	69	73	273	187	68
Stage IV	27	19	70	82	59	72

Table 5 summarizes the results of adjusted logistic regression models assessing associations between patients with early-onset colorectal cancer and stage at diagnosis, tumor treatment (neoadjuvant, adjuvant), smoking, and BMI categories. All the results described below are from a model (Model 3) which is mutually adjusted for sex, race, tumor site, stage at diagnosis, BMI, smoking, and study site. The odds of being diagnosed with a more advanced stage for early-onset patients was approximately two times that of late-onset patients (stage III: 1.99 (1.39–2.87), stage IV: 2.50 (1.69–3.72)). Among rectal cancer patients, the odds of receiving neoadjuvant treatment was 2.31-fold (1.43–3.70) higher for early-onset compared to late-onset patients. Similar results were observed for adjuvant treatment. Early-onset colorectal cancer patients were less likely to be overweight and obese compared to patients with late-onset colorectal cancer (OR (95% CI) comparing early- to late-onset = 0.56 (0.41–0.76) and 0.66 (0.48–0.90), for overweight and obese patients, respectively). Early-onset patients were more likely to be never smokers compared to late-onset patients (OR (95% CI) = 1.55 (1.21–1.98)).

Table 5. Logistic regression OR (95% confidence interval) comparing tumor, clinical, and behavioral characteristics between early- vs. late-onset colorectal cancer patients.

Exposure Variable		Age of Onset N		Model 1 [a]	Model 2 [b]	Model 3 [c]
		Early	Late			
Neoadjuvant treatment (rectal cancer only)	No	134	721	1.00	1.00	1.00
	Yes	319	524	2.45 (1.60–3.75)	2.25 (1.41–3.57)	2.30 (1.43–3.70)
Adjuvant treatment	No	133	453	1.00	1.00	1.00
	Yes	232	704	2.00 (1.53–2.62)	1.69 (1.25–2.28)	2.00 (1.43–2.81)
Stage at diagnosis	0	7	61	0.75 (0.33–1.74)	–	1.00 (0.46–2.17)
	I	50	322	1.00	–	1.00
	II	93	436	1.36 (0.93–1.98)	–	1.44 (0.97–2.13)
	III	185	597	1.98 (1.40–2.78)	–	1.99 (1.39–2.87)
	IV	107	291	2.31 (1.59–3.37)	–	2.50 (1.69–3.72)
Smoking	Ever	159	846	1.00	1.00	1.00
	Never	207	679	1.60 (1.27–2.03)	1.56 (1.23–1.99)	1.55 (1.21–1.98)
BMI	Underweight	62	95	1.26 (0.61–2.62)	1.02 (0.46–2.24)	1.08 (0.49–2.41)
	Normal weight	142	343	1.00	1.00	1.00
	Overweight	116	617	0.58 (0.44–0.77)	0.60 (0.45–0.80)	0.56 (0.41–0.76)
	Obese	128	561	0.72 (0.55–0.94)	0.78 (0.59–1.03)	0.66 (0.48–0.90)

[a] adjusted for sex and race; [b] adjusted for sex, race, tumor site and stage; [c] mutually adjusted for sex, race, tumor site and stage, BMI, smoking, and study site.

Some studies have suggested a varying risk for intermediate onset colorectal cancers [25]; therefore, we conducted further subgroup analyses categorizing patients into early- (<50 years), intermediate (50–55 years), and late-onset (>55 years) colorectal cancer (Supplementary Table S1). Similar to early-onset patients, the odds of receiving adjuvant treatment were 1.54-fold (1.15–2.05) for patients with intermediate onset disease as compared to late-onset disease. Intermediate onset patients were more likely to be diagnosed with stage IV disease (1.79-fold (1.16–2.78)) compared to late-onset patients. No differences were observed for stage 0–III. Similar to early-onset patients, the odds of being a never smoker were 1.54-fold (1.19–2.01) for patients with intermediate onset disease in contrast with late-onset disease. No differences between intermediate and late-onset patients were observed for neoadjuvant treatment or BMI. These results indicate that cancers developing early in life may have distinct risk factors compared to those developing later in life.

4. Discussion

This study describes demographic, clinical, and behavioral characteristics of participants in the ColoCare Study, an international multicenter cohort of patients with newly diagnosed colorectal cancer. Patients with early-onset colorectal cancer were observed to be diagnosed at a higher stage compared to their late-onset counterparts. Additionally, regardless of stage at diagnosis and tumor site, early-onset patients were more likely to receive a more aggressive treatment regimen than the recommended standard of care compared to late-onset patients, e.g., stage I rectal cancer patients received neoadjuvant treatment when not indicated by National Comprehensive Cancer Network (NCCN) guidelines. Early-onset patients were generally "healthier" and were less likely to be smokers or overweight/obese.

The most recently updated colorectal cancer treatment guidelines from NCCN do not include different recommended regimens for early- vs. late-onset colorectal cancers [14]. Yet, it has been observed that early-onset patients are generally subjected to more aggressive treatment regimens [15–18]. A large cohort study of 1424 patients with early-onset and 10,810 with late-onset colorectal cancer recently reported that 12% of patients with stage I colorectal cancer in their cohort received systemic treatments [15], despite the fact that the NCCN guidelines do not recommend any systemic treatment for patients with stage I colorectal cancer [14]. This observation was also reported in other large population-based studies [16,18]. One study particularly observed a higher prescription of adjuvant chemotherapy among early-onset patients at all stages without gaining any survival benefit [16]. Results from our study support these observations and indicate that (1) early-onset patients—regardless of stage at diagnosis or tumor site—are more likely to receive systemic treatment, and (2) stage I rectal cancer patients seem to receive neoadjuvant and/or adjuvant treatment regardless of age of onset. Occasionally, multidisciplinary treatment teams espouse applications for neoadjuvant chemoradiation beyond locally advanced stage II and III rectal cancers. One such indication is for earlier stage (e.g., stage I, T2N0) distal rectal cancers for which response may increase the likelihood of sphincter preservation. Younger patients are often the ideal candidates for this approach due to multifactorial reasons, including aggressive interest in avoiding permanent colostomy, ability to tolerate multimodality therapy, and strong pre-existing baseline bowel function that would translate to acceptable function/continence following aggressive sphincter-preserving surgery. Systemic treatments, however, are highly toxic and may cause severe short- and long-term complications including cumulative neuropathy and liver toxicity [26]. Understanding patterns of treatments among this high-risk subgroup will aid further evaluation and appropriate adjustment of treatment guidelines.

Modifiable risk factors for early-onset colorectal cancer have yet to be established. Given the strong evidence for the obesity–colorectal cancer relationship, studies on colorectal cancer in young individuals have early on investigated the impact of obesity on the observed increased incidence in this population [10,27]. To date, results remain limited and inconclusive. We observed a lower proportion of overweight and obese patients within our early-onset cancers compared to late-onset cancers. However, a recently published study comparing BMI of 269 patients with early-onset and 2809 with late-onset colorectal cancer did not support our findings, and reported similar BMI distributions in the early- and late-onset groups [10]. While BMI is an established risk factor for colorectal cancer overall, our data does not identify BMI as the driver for the increased incidence of early-onset colorectal cancer. Underlying reasons may be that BMI has been more strongly associated with colon cancer, and the observed association seems to be stronger for men than for women [28].

Smoking has been strongly associated with increased overall colorectal cancer risk in previous studies [29,30]. Zisman et al. observed that smokers were on average 5.2 years (95% CI: 4.9–5.5. years) younger at their colorectal cancer diagnosis than non-smokers. Two studies have investigated smoking as a driver for early-onset colorectal cancer [10,31]. While one study did not observe differences in smoking behavior, a more recent study supports our findings of early-onset patients being less likely to be smokers [10,31]. Taken together, our results suggest that the traditional risk factors for CRC such as BMI and smoking may not explain the recent increase in early-onset cancers, demonstrating the need to identify other risk factors that may explain this increasing trend of early-onset cancers.

The observed rise in the incidence of patients with early-onset colorectal cancer has been reported to be largely driven by rectal and left-sided colon cancers [4,15]. Burnett-Hartman et al. reported a higher proportion of rectal cancers in patients under the age of 39 years [15]. However, underlying reasons for such an increase remain unknown. We did not observe such an increase in rectal cancers in younger patients in our cohort, although we observed a trend for a higher incidence of colon cancer among female early-onset patients.

Our results are aligned with previous studies reporting that patients with early-onset colorectal cancer are characterized by more advanced disease stage at diagnosis [4,12,32]. Delayed diagnosis or misdiagnosis with other related colorectal diseases in the younger population, no existing recommended guidelines for targeted screening, varying symptoms, as well as other unknown molecular factors are hypothesized to underlie this observation [4,12,32,33]. Recently, societies, including the American Cancer Society and the USPSTF [6,7], updated their guidelines to lower the colorectal cancer screening initiation age to 45 years, which may help reduce the number of cases with advanced stage disease among the early-onset colorectal cancer population.

Compared to the general US population, our study population consisted of both a higher proportion of early-onset (21%) and rectal (47%) cancers, making the ColoCare Study cohort a great resource to study these high-risk subgroups. In comparison, out of the expected new patients with colorectal cancer in the US in 2020, approximately 12% will be early-onset, and 29% will be rectal cancers [34]. Our study population was largely recruited at National Comprehensive Cancer Centers and University clinics. Some of these specialized centers are more likely to treat referrals and complex surgeries, which may partly explain the higher proportion of rectal and early-onset patients in our cohort. In the US, on average, over 40% of individuals across all age groups are obese (BMI ≥ 30 kg/m^2) [35]. Our study population had slightly lower rates of obesity for patients under and over the age of 50 years.

This study has several strengths and limitations. The ColoCare Study is an observational cohort and the reported associations may be influenced by unmeasured confounding. Our study population had a higher proportion of rectal and early-onset patients as compared to the general population, making it an ideal research environment to study these high-risk subgroups, including patients with early-onset cancer. Previous research assessing treatment differences by age of onset in patients with colorectal cancer were limited to data from the United States [9,15,33]; having an international study site is particularly unique to our cohort, and allows comparisons between treatment trends in patients with early-onset colorectal cancer. Tumor and clinical characteristics were abstracted from medical records, ensuring accurate classifications of the study population. Family history—as well as other molecular tumor features including MSI status, which have previously been associated with early-onset disease—could not be included in the present study due to pending medical chart abstractions on a larger proportion of our study participants. As smoking behavior is self-reported in the questionnaires, there may be misclassification of smoking status due to social desirability or recall bias.

5. Conclusions

This study of a large prospectively followed colorectal cancer cohort revealed differences in stage at diagnosis and site, neo and adjuvant treatment, BMI, and smoking behavior among patients with early-onset colorectal cancer compared to late-onset patients. Studies comparing treatment differences in patients with early- and late-onset colorectal cancer are needed to test the risk-benefit of more aggressive treatment regimens for patients with early-onset colorectal cancer. Future research involving a more comprehensive assessment of newer modalities of tobacco use, including the use of e-cigarettes, are needed to completely understand the contribution of tobacco use to the recent increase of colorectal cancer in younger patients. More accurate assessments of body composition, including the proportion of visceral and subcutaneous adipose tissues, trends over time in body composition measures, and childhood obesity and weight fluctuations should be considered over BMI when investigating the impact of obesity on early-onset colorectal cancer.

Supplementary Materials: The following are available online at https://www.mdpi.com/article/10.3390/cancers13153817/s1, Table S1: Logistic regression OR (95% confidence interval) comparing tumor, clinical, and behavioral characteristics between early- (≤50 years), intermediate (50–55 years), and late-onset (≥55 years) colorectal cancer patients.

Author Contributions: Conceptualization: C.H., D.S., S.H., J.O., C.M.U.; formal analysis: C.H., S.H., J.O., T.L., L.C.H., C.M.U.; investigation: C.H., S.H., C.M.U.; methodology: C.H., D.S., S.H., C.M.U., L.C.H., C.M.U.; writing—original draft preparation: C.H., J.C.F., S.H., C.M.U.; project administration: J.O., B.G., M.S., A.B.U., A.T.T., E.M.S., C.I.L., S.H., C.M.U.; funding acquisition: J.C.F., C.M.U., D.S., J.O., B.G., M.S., A.B.U., A.T.T., E.M.S., C.I.L., C.M.U.; writing—review and editing: D.S., J.O., L.C.H., A.R.P., C.L.S., B.P., L.L., J.N.C., M.B., S.F., J.S., S.D., D.C. (Domenico Coppola), D.M.H., Y.F.N., R.W.D., K.Z., Z.A.M., A.H., J.G., E.F., A.G., B.A.M., K.G.C., M.S.E.-M., N.H., J.M., M.M., C.B., D.C. (Deyali Chatterjee), M.S., S.A.C., U.W., W.M.G., P.D.L., R.W.D., M.K. (Mukta Krane), A.F., R.M., E.H., P.S., M.K. (Matthias Kloor), M.v.K.-D., J.N., H.-U.K., E.M.S., J.J., S.L.S., B.G., M.S., A.B.U., A.T.T., E.M.S., C.I.L., C.M.U., D.R., E.S. All authors have read and agreed to the published version of the manuscript.

Funding: Hardikar, Ulrich, Ose, Siegel, Toriola, Colditz, Li, Figueiredo are supported by U01206110. Hardikar is funded by K07 222060. Ulrich and Ose, and C. Himbert are funded by the Huntsman Cancer Foundation and R01 CA189184, R01 CA207371. Ulrich is also funded by P30 CA042014. C.Himbert is funded by R01 CA211705 and the Stiftung LebensBlicke. Gigic is funded by the Lackas Foundation, the ERA-NET on Translational Cancer Research (TRANSCAN) project 01KT1503, R01 CA189184, and the Stiftung Lebensblicke. Dr. Grady is funded by the Fred Hutchinson Cancer Research Center, the Seattle Translational Tumor Research Program, the Cottrell Family, and P30CA015704, U01CA152756, R01CA194663, and R01CA220004. Dr. Siegel is funded by the Florida Department of Health Bankhead Coley New Investigator Award (09BN-13) and R01 CA189184, R01 CA207371. ColoCare Moffitt has been supported in part by P30 CA076292. Toriola and Colditz are also supported by P30 CA091842.

Institutional Review Board Statement: The study was conducted according to the guidelines of the Declaration of Helsinki, and approved by the Institutional Review Boards of Fred Hutchinson Cancer Center (6407, 18 October 2006), Moffitt Cancer Center (USF 104189, 20 October 2009), University of Tennessee (16-04626-FB, 23 September 2016), Washington University School of Medicine (201610032, 18 October 2006), University of Utah (IRB_00077147, 20 May 2015), Cedars Sinai Center (Pro00046423, 1 December 2016), and University of Heidelberg (310/2001, 5 May 2010).

Informed Consent Statement: Informed consent was obtained from all subjects involved in the study.

Data Availability Statement: The data presented in this study are available in this article (and Supplementary Materials).

Acknowledgments: The authors thank all ColoCare Study participants and the ColoCare Study teams as multiple locations, specifically: Fred Hutchinson Cancer Research Center: George McDonald, Karen Makar, Meredith Hullar, Chris Velicer, and also Kathy Vickers, and Shannon Rush. National Center for Tumor Diseases and University Hospital of Heidelberg: Petra Schrotz-King, Clare Abbenhardt-Martin, Nina Habermann, Dominique Scherer, Robert W. Owen, Romy Kirsten, Peter Schirmacher, Esther Herpel, Magnus von Knebel Doeberitz, Matthias Kloor, Hans-Ulrich Kauczor, Johanna Nattenmüller, Nikolaus Becker, Hermann Brenner, Jenny Chang-Claude, Michael Hoffmeister, Stephanie Skender, Werner Diehl, and also Susanne Jakob, Judith Kammer, Lin Zielske, Anett Brendel, Marita Wenzel, Renate Skatula, Rifraz Farook, and Torsten Kölsch. Huntsman Cancer Institute: John Weis, Ute Gawlick, Mark Lewis, June Round, Zac Stephenson, James Cox, Chris Fillmore, Kenneth Boucher, and also Debra Ma, Samir Courdy, Therese Berry, Karen Salas, Anjelica Ashworth, Christy Warby, Bailee Rushton, Darren Walker, and Marissa Grande. Moffitt Cancer Center: Paul Jacobsen, Christine Pierce, Heather Jim and also Gazelle Rouhani, Maria Gomez, Kristen Maddox, Amanda DeRenzis, Gillian Trujillo, Amanda Bloomer, Paige Parkinson, Bianca Nguyen, Alina Hoehn, Bridget Riggs. Cedars-Sinai Medical Center: Phillip Fleshner, Solomon Hamburg, David Magner, Sepehr Rokhsar, Samuel Klempner, Joshua Ellenhorn, Thomas Sokol, Eiman Firoozmand, and also Julissa Ramirez, Sarah Villeda, Cindy Miao, Blair Carnes, Dogra Khushi, Carissa Huynh, and Nathalie Nguyen. Washington University School of Medicine: Matthew G. Mutch, Cory Bernadt, and also

Sonya Izadi, Michelle Sperry, June Smith, and Esinam Wash. Center for Cancer Research, Memphis: Scott Daugherty, Holly Hilsenbeck, Thomas O'Brien, Leah Hendrick, and also Nuzhat Ali, Meghana Karchi, and Demi Ajidhahun.

Conflicts of Interest: As Cancer Center Director, C.M.U. has oversight over research funded by several pharmaceutical companies, but has not received funding directly herself. Other authors have no conflict of interest.

References

1. Murphy, C.C.; Singal, A.G.; Baron, J.A.; Sandler, R.S. Decrease in Incidence of Young-Onset Colorectal Cancer Before Recent Increase. *Gastroenterology* **2018**, *155*, 1716–1719.e4. [CrossRef]
2. Siegel, R.L.; Fedewa, S.A.; Anderson, W.F.; Miller, K.D.; Ma, J.; Rosenberg, P.S.; Jemal, A. Colorectal Cancer Incidence Patterns in the United States, 1974–2013. *J. Natl. Cancer Inst.* **2017**, *109*. [CrossRef] [PubMed]
3. Abualkhair, W.H.; Zhou, M.; Ahnen, D.; Yu, Q.; Wu, X.C.; Karlitz, J.J. Trends in Incidence of Early-Onset Colorectal Cancer in the United States Among Those Approaching Screening Age. *JAMA Netw. Open* **2020**, *3*, e1920407. [CrossRef] [PubMed]
4. Mauri, G.; Sartore-Bianchi, A.; Russo, A.G.; Marsoni, S.; Bardelli, A.; Siena, S. Early-onset colorectal cancer in young individuals. *Mol. Oncol.* **2019**, *13*, 109–131. [CrossRef] [PubMed]
5. Bailey, C.E.; Hu, C.Y.; You, Y.N.; Bednarski, B.K.; Rodriguez-Bigas, M.A.; Skibber, J.M.; Cantor, S.B.; Chang, G.J. Increasing disparities in the age-related incidences of colon and rectal cancers in the United States, 1975–2010. *JAMA Surg.* **2015**, *150*, 17–22. [CrossRef]
6. Wolf, A.M.D.; Fontham, E.T.H.; Church, T.R.; Flowers, C.R.; Guerra, C.E.; LaMonte, S.J.; Etzioni, R.; McKenna, M.T.; Oeffinger, K.C.; Shih, Y.T.; et al. Colorectal cancer screening for average-risk adults: 2018 guideline update from the American Cancer Society. *CA Cancer J. Clin.* **2018**, *68*, 250–281. [CrossRef]
7. U.S. Preventive Services Task Force. U.S. Preventive Services Task Force Issues Draft Recommendation on Screening for Colorectal Cancer. 2020. Available online: https://uspreventiveservicestaskforce.org/uspstf/recommendation/colorectal-cancer-screening (accessed on 5 July 2021).
8. World Cancer Research Fund. Diet, Nutrition, Physical Activity and Colorectal Cancer; American Institute for Cancer Research. 2018. Available online: https://www.wcrf.org/wp-content/uploads/2021/02/Colorectal-cancer-report.pdf (accessed on 5 July 2021).
9. Low, E.E.; Demb, J.; Liu, L.; Earles, A.; Bustamante, R.; Williams, C.D.; Provenzale, D.; Kaltenbach, T.; Gawron, A.J.; Martinez, M.E.; et al. Risk Factors for Early-Onset Colorectal Cancer. *Gastroenterology* **2020**, *159*, 492–501.e7. [CrossRef]
10. Gausman, V.; Dornblaser, D.; Anand, S.; Hayes, R.B.; O'Connell, K.; Du, M.; Liang, P.S. Risk Factors Associated With Early-Onset Colorectal Cancer. *Clin. Gastroenterol. Hepatol.* **2020**, *18*, 2752–2759.e2752. [CrossRef]
11. Syed, A.R.; Thakkar, P.; Horne, Z.D.; Abdul-Baki, H.; Kochhar, G.; Farah, K.; Thakkar, S. Old vs. new: Risk factors predicting early onset colorectal cancer. *World J. Gastrointest. Oncol.* **2019**, *11*, 1011–1020. [CrossRef]
12. Hofseth, L.J.; Hebert, J.R.; Chanda, A.; Chen, H.; Love, B.L.; Pena, M.M.; Murphy, E.A.; Sajish, M.; Sheth, A.; Buckhaults, P.J.; et al. Early-onset colorectal cancer: Initial clues and current views. *Nat. Rev. Gastroenterol. Hepatol.* **2020**, *17*, 352–364. [CrossRef] [PubMed]
13. Holowatyj, A.N.; Gigic, B.; Herpel, E.; Scalbert, A.; Schneider, M.; Ulrich, C.M. Distinct Molecular Phenotype of Sporadic Colorectal Cancers Among Young Patients Based on Multiomics Analysis. *Gastroenterology* **2020**, *158*, 1155–1158.e2. [CrossRef]
14. Benson, A.B., 3rd.; Venook, A.P.; Cederquist, L.; Chan, E.; Chen, Y.J.; Cooper, H.S.; Deming, D.; Engstrom, P.F.; Enzinger, P.C.; Fichera, A.; et al. Colon Cancer, Version 1.2017, NCCN Clinical Practice Guidelines in Oncology. *J. Natl. Compr. Cancer Netw. JNCCN* **2017**, *15*, 370–398. [CrossRef]
15. Burnett-Hartman, A.N.; Powers, J.D.; Chubak, J.; Corley, D.A.; Ghai, N.R.; McMullen, C.K.; Pawloski, P.A.; Sterrett, A.T.; Feigelson, H.S. Treatment patterns and survival differ between early-onset and late-onset colorectal cancer patients: The patient outcomes to advance learning network. *Cancer Causes Control* **2019**, *30*, 747–755. [CrossRef]
16. Kneuertz, P.J.; Chang, G.J.; Hu, C.Y.; Rodriguez-Bigas, M.A.; Eng, C.; Vilar, E.; Skibber, J.M.; Feig, B.W.; Cormier, J.N.; You, Y.N. Overtreatment of young adults with colon cancer: More intense treatments with unmatched survival gains. *JAMA Surg.* **2015**, *150*, 402–409. [CrossRef]
17. Kolarich, A.; George, T.J., Jr.; Hughes, S.J.; Delitto, D.; Allegra, C.J.; Hall, W.A.; Chang, G.J.; Tan, S.A.; Shaw, C.M.; Iqbal, A. Rectal cancer patients younger than 50 years lack a survival benefit from NCCN guideline-directed treatment for stage II and III disease. *Cancer* **2018**, *124*, 3510–3519. [CrossRef] [PubMed]
18. Abdelsattar, Z.M.; Wong, S.L.; Regenbogen, S.E.; Jomaa, D.M.; Hardiman, K.M.; Hendren, S. Colorectal cancer outcomes and treatment patterns in patients too young for average-risk screening. *Cancer* **2016**, *122*, 929–934. [CrossRef]
19. Cheng, E.; Blackburn, H.N.; Ng, K.; Spiegelman, D.; Irwin, M.L.; Ma, X.; Gross, C.P.; Tabung, F.K.; Giovannucci, E.L.; Kunz, P.L.; et al. Analysis of Survival Among Adults with Early-Onset Colorectal Cancer in the National Cancer Database. *JAMA Netw. Open* **2021**, *4*, e2112539. [CrossRef] [PubMed]
20. Ulrich, C.M.; Gigic, B.; Böhm, J.; Ose, J.; Viskochil, R.; Schneider, M.; Colditz, G.A.; Figueiredo, J.C.; Grady, W.M.; Li, C.I.; et al. The ColoCare Study: A Paradigm of Transdisciplinary Science in Colorectal Cancer Outcomes. *Cancer Epidemiol. Biomark. Prev.* **2019**, *28*, 591–601. [CrossRef] [PubMed]

21. Gigic, B.; Boeing, H.; Toth, R.; Bohm, J.; Habermann, N.; Scherer, D.; Schrotz-King, P.; Abbenhardt-Martin, C.; Skender, S.; Brenner, H.; et al. Associations Between Dietary Patterns and Longitudinal Quality of Life Changes in Colorectal Cancer Patients: The ColoCare Study. *Nutr. Cancer* **2018**, *70*, 51–60. [CrossRef] [PubMed]
22. Gigic, B.; Nattenmüller, J.; Schneider, M.; Kulu, Y.; Syrjala, K.L.; Böhm, J.; Schrotz-King, P.; Brenner, H.; Colditz, G.A.; Figueiredo, J.C.; et al. The Role of CT-Quantified Body Composition on Longitudinal Health-Related Quality of Life in Colorectal Cancer Patients: The Colocare Study. *Nutrients* **2020**, *12*, 1247. [CrossRef]
23. Himbert, C.; Ose, J.; Lin, T.; Warby, C.A.; Gigic, B.; Steindorf, K.; Schrotz-King, P.; Abbenhardt-Martin, C.; Zielske, L.; Boehm, J.; et al. Inflammation- and angiogenesis-related biomarkers are correlated with cancer-related fatigue in colorectal cancer patients: Results from the ColoCare Study. *Eur. J. Cancer Care (Engl.)* **2019**, *28*, e13055. [CrossRef]
24. Ose, J.; Gigic, B.; Lin, T.; Liesenfeld, D.B.; Bohm, J.; Nattenmuller, J.; Scherer, D.; Zielske, L.; Schrotz-King, P.; Habermann, N.; et al. Multiplatform Urinary Metabolomics Profiling to Discriminate Cachectic from Non-Cachectic Colorectal Cancer Patients: Pilot Results from the ColoCare Study. *Metabolites* **2019**, *9*, 178. [CrossRef]
25. Sehgal, M.; Ladabaum, U.; Mithal, A.; Singh, H.; Desai, M.; Singh, G. Colorectal Cancer Incidence After Colonoscopy at Ages 45–49 or 50–54 Years. *Gastroenterology* **2021**, *160*, 2018–2028.e3. [CrossRef]
26. Dekker, E.; Tanis, P.J.; Vleugels, J.L.A.; Kasi, P.M.; Wallace, M.B. Colorectal cancer. *Lancet* **2019**, *394*, 1467–1480. [CrossRef]
27. Liu, P.H.; Wu, K.; Ng, K.; Zauber, A.G.; Nguyen, L.H.; Song, M.; He, X.; Fuchs, C.S.; Ogino, S.; Willett, W.C.; et al. Association of Obesity With Risk of Early-Onset Colorectal Cancer Among Women. *JAMA Oncol.* **2019**, *5*, 37–44. [CrossRef]
28. Bull, C.J.; Bell, J.A.; Murphy, N.; Sanderson, E.; Davey Smith, G.; Timpson, N.J.; Banbury, B.L.; Albanes, D.; Berndt, S.I.; Bézieau, S.; et al. Adiposity, metabolites, and colorectal cancer risk: Mendelian randomization study. *BMC Med.* **2020**, *18*, 396. [CrossRef] [PubMed]
29. Botteri, E.; Iodice, S.; Bagnardi, V.; Raimondi, S.; Lowenfels, A.B.; Maisonneuve, P. Smoking and colorectal cancer: A meta-analysis. *JAMA* **2008**, *300*, 2765–2778. [CrossRef]
30. Acott, A.A.; Theus, S.A.; Marchant-Miros, K.E.; Mancino, A.T. Association of tobacco and alcohol use with earlier development of colorectal cancer: Should we modify screening guidelines? *Am. J. Surg.* **2008**, *196*, 915–918, discussion 918–919. [CrossRef] [PubMed]
31. Di Leo, M.; Zuppardo, R.A.; Puzzono, M.; Ditonno, I.; Mannucci, A.; Antoci, G.; Russo Raucci, A.; Patricelli, M.G.; Elmore, U.; Tamburini, A.M.; et al. Risk factors and clinical characteristics of early-onset colorectal cancer vs. late-onset colorectal cancer: A case-case study. *Eur. J. Gastroenterol. Hepatol.* **2020**. [CrossRef]
32. You, Y.N.; Xing, Y.; Feig, B.W.; Chang, G.J.; Cormier, J.N. Young-onset colorectal cancer: Is it time to pay attention? *Arch. Intern. Med.* **2012**, *172*, 287–289. [CrossRef]
33. Willauer, A.N.; Liu, Y.; Pereira, A.A.L.; Lam, M.; Morris, J.S.; Raghav, K.P.S.; Morris, V.K.; Menter, D.; Broaddus, R.; Meric-Bernstam, F.; et al. Clinical and molecular characterization of early-onset colorectal cancer. *Cancer* **2019**, *125*, 2002–2010. [CrossRef] [PubMed]
34. Siegel, R.L.; Miller, K.D.; Goding Sauer, A.; Fedewa, S.A.; Butterly, L.F.; Anderson, J.C.; Cercek, A.; Smith, R.A.; Jemal, A. Colorectal cancer statistics, 2020. *CA Cancer J. Clin.* **2020**, *70*, 145–164. [CrossRef] [PubMed]
35. Hales, C.M.; Carroll, M.D.; Fryar, C.D.; Ogden, C.L. *Prevalence of Obesity Among Adults and Youth: United States, 2015–2016*; NCHS Data Brief No 288; National Center for Health Statistics: Hyattsville, MD, USA, 2017; pp. 1–8.

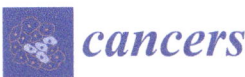

Article

Influence of Gender on Radiosensitivity during Radiochemotherapy of Advanced Rectal Cancer

Barbara Schuster [1,2,†], Markus Hecht [1,2,†], Manfred Schmidt [1,2], Marlen Haderlein [1,2], Tina Jost [1,2], Maike Büttner-Herold [2,3], Klaus Weber [2,4], Axel Denz [2,4], Robert Grützmann [2,4], Arndt Hartmann [2,5], Hans Geinitz [6], Rainer Fietkau [1,2] and Luitpold V. Distel [1,2,*]

1. Department of Radiation Oncology, Universitätsklinikum Erlangen, Friedrich-Alexander-Universität Erlangen-Nürnberg, 91054 Erlangen, Germany; schuster-barbara@gmx.net (B.S.); Markus.Hecht@uk-erlangen.de (M.H.); Manfred.Schmidt@uk-erlangen.de (M.S.); Marlen.Haderlein@uk-erlangen.de (M.H.); Tina.Jost@uk-erlangen.de (T.J.); Rainer.Fietkau@uk-erlangen.de (R.F.)
2. Comprehensive Cancer Center Erlangen-EMN (CCC ER-EMN), Universitätsklinikum Erlangen, Friedrich-Alexander-Universität Erlangen-Nürnberg, 91054 Erlangen, Germany; Maike.Buettner-Herold@uk-erlangen.de (M.B.-H.); Klaus.Weber@uk-erlangen.de (K.W.); Axel.Denz@uk-erlangen.de (A.D.); Robert.Gruetzmann@uk-erlangen.de (R.G.); Arndt.Hartmann@uk-erlangen.de (A.H.)
3. Department of Nephropathology, Institute of Pathology, Universitätsklinikum Erlangen, Friedrich-Alexander-University Erlangen-Nuremberg (FAU), 91054 Erlangen, Germany
4. Department of General and Visceral Surgery, Friedrich Alexander University, Krankenhausstraße 12, 91054 Erlangen, Germany
5. Institute of Pathology, Universitätsklinikum Erlangen, Friedrich-Alexander-Universität Erlangen-Nürnberg, 91054 Erlangen, Germany
6. Department of Radiation Oncology, Ordensklinikum Linz, Barmherzige Schwestern, 4010 Linz, Austria; Hans.Geinitz@ordensklinikum.at
* Correspondence: Luitpold.distel@uk-erlangen.de; Tel.: +49-9131-85-32312
† These authors contributed equally to this work.

Simple Summary: In radiotherapy for rectal cancer, the treatment is identical for women and men. In recent years, the question has arisen whether there are gender differences in radiochemotherapy. We have investigated, in detail, differences between men and women, especially with regard to radiation sensitivity. We found no evidence for a difference in radiosensitivity between the sexes. Nevertheless, during radiochemotherapy, women experienced increased impairments in the quality of life, which, however, are restored in the subsequent period. One possibility is an increased sensitivity of women to chemotherapy.

Abstract: Gender is increasingly recognized as an important factor in medicine, although it has long been neglected in medical research in many areas. We have studied the influence of gender in advanced rectal cancer with a special focus on radiosensitivity. For this purpose, we studied a cohort of 495 men (84.1% ≥ T3, 63.6% N1, 17.6%, M1) and 215 women (84.2% ≥ T3, 56.7% N1, 22.8%, M1) who all suffered from advanced rectal cancer and were treated with radiochemotherapy. The energy deposited, DNA double-strand break (dsb) repair, occurrence of chromosomal aberrations, duration of therapy, tumor regression and tumor-infiltrating lymphocytes, laboratory parameters, quality of life and survival were assessed. The residual DNA dsb damage 24 h after irradiation in lymphocytes was identical in both sexes. Furthermore, chromosomal aberrations accurately reflecting radiosensitivity, were similar in both sexes. There were no gender-dependent differences in tumor regression, tumor-infiltrating lymphocytes and outcome indicating no differences in the radiosensitivity of cancer cells. The irradiated tumor volume in women was slightly lower than in men, related to body weight, no difference was observed. However, when the total energy deposited was calculated and related to the body weight, women were exposed to higher amounts of ionizing radiation. During radiochemotherapy, decreases in blood lymphocyte counts and albumin and several quality-of-life parameters such as nausea and vomiting, loss of appetite, and diarrhea were significantly worse in women. There is no difference in radiation sensitivity between men and women in both normal tissue and tumors. During radiochemotherapy, the quality of life deteriorates more in women than in men. However, women also recover quickly and there are no long-term differences in quality of life.

Keywords: gender; rectal cancer; radiochemotherapy; radiosensitivity; DNA double-strand breaks; radiosensitivity; deposited energy; quality of life; blood values

1. Introduction

In medicine, gender differences are receiving more and more attention both with regard to the choice of therapy and side effects [1,2]. In oncology, the gender-dependent induction of cancer is also an important topic and clear sex differences are observed. For the vast majority of cancers, men have a significantly increased risk of developing malignancies [3]. In colorectal carcinoma, men have 30% higher incidence rates than women [3]. Causes of colon and rectal cancer seem to be different, and in the case of rectal cancer, alcohol and smoking are clearly of importance as to what might explain the difference. Additionally, there are clear differences depending on the sex with regard to response to cancer therapy and the occurrence of undesirable therapy-related side effects [2,4,5].

From a molecular point of view, several findings support a clear difference in carcinogenesis and therapeutic response. Gender-dependent differences in epigenetic regulation, metabolism, expression of tumor suppressor genes such as p53, cellular senescence, anti-tumor immune reaction and angiogenesis are described [3]. However, the most important differences are probably the hormonal differences and the resulting different effects [6].

Locally advanced rectal cancer is commonly treated with neoadjuvant radiochemotherapy (RCT) or short course radiotherapy alone, followed by total mesorectal excision and adjuvant chemotherapy. New treatment strategies comprise total neoadjuvant treatment or a watch and wait strategy after clinically complete remission following neoadjuvant treatment. RCT carries a certain risk of adverse therapeutic effects both during therapy and in the long term. It is extremely important that acute side effects are well tolerated and do not lead to therapy discontinuation thus comprising oncologic outcome. Long-term therapy consequences can only be experienced if the therapy was successful but might be associated with debilitating symptoms and reduced quality of life. However, judgement on the tolerability of RCT is based on results looking at the average patient population, but does not consider gender [7]. We searched for indicators of differences in men and women in terms of altered efficacy of therapy or side effects. In particular, we were interested as to whether there are gender differences between the radiosensitivity of both normal and tumor tissue and whether this could lead to adverse radiation or chemotherapeutic effects in one sex or an altered tumor response.

2. Materials and Methods

2.1. Rectal Cancer Cohort and Healthy Individuals

This advanced rectal cancer cohort of 495 males and 215 females was originally derived from three studies on radiosensitivity, tumor-infiltrating lymphocytes and quality of life analyses. The study period was between 2005 and 2018 and represented a consecutive cohort. The fourth cohort of laboratory values is composed of the first three cohorts, including patients who were scheduled for one of the other studies but from whom blood, tissue, or questionnaires were not available and therefore could not be included in these studies. In the radiosensitivity cohort, besides 400 rectal cancer patients, an additional 187 healthy individuals were included as a control group. The γH2AX cohort of 137 rectal cancer patients and 59 healthy individuals was a subgroup of the radiosensitivity cohort. The tumor-infiltrating lymphocytes study consists of 209 patients and the quality of life group consists of 357 patients. Lab data are derived in maximum from 616 patients (Figure 1).

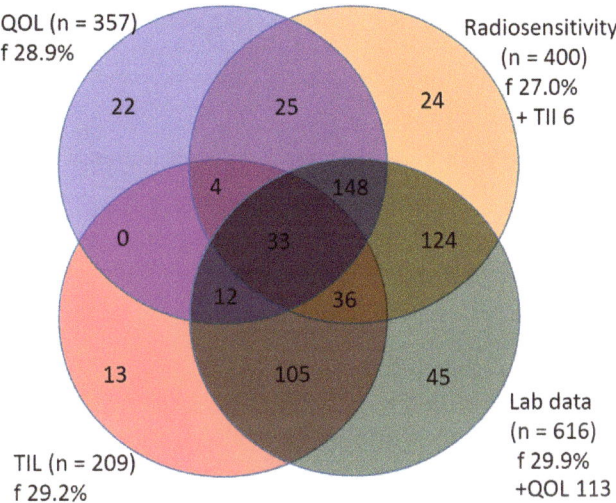

Figure 1. Members of the cohort from four subgroups. The number in the four overlapping circles indicates the number of participants from all four subgroups, corresponding to the three, two and single subgroups. The numbers "+TIL" stand for the intersection of the patient numbers from the radiosensitivity group and the TIL group or "+QOL" for the intersection of the QOL group and the laboratory data group. m = male, f = female, QOL = quality of life cohort, TIL = tumor-infiltrating lymphocytes cohort.

All patients were intended to receive a neoadjuvant RCT consisting of a conventional radiotherapy of 28 fractions with 1.8 Gy each, up to a total dose of 50.4 Gy. Simultaneous chemotherapy was 5-fluorouracil-based. The most commonly used concurrent chemotherapy combination was 5-FU and oxaliplatin. The remaining patients received similar treatment regimens, including 5-FU alone, capecitabine, 5-FU + antibody, 5-FU + cisplatin, or 5-FU + irinotecan. Metastatic patients usually received FOLFOX, FOLFIRI, or FOLFOX-IRI; in some cases, in combination with antibodies. After completion of radiochemotherapy, patients were treated with a total mesorectal resection.

2.2. Deposited Energy Calculation

The 95%, 90%, 80%, 60%, 40%, 30% and 20% isodose volumes were derived from the treatment planning software (TPS) Pinnacle (Philips Radiation Oncology Systems, Fitchburg, WI, USA). Deposited energy values were calculated according to the equation described previously (Figure 3B) [8].

2.3. γH2AX Detection of DNA Double-Strand Breaks

EDTA blood was drawn before RCT was started and divided into three samples. The background was the initial damage of 0.5 Gy and 30 min repair time and the remaining residual damage 24 h after a dose of 2 Gy IR (Isovolt 160, General electrics, Ahrensburg, Germany). Lymphocytes were then prepared on a slide by cytospin centrifuge and immunostaining with γH2AX (abcam, Cambridge, UK) and counterstained with dapi [9]; 1000 lymphocytes were counted in each group for the average number of foci [10].

2.4. Chromosomal Aberrations by Three Color Fluorescence In Situ Hybridization

Before starting the RCT, heparinized blood was drawn and half of it was irradiated with 2 Gy 6-MV ionizing radiation (Oncor, Siemens, Erlangen, Germany) and the other half was taken as background. Lymphocytes were stimulated with phytohemagglutinin and incubated at 37 °C for 48 h. Colcemid was added for 3 h and then the chromosomes were prepared. Chromosomes #1, #2 and #4 were stained with fluorescent probes in red, green and yellow and counterstained with dapi. Metaphases were imaged automatically using a fluorescence microscope (Zeiss, Axioplan 2, Göttingen, Germany) and a specialized software (Metafer 4 V3.10.1, Altlussheim, Germany). An image analysis software (Biomas, Erlangen, Germany) was used to determine the breaks per metaphase. The background value was subtracted from the 2 Gy irradiated values [11,12].

2.5. Therapy Duration and Regression Grade

Therapy duration, total dose, and fractions were derived from patient records. The Dworak regression grade was derived from the pathological reports.

2.6. Blood Values

Blood values of leucocytes, thrombocytes, monocytes, eosinophils, erythrocytes, hemoglobin, albumin, LDH, creatinine, alkaline phosphatase, C-reactive protein (CRP), glutamic oxaloacetic transaminase (GOT), glutamate pyruvate transaminase (GPT), potassium, thyroid-stimulating hormone and 25-hydroxyvitamin D were obtained from the hospital database. In each case, the value immediately before the start of therapy and before each start of the following therapy weeks was selected. Blood values for thyroid-stimulating hormone and 25-hydroxyvitamin D were only available prior to the start of RCT.

2.7. Tumor-Infiltrating Lymphocytes

Paraffin-embedded tissues from biopsies ($n = 103$) and tumor resections ($n = 173$) were repunched into tissue micro arrays of 2 mm diameter. Immunohistochemical double-staining for FoxP3+ (Ab20034, abcam, Cambridge, UK) and CD8+ (M7103, Agilent, Santa Clara, CA, USA) was performed. Visualization was performed using a Polymer Kit and Fast Red and Polymer Kit and Fast Blue (POLAP-100 Zytomed Systems, Berlin, Germany). Images of each spot were acquired at 400× magnification (Imager Z2, Zeiss, Göttingen, Germany) combined with a Metafer software (Metasystems, Altlussheim, Germany). The number of lymphocytes per square mm were counted separately for tumoral stroma and tumoral epithelium using an image analysis software (Biomas, Erlangen, Germany) [13,14].

2.8. Quality of Life

Quality of life was prospectively assessed using the EORTC QLQ C30 and CR38 questionnaires. Time points were before the start of the RCT ($n = 357$), during the RCT at week 2 ($n = 218$) and at the end of the RCT at week 5 ($n = 195$), and after 10 weeks ($n = 208$) immediately prior to surgery. From then on, the questionnaire was answered annually (1 year = 185; 2 years = 105; 3 years = 71; 4 years = 68; 5 years = 48). Scores were calculated according to the official EORTC manual. In the function scales, a higher score means that the patient is doing well in this category. In contrast, a higher score in the symptom category means that the patient has more complaints [15]. Clinical significance for QOL data was assumed at a change of 10% or more.

2.9. Survival Curves

Overall survival is calculated as the time from diagnosis to the time of death. Tumor-specific survival was defined as the duration from the date of diagnosis until death due to rectal cancer. Recurrence-free survival was measured from the time of diagnosis to the date of recurrence or death from any cause. Metastasis-free survival was measured from the time of diagnosis to the date of distant metastasis or death from any cause. Local recurrence was defined as recurrent disease within locoregional area and distant recurrence was defined as recurrence beyond the locoregional area. Progression was defined as locoregional failure or distant metastasis. Patients lost to follow-up or who have no events are censored at this time. Median time to follow-up was 49.5 months.

2.10. Statistics

All statistical analyses were performed using SPSS version 24 (IBM Inc., Chicago, IL, USA). Student's *t*-test was used for independent samples and Pearson's Chi-squared test was used to compare the TNM stages of women and men. Survival plots were generated according to the Kaplan–Meier method [16] and compared using the log-rank test; *p*-values < 0.05 were considered to be statistically significant.

3. Results

3.1. Patient and Treatment Characteristics

We studied the influence of gender on therapy-related effects in a cohort of 710 patients suffering from rectal cancer; 495 patients were male (69.7%) and 215 female (30.3%). The cohort consisted of four sub-cohorts, namely a cohort testing radiosensitivity (n = 400), a quality of live cohort (n = 357), a tumor-infiltrating lymphocytes cohort (n = 209) and a lab data cohort (n = 616). Patients were consecutively included.

Data of all four endpoints (radiosensitivity, tumor-infiltrating lymphocytes, lab data and quality of life analyses) were available in 33 patients, of three endpoints in 200 patients and of two endpoints in 373 patients (Figure 1). TNM stages were slightly different between females and males (p = 0.048) (Table 1). The mean age of female (62.2 years) and male (62.8) patients was nearly identical (p = 0.554) (Figure 2A). Body weight (p < 0.001) (Figure 2B) and height (p < 0.001) (Figure 2C) was significantly higher in males. Nevertheless, the body mass index was comparable (p = 0.409) (Figure 2D).

Table 1. Tumor stage according to gender of the entire cohort.

Stage		Male (%)	Female (%)	Significance (p)
cT-stage	1	13 (2.6%)	8 (3.7%)	
	2	66 (13.3%)	26 (12.1%)	
	3	332 (67.1%)	127 (59.1%)	
	4	84 (17.0%)	54 (25.1%)	0.011
pN-stage	0	180 (36.4%)	93 (43.3%)	
	1	315 (63.6%)	122 (56.7%)	0.093
cM-stage	0	408 (82.4%)	166 (77.2%)	
	1	87 (17.6%)	49 (22.8%)	0.144

Significance calculated by Pearson's Chi-squared test. For the cT-stages, only stage 3 and 4 were used for the statistical calculation.

We assessed whether there was a difference in the total deposited energy between males and females. We used the isodose volumes of the radiation planning system and calculated a deposited energy of each patient (Figure 3A). The deposited energy is defined as the sum of the isodose dose values multiplied by the volume of this dose level and the mass density (Figure 3B). Equal amounts of energy were deposited in males and females (Figure 3C). However, taking into account that females have a lower mass, the mean dose related to the total body is significantly higher in females (p < 0.001) (Figure 3D). The 95% isodose volume to treat the tumor, however, tended to be smaller in women than in men (p = 0.088). In terms of body weight, there was no difference, indicating that the tumor region was treated equally in men and women (p = 0.488), as shown in Supplementary Figure S1. Chemotherapy given simultaneously was 5-FU based in males in 90.9% and in females in 85.6% of the cases. The healthy control cohort consisted of 79 men and 108 women with mean ages of 51 years and 49.4 years, respectively.

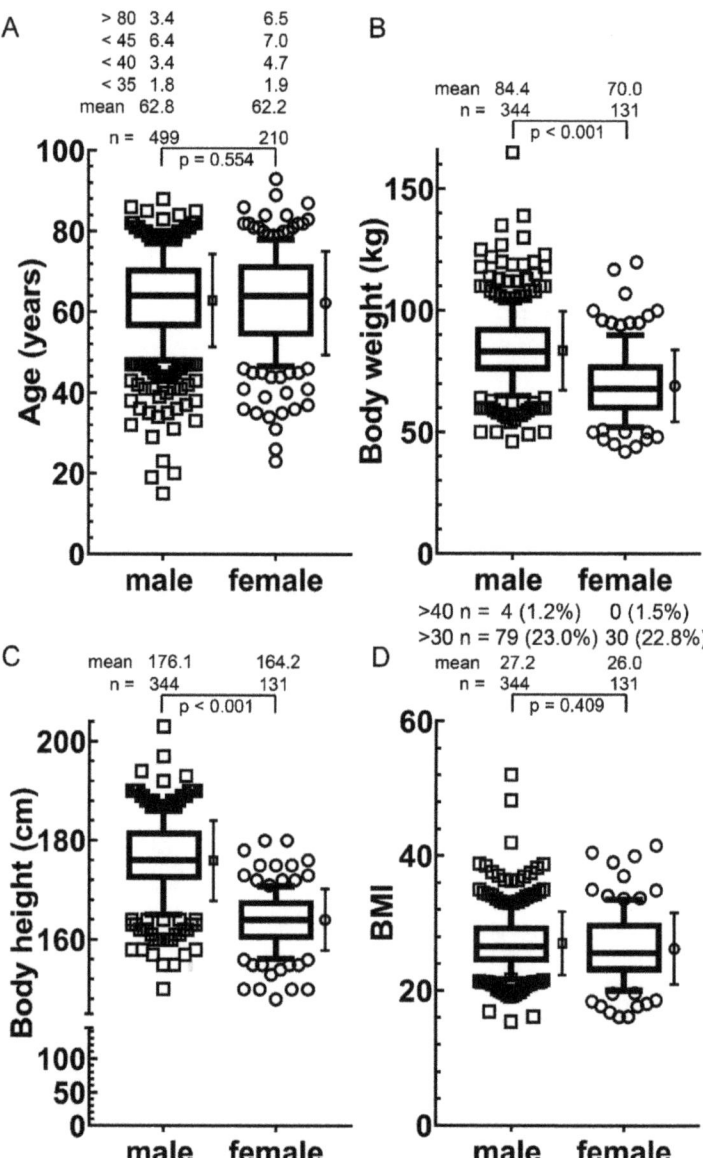

Figure 2. Age, body weight, height and body mass index compared between women and men in the entire cohort. Indicated are the number of individuals: (**A**) Age; (**B**) Body weight; (**C**) Height and (**D**) Body mass index. The box represents the median, the 25th to 75th percentiles and the whiskers of the 10th to 90th percentiles. The mean and standard deviation are shown to the right of the box; *p*-values were calculated by the Student's *t*-test.

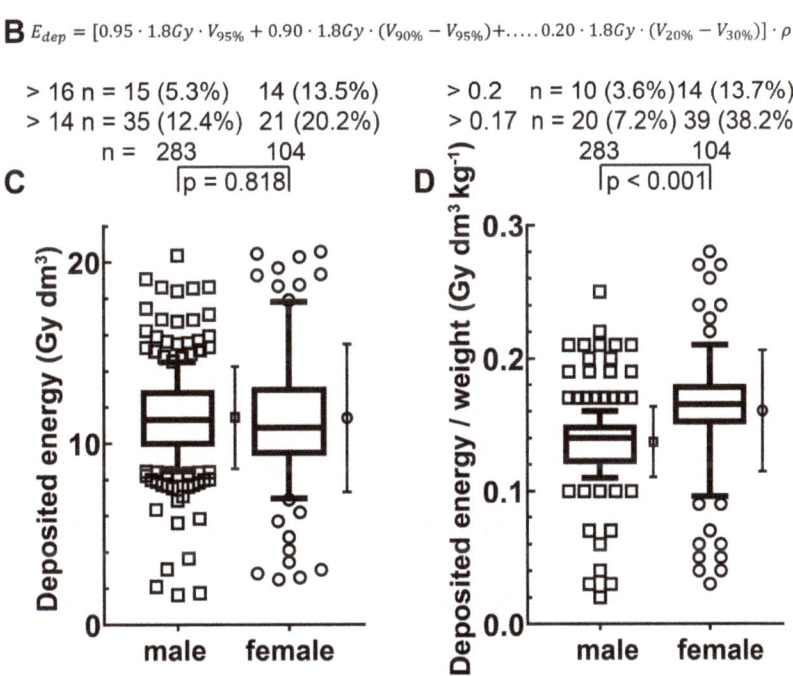

Figure 3. Deposited energy in patients with rectal cancer (radiosensitivity cohort): (**A**) Treatment plan of a patient with rectal cancer where the isodose ranges are marked with different color wash. The magenta line represents the gross target volume; the inner yellow line represents the planning target volume; (**B**) The deposited energy (Edep) is calculated using the equation given, where V is the volume and ρ is the density; (**C**) The deposited energy and (**D**) The deposited energy related to body mass in the cohort. The box represents the 25th to 75th percentiles and the whiskers represent the 10th to 90th percentiles. The mean and standard deviation are shown to the right of the box; *p*-values were calculated by the Student's *t*-test.

3.2. DNA Double-Strand Breaks and Chromosomal Aberrations

A key question of our analyses was whether a gender difference in the DNA double-strand break (dsb) repair and chromosomal aberrations induction exists. DNA dsb were analyzed by γH2AX staining (Figure 4A) in blood lymphocytes obtained prior to RCT. DNA dsb background rates in men were slightly higher in both healthy individuals ($p = 0.021$) and patients with rectal cancer ($p = 0.017$) (Figure 4B). The initial dsbs 30 min after an ex vivo dose of 0.5 Gy ionizing radiation were equal in healthy individuals and slightly higher in males with rectal cancer (Figure 4C). The remaining DNA DSB after a dose of

2 Gy and 24 h of repair time were identical between genders in healthy subjects ($p = 0.684$) and patients with rectal cancer ($p = 0.507$) (Figure 4D).

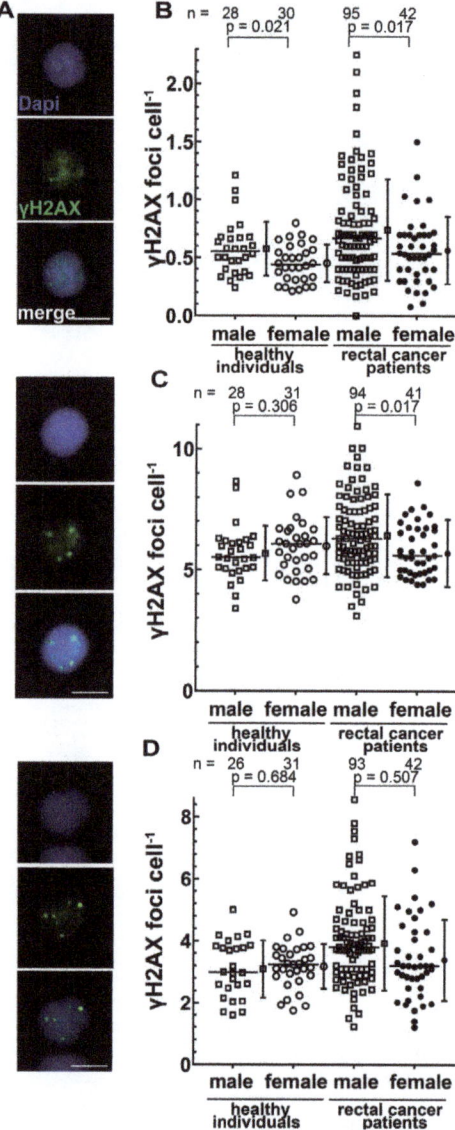

Figure 4. Number of DNA double-strand breaks per lymphocyte quantified by γH2AX after immunostaining of lymphocytes from healthy individuals and patients with rectal cancer (radiosensitivity cohort): (**A**) Representative images of an unirradiated cell, a 0.5 Gy irradiated cell with 30 min and a 2 Gy irradiated cell with 24h repair time. Blue staining is dapi and green staining is γH2AX; (**B**) Pre-existing γH2AX foci; (**C**) Initially formed γH2AX foci 30 min after an IR dose of 0.5 Gy and (**D**) γH2AX foci after an IR dose of 2 Gy and a repair time of 24 h. The mean and standard deviation are shown to the right of the dot plots; *p*-values were calculated by the Student's *t*-test.

Chromosomal aberrations were analyzed by three color fluorescence in situ hybridization (Figure 5A). Background levels of both genders in rectal cancer patients were clearly higher compared to healthy individuals, yet between genders no difference was observed (Figure 5B). After 2 Gy ex vivo irradiation, there was no difference in between healthy individuals and rectal cancer patients between sexes. The same was observed when only stable or unstable or complex aberrations were compared (Supplementary Figure S2A–C).

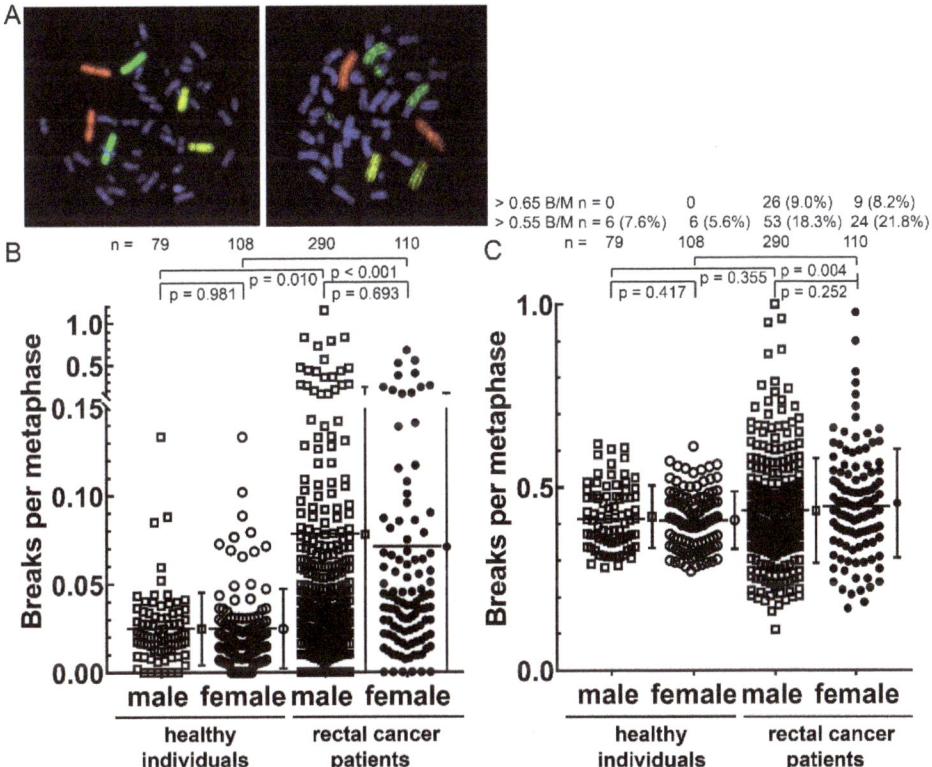

Figure 5. Radiosensitivity testing by three color fluorescence in situ hybridization of chromosomes #1, #2 and #4 (radiosensitivity cohort and healthy individuals). Metaphase spreads of human blood lymphocytes with chromosomes #1 (red), #2 (green) and #4 (yellow) stained. DNA was counterstained with DAPI (blue): (A) Normal metaphase spread in comparison to a metaphase spread with a translocation and a dicentric aberration each in chromosome #2, in sum scored with 4 breaks. Chromosomal aberrations in 179 healthy individuals and 400 patients suffering from rectal cancer; (B) Individual background B/M rates for both cohorts; (C) After ex vivo IR of 2 Gy. The mean and standard deviation are shown to the right of the dot plots; p-values were calculated by the Student's t-test.

3.3. Total Treatment Time, Tumor Regression, Blood Counts and Serum Parameters

During radiotherapy, higher energy per mass was deposited in females. In addition, there was only marginal difference in DNA DSB repair and chromosomal aberrations. Therefore we examined indicators of higher toxicity. An interruption of RCT and thus a prolongation of total radiation treatment time can be an indicator of a stronger toxic effect of the RCT. Therapy length was slightly longer by nearly one day in women as compared to men (38.4 day versus 37.8day, $p = 0.063$) (Figure 6A). Total dose (49.9 Gy versus 49.2 Gy $p = 0.634$) and fractions (27.5 versus 26.8 $p = 0.672$) were comparable between both genders

(Figure 6B,C). An indicator of radiation sensitivity is histological tumor regression after RCT. For this purpose, Dworak grading was used that indicated a mean value of 2.59 for men and 2.56 for women, which did not show a significant difference ($p = 0.778$) (Figure 6D).

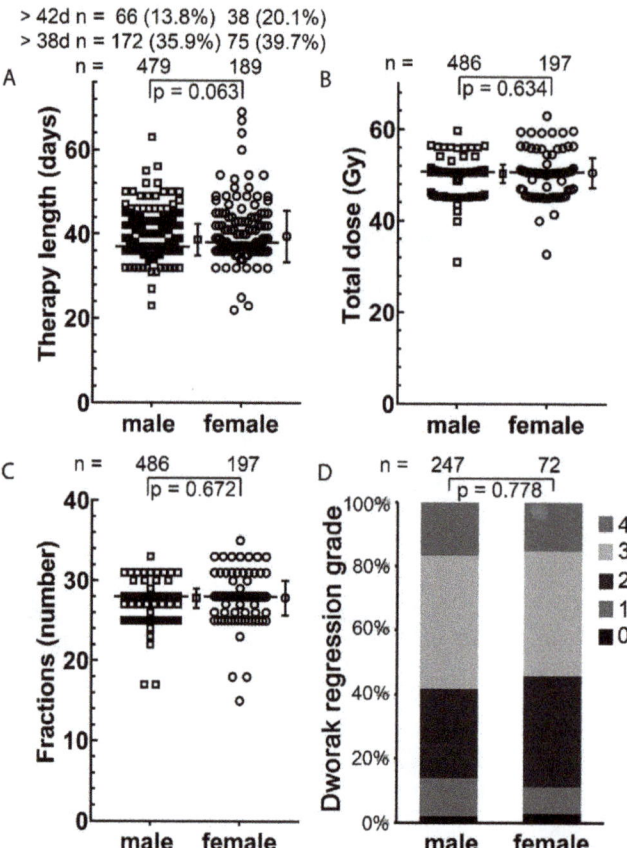

Figure 6. Therapy length, total dose and number of fractions of the entire cohort: (**A**) Length of therapy in days of 479 men and 189 women; (**B**) Total dose applied in Gy; (**C**) Number of fractions irradiated. The line indicates the median; (**D**) Regression of the cancer cells after RCT of the radiosensitivity cohort. Dworak regression grade means 0 is no regression and 4 is no remaining cancer cells. The mean and standard deviation are shown to the right of the dot plots; p-values were calculated by the Student's t-test and the Fisher's exact test were used for regression.

Changes in leukocyte blood counts may indicate differences in toxicity and were studied during RCT. Leucocyte decrease was mildly enhanced in females compared to males, while thrombocytes, monocytes, eosinophils (Figure 7A–D) and erythrocytes did not differ between the two groups. Hemoglobin decreased constantly in both groups (Figure 7E) while albumin decreased slightly more in females (Figure 7F). There was no gender specific difference in thyroid-stimulating hormone prior to therapy ($p = 0.537$), yet women had slightly higher levels in 25-hydroxyvitamin D ($p = 0.043$). Erythrocytes, LDH, creatinine, alkaline phosphatase, CRP, GOT, GPT and potassium did not clearly differ during RCT between both genders (Supplementary Figures S3–S5).

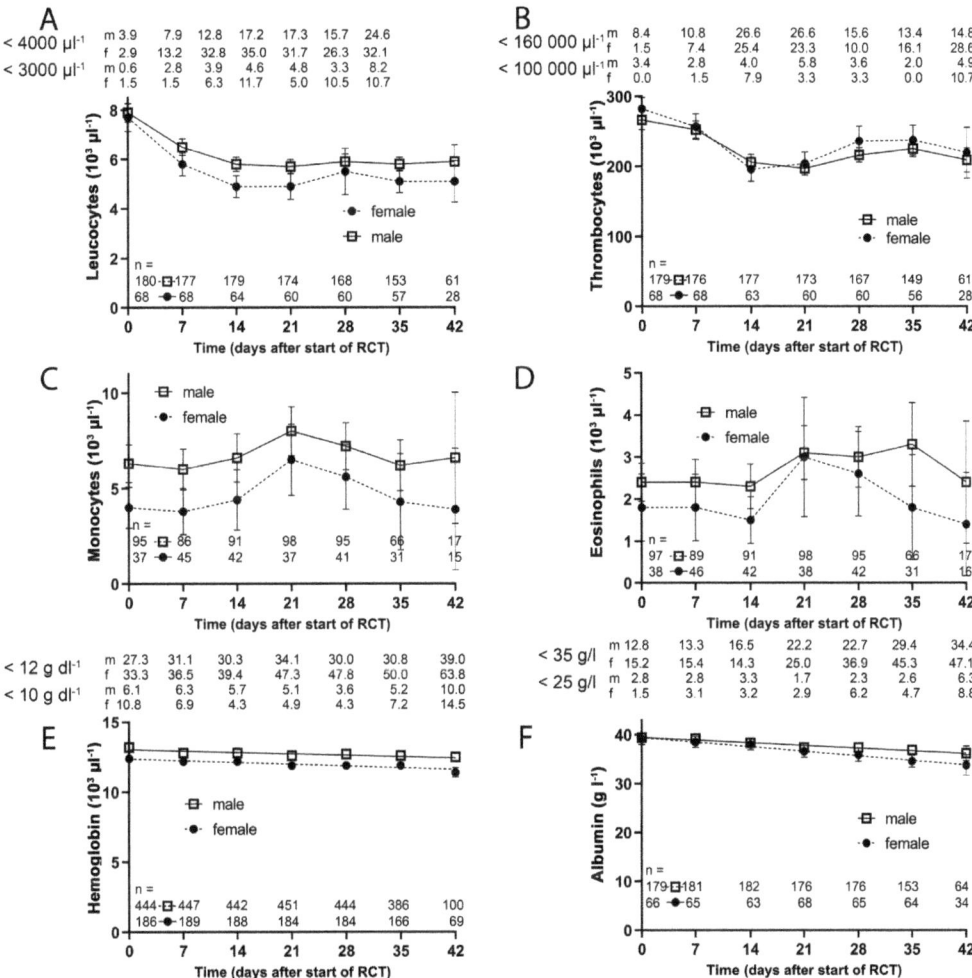

Figure 7. Blood values prior to and during the RCT of the lab data cohort. The filled dots represent women and the open rectangles represent men. The number of people with blood samples is indicated. The number of (**A**) Leukocytes; (**B**) Platelets; (**C**) Monocytes; (**D**) Eosinophils and the amount of (**E**) hemoglobin and (**F**) Albumin were given. Length of the error bars is the 95% confidence interval for the mean. m = male, f = female.

3.4. Tumor-Infiltrating Lymphocytes

The immune response against the tumor could differ depending on sex, so that tumor-infiltrating CD8+ cytotoxic lymphocytes and FoxP3+ regulatory T lymphocytes prior to RCT in the biopsy and about 55 days after RCT in the surgical specimen were compared between sexes. Lymphocyte counts were analyzed in the stromal and epithelial compartment of the tumors. No differences were found between genders with the exception of lower counts of CD8+ cytotoxic lymphocytes in the epithelial compartment after RCT in women (Figure 8).

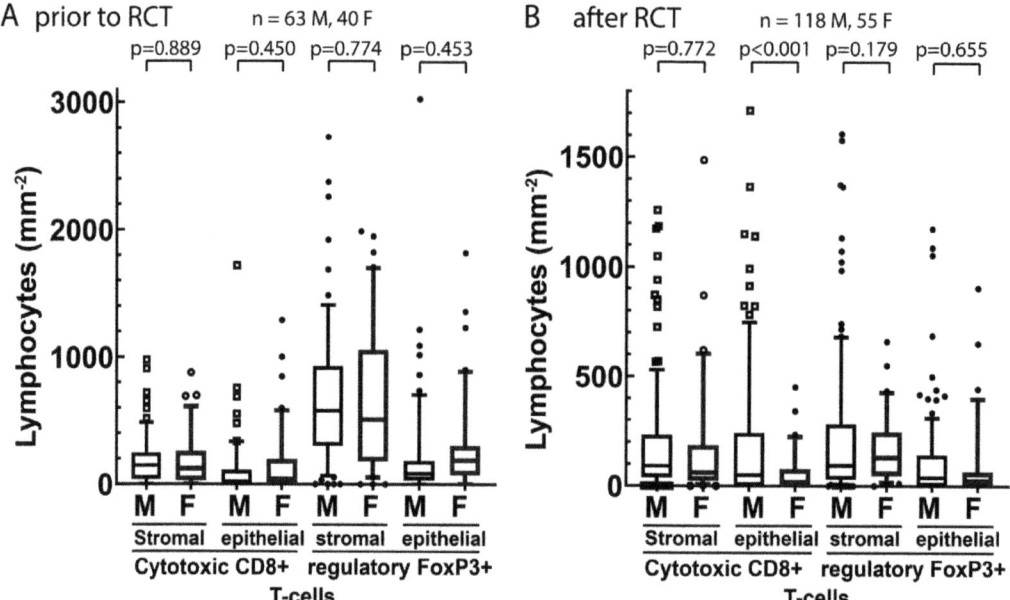

Figure 8. Stromal and intraepithelial cell density distributions of CD8+ and FoxP3+ regulatory T cells from samples (**A**) prior to RCT and, on average, (**B**) 55 days after RCT (tumor-infiltrating lymphocytes cohort). The center line represents the median value, while the box indicates the interquartile range (IQR). The whiskers represent 1.5 times the IQR or the minimum/maximum. Outliers are indicated by symbols; p-values were calculated by the Student's t-test. The box represents the 25th to 75th percentiles and the whiskers represent the 10th to 90th percentiles. M = male, F = female, RCT = radiochemotherapy.

3.5. Health-Related Quality of Life

Furthermore, we analyzed quality of life to study therapy-related side effects during therapy and for a long follow-up period of up to 5 years after RCT. The QLQ-C30 and C38 questionnaires were used. In nearly all function and symptom scores, the females' baselines tended to be worse or were 10% points below the males' scores and were therefore regarded as significantly inferior. During RCT, females tend to deteriorate more than males in several scores. This was most pronounced for nausea and vomiting, appetite loss and diarrhea (Figure 9). However, already ten weeks after the beginning of RCT, most symptoms returned to baseline. One year after beginning the RCT or later, there was even an improvement in the state of women compared to men of 10% or more with regard to body image, fatigue, dyspnea and diarrhea. This was true for most of the other functional scores (Supplementary Figures S6–S9).

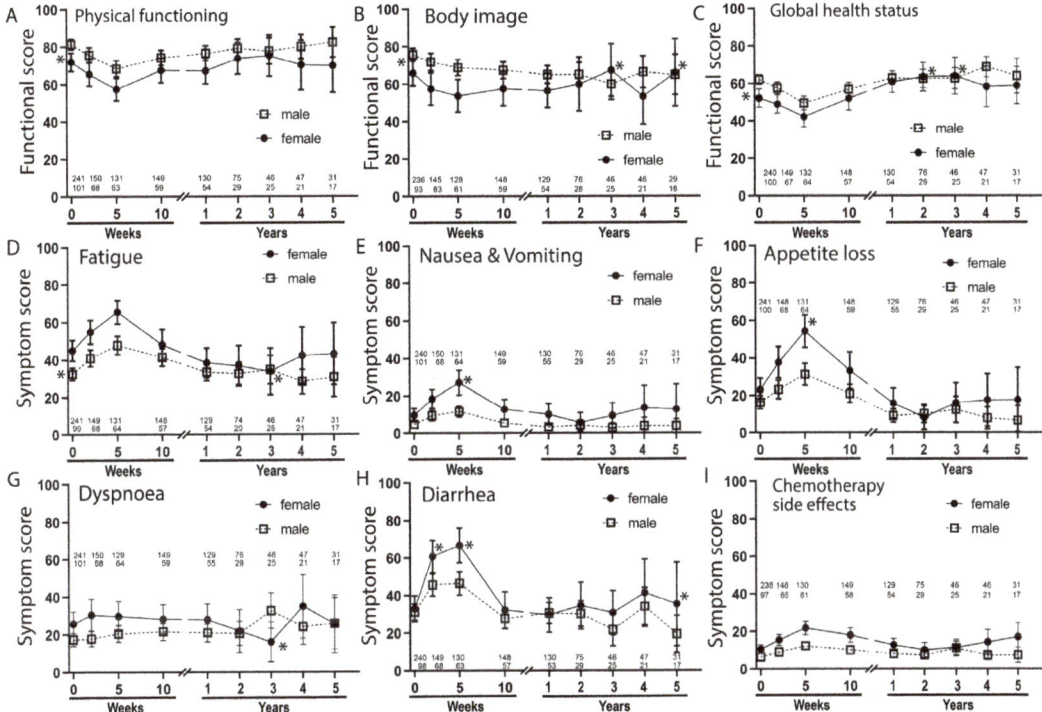

Figure 9. Quality of life by QLQ C30 and CR38 questionnaires of the quality of life cohort. Data points are baseline, during RCT (2nd and 3rd point), directly prior to surgery (4th point) and 1 to 5 years after beginning of RCT. Functional scores (**A–C**) and symptom scores (**D–I**). The scores are: (**A**) Physical functioning (**B**) Body image (**C**) Global health status (**D**) Fatigue (**E**) Nausea & Vomiting (**F**) Appetite loss (**G**) Dyspnoea (**H**) Diarrhea (**I**) Chemotherapy side effects. Asterisks to the left of the abscissa mark differences of more than 10% in the baseline, and asterisks (*) in the time data mark a change of more than 10 percentage points from the baseline. The length of the error bars corresponds to the 95% confidence interval for the mean. The number of patients who answered the questionnaires is given.

3.6. Survival and Oncologic Outcome

Finally, we analyzed the difference in survival between men and women. We found no differences in overall survival ($p = 0.596$), tumor-specific survival ($p = 0.199$), local recurrence free survival ($p = 0.621$), distant metastasis free survival ($p = 0.306$) or progression- free survival ($p = 0.423$) (Figure 10). Cumulative incidence of local recurrence ($p = 0.375$), metastatic disease ($p = 0.804$) and progression ($p = 0.657$) was not different between men and women.

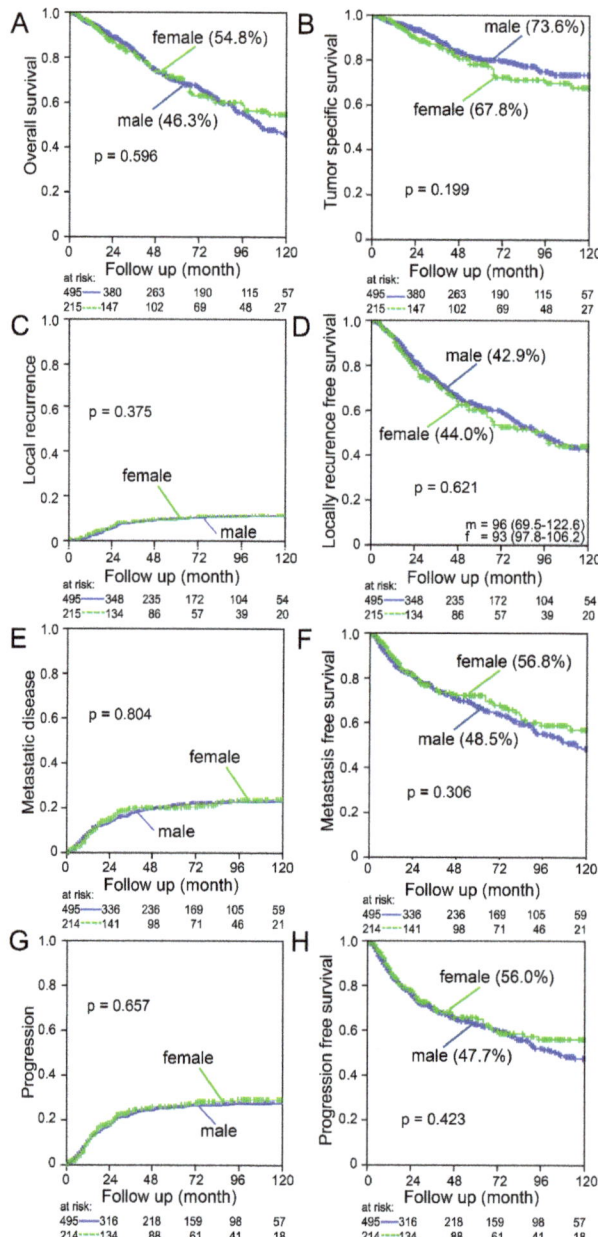

Figure 10. Ten year follow-up of male and female patients suffering from rectal cancer of the entire cohort: (**A**) Overall survival; (**B**) Tumor-specific survival; (**C**) Cumulative incidence of local recurrence; (**D**) Local recurrence-free survival; (**E**) Cumulative incidence of metastatic disease; (**F**) Metastasis-free survival; (**G**) Cumulative incidence of any recurrence and (**H**) Progression-free survival. The 10-year survival is given in brackets. Log-rank test was used to calculate *p*-values.

4. Discussion

The most significant finding of this study was an only minor difference in DNA repair between genders in normal tissue but no difference in the occurrence of chromosomal aberrations. This data were derived from a large number (n = 587) of rectal cancer patients and healthy individuals. In the repair examined with γH2AX, the accuracy of the repair plays an important role in addition to the reconnection, but this can only be checked to a limited extent with γH2AX [17]. In contrast, chromosomal aberrations reflect not only the repair but also the mutation frequency and thus, to a certain extent, the correctness of the repair. Additionally, chromosomal aberrations reflect individual radiosensitivity very well [18]. Therefore, this finding reveals that DNA repair and DNA damage processing is not different between males and females. Since there is a notion that instable aberrations predominantly reflect the occurrence of cell death and thus side effects, and stable aberrations represent more the stochastic risk [19], these parameters were also studied. There were no identifiable differences between both sexes. In epidemiological observations from the Hiroshima and Nagasaki atomic bomb studies, the stochastic risk of cancer development was significantly higher in women [20]. In the context of our data, this would suggest that the increased stochastic risk of the Hiroshima and Nagasaki cohort is not indicative of poorer repair or damage processing, but later processes of carcinogenesis where hormonal differences then lead to the development of cancer [3].

On the contrary, in a study with fibroblast cell lines from 89 women and 63 men, a higher sensitivity of the female cell lines was found despite a very strong variation in the colony-forming assay. Likewise, significant gender differences were found in 10 radiation responsive genes [21]. A review on Sex Difference of Radiation Response reports that long-term radiosensitivity in females is higher than that in males. The same paper also states that data are still insufficient [22].

To investigate the radiation sensitivity of the tumor, we measured the regression of tumor cells after RCT in surgical tumor specimens, on average, 55 days after the end of RCT. We found no sex-dependent difference in tumor regression grades. In addition, no differences in the amount of tumor-infiltrating CD8+ and FoxP3+ lymphocytes were detected. This indicates that there is no differential immune response between the sexes in these two lymphocyte types. Finally, no difference in the therapy outcome was found. This also indicates that the radiosensitivity of the tumor is not different between males and females.

The clearest difference between men and women during the RCT was seen in quality of life. Already at baseline, women often had worse scores than men. There was a general trend for these scores to worsen during therapy and to improve significantly after RCT. In long-term follow-up, even an improved state in women compared to men as opposed to the baseline was shown. This suggests an increased acute sensitivity to RCT. It is not clear whether this is more an effect of radiotherapy or chemotherapy. Most blood parameters proceeded similarly between sexes. However, leukocytes and albumin decrease more in women than in men.

One possible explanation for these effects, as we have shown, could be the relatively higher deposited energy of radiation in women. Although the 95% isodose volume is smaller in women than in men, no difference can be seen in relation to body weight. If the total deposited energy is calculated in relation to body weight, then 17% more energy per mass is deposited in women. The reason for this is probably the different anatomical situation in women compared to men. Since the BMI was the same in both groups, overweightness in women cannot be the reason for this difference. Toxicity of chemotherapeutic agents could be an alternative explanation for the increased side effects in women. Women have an increased risk of therapy-related side effects after application of chemotherapeutic agents [23,24]. This has been reported for colorectal cancer [25] and rectal cancer [26]. Fluorouracil as the main component of therapy causes higher toxicity in women [27]. This could be due to the lower concentration of the 5-FU degrading enzyme dihydropyridine dehydrogenase [2] or more frequent polymorphisms in women's enzyme [28,29]. Moreover, the gender-specific heterogeneous body fat composition could have an influence [26,29]. In addition, the calculation of body surface area in women leads to a relatively high dose, since the percentage of fat in women is higher [30]. A combination of both the increased deposited energy per mass and the increased side effects of chemotherapy might also be operational. It was suggested to use lean body mass instead of body surface area to calculate the 5-FU dose [30].

In general, increased side effects in women were limited to the duration of therapy and disappeared in the long-run. In terms of quality of life, women tended to achieve better values in the long-term. Finally, there was no observed difference between men and women in the incidence of local recurrences or distant metastases, or in progression-free, tumor-specific, or overall survival. This is in line with multiple observations of no difference between men and women in survival parameters [26,31].

5. Conclusions

Radiation sensitivity of normal tissue and tumor appears to be the same in males and females in this large set of rectal cancer patients and healthy individuals. During radiochemotherapy, QoL deteriorates more in women than in men, and women also experience larger depletions in leucocyte counts during treatment. We postulate that increased chemotherapy-derived toxicity and a slightly higher deposited energy is the underlying cause for these phenomena.

Supplementary Materials: The following supporting information can be downloaded at: https://www.mdpi.com/article/10.3390/cancers14010148/s1, Figure S1: Irradiated volume of the radiosensitivity cohort; Figure S2: Different types of chromosomal aberrations in females and males of the radiosensitivity cohort; Figure S3: Blood values prior to and during the RCT; Figure S4: Blood values prior to and during the RCT; Figure S5: Blood values prior to and during the RCT; Figure S6: Functional scores of quality of life by QLQ C30 questionnaires; Figure S7: Functional scores of quality of life by QLQ CR38 questionnaires; Figure S8: Symptom scores of quality of life by QLQ C30 questionnaires; Figure S9: Symptom scores of quality of life by QLQ C30 questionnaires.

Author Contributions: Conceptualization, L.V.D., H.G. and R.F.; methodology, B.S., M.H. (Markus Hecht), M.S., T.J., M.B.-H. and L.V.D.; software, L.V.D.; validation, B.S., M.H. (Markus Hecht), M.H. (Marlen Haderlein), M.S. and T.J.; formal analysis, B.S., M.H. (Markus Hecht), M.S., A.D., K.W. and T.J.; investigation, B.S., M.H. (Marlen Haderlein), M.S., A.D., K.W., R.G. and T.J.; resources, L.V.D. and R.F.; data curation, M.H. (Marlen Haderlein), T.J. and L.V.D.; writing—original draft preparation, B.S. and L.V.D.; writing—review and editing, B.S., H.G., M.B.-H., A.H. and L.V.D.; visualization, B.S., M.H. (Markus Hecht) and L.V.D.; supervision, L.V.D. and R.F.; project administration, R.F. and L.V.D. All authors have read and agreed to the published version of the manuscript.

Funding: This research received no external funding.

Institutional Review Board Statement: The Ethics Review Committee of the University Hospital Erlangen approved the study including the use of individual patient data. Ethics committee approval numbers 2725, 3745 and 21_19 B.

Informed Consent Statement: All patients and healthy individuals gave their written informed consent to the scientific processing of their material and data.

Data Availability Statement: The datasets used and/or analyzed during the current study are available from the corresponding author on reasonable request.

Conflicts of Interest: The authors declare no conflict of interest.

References

1. Buoncervello, M.; Marconi, M.; Care, A.; Piscopo, P.; Malorni, W.; Matarrese, P. Preclinical models in the study of sex differences. *Clin. Sci.* **2017**, *131*, 449–469. [CrossRef] [PubMed]
2. Ozdemir, B.C.; Csajka, C.; Dotto, G.P.; Wagner, A.D. Sex Differences in Efficacy and Toxicity of Systemic Treatments: An Undervalued Issue in the Era of Precision Oncology. *J. Clin. Oncol.* **2018**, *36*, 2680–2683. [CrossRef]

3. Rubin, J.B.; Lagas, J.S.; Broestl, L.; Sponagel, J.; Rockwell, N.; Rhee, G.; Rosen, S.F.; Chen, S.; Klein, R.S.; Imoukhuede, P.; et al. Sex differences in cancer mechanisms. *Biol. Sex Differ.* **2020**, *11*, 17. [CrossRef]
4. Dobie, S.A.; Baldwin, L.M.; Dominitz, J.A.; Matthews, B.; Billingsley, K.; Barlow, W. Completion of therapy by Medicare patients with stage III colon cancer. *J. Natl. Cancer Inst.* **2006**, *98*, 610–619. [CrossRef] [PubMed]
5. van der Geest, L.G.; Portielje, J.E.; Wouters, M.W.; Weijl, N.I.; Tanis, B.C.; Tollenaar, R.A.; Struikmans, H.; Nortier, J.W. All Nine Hospitals in the Leiden Region of the Comprehensive Cancer Centre The, N. Complicated postoperative recovery increases omission, delay and discontinuation of adjuvant chemotherapy in patients with Stage III colon cancer. *Colorectal Dis.* **2013**, *15*, e582–e591. [CrossRef]
6. Kim, S.E.; Paik, H.Y.; Yoon, H.; Lee, J.E.; Kim, N.; Sung, M.K. Sex- and gender-specific disparities in colorectal cancer risk. *World J. Gastroenterol.* **2015**, *21*, 5167–5175. [CrossRef]
7. De Courcy, L.; Bezak, E.; Marcu, L.G. Gender-dependent radiotherapy: The next step in personalised medicine? *Crit. Rev. Oncol. Hematol.* **2020**, *147*, 102881. [CrossRef]
8. Mayo, T.; Schuster, B.; Ellmann, A.; Schmidt, M.; Fietkau, R.; Distel, L.V. Individual Radiosensitivity in Lung Cancer Patients Assessed by G0 and Three Color Fluorescence in Situ Hybridization. *OBM Genet.* **2019**, *3*, 13. [CrossRef]
9. Huang, A.; Xiao, Y.; Peng, C.; Liu, T.; Lin, Z.; Yang, Q.; Zhang, T.; Liu, J.; Ma, H. 53BP1 expression and immunoscore are associated with the efficacy of neoadjuvant chemoradiotherapy for rectal cancer. *Strahlenther. Onkol.* **2020**, *196*, 465–473. [CrossRef] [PubMed]
10. Kroeber, J.; Wenger, B.; Schwegler, M.; Daniel, C.; Schmidt, M.; Djuzenova, C.S.; Polat, B.; Flentje, M.; Fietkau, R.; Distel, L.V. Distinct increased outliers among 136 rectal cancer patients assessed by gammaH2AX. *Radiat. Oncol.* **2015**, *10*, 36. [CrossRef]
11. Schuster, B.; Ellmann, A.; Mayo, T.; Auer, J.; Haas, M.; Hecht, M.; Fietkau, R.; Distel, L.V. Rate of individuals with clearly increased radiosensitivity rise with age both in healthy individuals and in cancer patients. *BMC Geriatr.* **2018**, *18*, 105. [CrossRef]
12. Mayo, T.; Haderlein, M.; Schuster, B.; Wiesmuller, A.; Hummel, C.; Bachl, M.; Schmidt, M.; Fietkau, R.; Distel, L. Is in vivo and ex vivo irradiation equally reliable for individual Radiosensitivity testing by three colour fluorescence in situ hybridization? *Radiat. Oncol.* **2019**, *15*, 2. [CrossRef]
13. Echarti, A.; Hecht, M.; Buttner-Herold, M.; Haderlein, M.; Hartmann, A.; Fietkau, R.; Distel, L. CD8+ and Regulatory T cells Differentiate Tumor Immune Phenotypes and Predict Survival in Locally Advanced Head and Neck Cancer. *Cancers* **2019**, *11*, 1398. [CrossRef] [PubMed]
14. Posselt, R.; Erlenbach-Wunsch, K.; Haas, M.; Jessberger, J.; Buttner-Herold, M.; Haderlein, M.; Hecht, M.; Hartmann, A.; Fietkau, R.; Distel, L.V. Spatial distribution of FoxP3+ and CD8+ tumour infiltrating T cells reflects their functional activity. *Oncotarget* **2016**, *7*, 60383–60394. [CrossRef]
15. Frank, F.; Hecht, M.; Loy, F.; Rutzner, S.; Fietkau, R.; Distel, L. Differences in and Prognostic Value of Quality of Life Data in Rectal Cancer Patients with and without Distant Metastases. *Healthcare* **2020**, *9*, 1. [CrossRef] [PubMed]
16. Kuncman, L.; Stawiski, K.; Maslowski, M.; Kucharz, J.; Fijuth, J. Dose-volume parameters of MRI-based active bone marrow predict hematologic toxicity of chemoradiotherapy for rectal cancer. *Strahlenther. Onkol.* **2020**, *196*, 998–1005. [CrossRef]
17. Alsbeih, G.; Al-Harbi, N.; Ismail, S.; Story, M. Impaired DNA Repair Fidelity in a Breast Cancer Patient with Adverse Reactions to Radiotherapy. *Front. Public Health* **2021**, *9*, 647563. [CrossRef] [PubMed]
18. Scott, D. Chromosomal radiosensitivity, cancer predisposition and response to radiotherapy. *Strahlenther. Onkol.* **2000**, *176*, 229–234. [CrossRef]
19. Ferlazzo, M.L.; Bourguignon, M.; Foray, N. Functional Assays for Individual Radiosensitivity: A Critical Review. *Semin. Radiat. Oncol.* **2017**, *27*, 310–315. [CrossRef]
20. Preston, D.L.; Ron, E.; Tokuoka, S.; Funamoto, S.; Nishi, N.; Soda, M.; Mabuchi, K.; Kodama, K. Solid cancer incidence in atomic bomb survivors: 1958–1998. *Radiat. Res.* **2007**, *168*, 1–64. [CrossRef] [PubMed]
21. Alsbeih, G.; Al-Meer, R.S.; Al-Harbi, N.; Bin Judia, S.; Al-Buhairi, M.; Venturina, N.Q.; Moftah, B. Gender bias in individual radiosensitivity and the association with genetic polymorphic variations. *Radiother. Oncol.* **2016**, *119*, 236–243. [CrossRef]
22. Narendran, N.; Luzhna, L.; Kovalchuk, O. Sex Difference of Radiation Response in Occupational and Accidental Exposure. *Front. Genet.* **2019**, *10*, 260. [CrossRef]
23. Nicolson, T.J.; Mellor, H.R.; Roberts, R.R. Gender differences in drug toxicity. *Trends Pharmacol. Sci.* **2010**, *31*, 108–114. [CrossRef]
24. Soldin, O.P.; Chung, S.H.; Mattison, D.R. Sex differences in drug disposition. *J. Biomed. Biotechnol.* **2011**, *2011*, 187103. [CrossRef]
25. Chua, W.; Kho, P.S.; Moore, M.M.; Charles, K.A.; Clarke, S.J. Clinical, laboratory and molecular factors predicting chemotherapy efficacy and toxicity in colorectal cancer. *Crit. Rev. Oncol. Hematol.* **2011**, *79*, 224–250. [CrossRef]
26. Diefenhardt, M.; Ludmir, E.B.; Hofheinz, R.D.; Ghadimi, M.; Minsky, B.D.; Rodel, C.; Fokas, E. Association of Sex with Toxic Effects, Treatment Adherence, and Oncologic Outcomes in the CAO/ARO/AIO-94 and CAO/ARO/AIO-04 Phase 3 Randomized Clinical Trials of Rectal Cancer. *JAMA Oncol.* **2020**, *6*, 294–296. [CrossRef] [PubMed]
27. Gusella, M.; Crepaldi, G.; Barile, C.; Bononi, A.; Menon, D.; Toso, S.; Scapoli, D.; Stievano, L.; Ferrazzi, E.; Grigoletto, F.; et al. Pharmacokinetic and demographic markers of 5-fluorouracil toxicity in 181 patients on adjuvant therapy for colorectal cancer. *Ann. Oncol.* **2006**, *17*, 1656–1660. [CrossRef]
28. Su, X.; Li, S.; Zhang, H.; Xiao, H.; Chen, C.; Wang, G. Thymidylate synthase gene polymorphism predicts disease free survival in stage II-III rectal adenocarcinoma patients receiving adjuvant 5-FU-based chemotherapy. *Chin. Clin. Oncol.* **2019**, *8*, 28. [CrossRef] [PubMed]

29. Wolff, H.A.; Conradi, L.C.; Schirmer, M.; Beissbarth, T.; Sprenger, T.; Rave-Frank, M.; Hennies, S.; Hess, C.F.; Becker, H.; Christiansen, H.; et al. Gender-specific acute organ toxicity during intensified preoperative radiochemotherapy for rectal cancer. *Oncologist* **2011**, *16*, 621–631. [CrossRef]
30. Prado, C.M.; Baracos, V.E.; McCargar, L.J.; Mourtzakis, M.; Mulder, K.E.; Reiman, T.; Butts, C.A.; Scarfe, A.G.; Sawyer, M.B. Body composition as an independent determinant of 5-fluorouracil-based chemotherapy toxicity. *Clin. Cancer Res.* **2007**, *13*, 3264–3268. [CrossRef] [PubMed]
31. Finlayson, E. Gender Influences Treatment and Survival in Colorectal Cancer Surgery INVITED COMMENTARY. *Dis. Colon Rectum* **2009**, *52*, 1991–1993. [CrossRef]